NOTIFIABLE DISEASES IN THE UNITED STATES

Acquired immune deficiency
  syndrome (AIDS)
Amebiasis*
Aseptic meningitis
Botulism (food-borne)
Botulism (infant)
Brucellosis
Chancroid*
Cholera
Diphtheria
Encephalitis (primary infection)
Encephalitis (postinfectious)
Gonorrhea
Granuloma inguinale*
Hepatitis A
Hepatitis B
Hepatitis non-A, non-B
Legionellosis
Leprosy
Leptospirosis
Lymphogranuloma venereum*
Malaria
Measles
Meningococcal infections
Mumps*
Pertussis
Plague
Poliomyelitis
Psittacosis
Rabies (animal)
Rabies (human)
Rheumatic fever*
Rubella
Rubella congenital syndrome
Salmonellosis
Shigellosis
Syphilis
Syphilis (congenital)
Tetanus
Toxic shock syndrome
Trichinosis
Tuberculosis
Tularemia
Typhoid fever
Typhus fever (Murine)
Typhus (Rocky Mountain spotted
  fever)*
Varicella (chickenpox)*

*Not notifiable in all states
Source: Centers for Disease Control. (1990,
October 5). Summary of notifiable diseases,
United States, 1989. *MMWR, 38*(54).

TABLE I RECOMMENDED SCHEDULE FOR ACTIVE [ ] OF NORMAL INFANTS AND CHILDREN.

Age	Vaccine	
2 mos.	Diphtheria, Tetanus, Pertussis (DTP) #1	DTP & OPV can be given
	Trivalent Oral Polio Vaccine (OPV #1)	earlier in highly endemic areas
4 mos.	DTP # 2 OPV #2	6 wks. to 2 mos. interval
6 mos.	DTP # 3 (Optional OPV)	Give OPV in epidemic areas
15 mos.	DTP #4, OPV #3	
	Measles, mumps, rubella (MMR)	Start at 12 mos. in high risk area
	Haemophilus influenzae b conjugate vaccine (Hib CV)	Conjugate preferred over polysaccharide
4–6 yrs.	DTP #5, OPV #4	
	2nd dose of measles vaccine	
14–15 yrs.	Td	Repeat every 10 years

TABLE II RECOMMENDED SCHEDULE FOR IMMUNIZATION OF INFANTS AND CHILDREN UP TO AGE SEVEN WHO HAVE NOT BEEN IMMUNIZED PREVIOUSLY.

Timing	Vaccine	Comments
First Visit	DTP #1, OPV #1	May be administered simultaneously
	MMR & Hib CV if child is over 15 mos.	
2 mos. after DTP #1	DTP #2, OPV #2	
2 mos. after DTP #2	DTP #3	
6–12 mos. after DTP #3	DTP #4, OPV #3	
4–6 yrs.	DTP #5, OPV #4	
	2nd dose of measles vaccine	
14–16 yrs.	TD	Repeat every 10 years

TABLE III RECOMMENDED SCHEDULE FOR PERSONS OVER 7 YEARS OF AGE AND NOT PREVIOUSLY IMMUNIZED.

Timing	Vaccine	Comments
First Visit	TD#1, OPV #1	OPV not routinely recommended for persons over 18 years.
2 mos. after TD & OPV #1	TD #2, OPV #2	OPV #2 may be given as soon as 6 wks. after OPV #1
6–12 mos. after TD & OPV #2	TD #3, OPV #3	OPV #3 may be given as soon as 6 wks. after OPV #1
10 yrs. after	TD	Repeat every 10 years throughout life

NB—Persons born after 1957 with no documentation of measles immunity should be vaccinated. This is especially important for health care workers and school aged children.

Sources:
Centers for Disease Control (Dec. 29, 1989). Measles prevention: Recommendations of the Immunization Practices Advisory Committee (ACIP). *MMWR, 38*(S-9).
Centers for Disease Control (April 7, 1989). ACIP: General recommendations on immunizations. *MMWR, 38*(13), 203–227.
Centers for Disease Control (April 13, 1990). ACIP: Supplementary statement: Change in administration schedule for hemophilus b conjugate vaccines. *MMWR, 39*(14), 232–233.

NATIONAL REFERENCE PHONE NUMBERS

AIDS
National AIDS Hotline: 1-800-342-AIDS
AIDS Information Line: 1-800-551-2728
Outreach Inc. Hotline: 1-800-441-2437

CENTERS FOR DISEASE CONTROL:

Information on Hepatitis, malaria, rabies, Rocky Mountain spotted fever and others: 1-404-332-4555
Information for international travelers: 1-404-332-4559
Information on influenza vaccine 1-404-639-1819

INFECTIOUS DISEASES

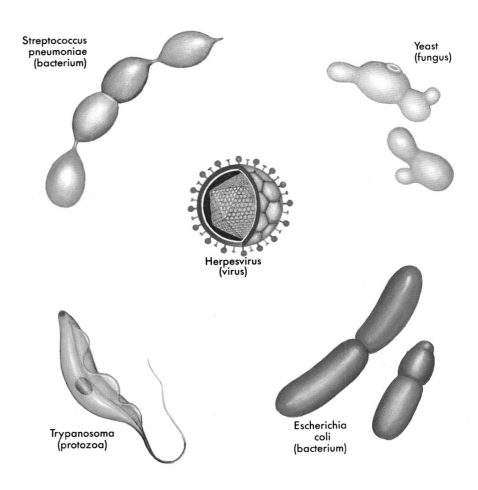

Streptococcus
pneumoniae
(bacterium)

Yeast
(fungus)

Herpesvirus
(virus)

Trypanosoma
(protozoa)

Escherichia
coli
(bacterium)

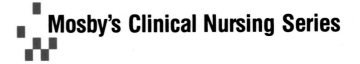

Mosby's Clinical Nursing Series

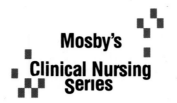

Mosby's Clinical Nursing Series

Cardiovascular Disorders

by Mary Canobbio

Respiratory Disorders

by Susan Wilson and June Thompson

Infectious Diseases

by Deanna Grimes

Orthopedic Disorders

by Leona Mourad

Renal Disorders

by Dorothy Brundage

Immunologic Disorders

by Christine Mudge-Grout

Neurologic Disorders

by Esther Chipps, Norma Clanin, and Victor Campbell

Cancer Disorders

by Anne Belcher

Gastrointestinal Disorders

by Dorothy Doughty and Debra Broadwell

Genitourinary Disorders

by Mikel Gray

INFECTIOUS DISEASES

DEANNA E. GRIMES, RN, DrPh

Associate Professor of Clinical Nursing
University of Texas Health Science Center
School of Nursing
Houston, Texas

*Chapter 8, "Acquired Immune Deficiency Syndrome (AIDS)
and HIV Infection," co–authored by*

RICHARD M. GRIMES, PhD

Associate Professor and Director, AIDS Education and Training Center
University of Texas Health Science Center
School of Public Health
Houston, Texas

Chapter 15, Antiinfective Agents, contributed by

MARK HAMELINK, MSN, CRNA, CCRN

Nurse Anesthetist
Morpheus Anesthesia Services, P.C.
South Haven, Michigan

Original illustrations by George J. Wassilchenko and Donald P. O'Connor

Original photography by Patrick Watson

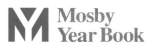
Mosby
Year Book

St. Louis Baltimore Boston Chicago London Philadelphia Sydney Toronto

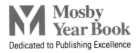
Mosby
Year Book
Dedicated to Publishing Excellence

Managing editor: Sally Adkisson
Developmental writer: Daphna Gregg
Project manager: Mark Spann
Designer: Liz Fett
Layout: Doris Hallas, Theresa Breckwoldt

Printed in the United States of America

Mosby–Year Book, Inc.
11830 Westline Industrial Drive
St. Louis, Missouri 63146

Library of Congress Cataloging-in-Publication Data

Grimes, Deanna.
    Infectious diseases/Deanna Grimes; original illustrations by
George J. Wassilchenko and Donald P. O'Connor; original photography
by Patrick Watson.
        p.   cm.—(Mosby's clinical nursing series)
    Includes index.
    ISBN 0-8016-2345-6
    1. Communicable diseases—Handbooks, manuals, etc.
  2. Communicable diseases—Nursing—Handbooks, manuals, etc.
  I. Title. II. Series.
    [DNLM: 1. Communicable Diseases—nursing.   WY 153 G862i]
RC111.G718   1991
616.9—dc20
DNLM/DLC
for Library of Congress   91-6272
                                                                   CIP

The authors and publisher have made a conscientious effort
to ensure that the drug information and recommended dosages
in this book are accurate and in accord with accepted standards
at the time of publication. However, pharmacology is a
rapidly changing science, so readers are advised to check
the package insert provided by the manufacturer before
administering any drug.

C/CD/VH   9 8 7 6 5 4 3 2

PREFACE

Infectious Diseases is the third volume in *Mosby's Clinical Nursing Series,* a new kind of resource for practicing nurses.

The *Series* is the result of the most elaborate market research ever undertaken by Mosby–Year Book, Inc. We first surveyed hundreds of working nurses to determine what kind of resources practicing nurses want in order to meet their advanced information needs. We then approached clinical specialists—proven authors and experts in 10 practice areas, from cardiovascular to ENT—and asked them to develop a common format that would meet the needs of nurses in practice, as specified by the survey respondents. This plan was then presented to 9 focus groups composed of working nurses over a period of 18 months. The plan was refined between each group, and in the later stages we published a 32-page full-color sample so that detailed changes could be made to improve the physical layout and appearance of the book, section by section and page by page.

The result is a new genre of professional books for nursing professionals.

Infectious Diseases begins with an innovative Color Atlas of Infectious Disease Pathophysiology. This is a complete and up–to–date review of the physiology of human defenses and immune system responses to infection. Color drawings enhance the presentation. Because of the increasing concern with prevention and control of infectious disease, the first chapter addresses transmission and control of infection.

Chapter 2 is a concise but comprehensive overview of nursing assessment for infection risks and signs of infection in all body systems. It includes detailed photographs of assessment techniques and drawings of skin lesions. Color plates of manifestations of specific infectious diseases on pages x to xvi complement this chapter.

Chapter 3, Diagnostic Procedures, is divided into two parts. The first describes the procedures for collection and handling of specimens and patient teaching for each procedure. Again, color photographs show proper equipment and technique in sharp detail. Part two describes the full range of diagnostic tests used to identify pathogens and antibodies against the pathogens.

Chapters 4 through 11 discuss various categories of infectious disease. Over 70 infectious diseases are grouped by chapter, either according to the body system where signs and symptoms are manifest or by mode of transmission or control. These chapters cover central nervous system infectious diseases, gastrointestinal infectious diseases, hepatitis and hematolymphatic infections, respiratory infectious diseases, AIDS, sexually transmitted diseases, vector-transmitted fevers, and childhood and vaccine-preventable diseases. With the exception of Chapter 11, which discusses the childhood and vaccine-preventable diseases, all other chapters combine diseases with similarities for nursing care.

Each disease chapter is presented in a similar format. Unique overview tables summarize the epidemiology for groups of similar diseases. Essential information is provided in these tables to enable nurses to quickly identify transmission risks and participate in control of infectious diseases. Pathophysiology is presented to answer the question that practicing nurses frequently ask. Disease complications are highlighted to alert nurses to prevent, observe, respond to, and report changes in the patient's condition. Definitive diagnostic tests and the physician's treatment plan are reviewed to facilitate interdisciplinary collaboration.

The nursing care for groups of diseases is presented according to the nursing process in easy-to-use tables. These pages are bordered in red to make them easy to find. Prevention and patient teaching are strongly emphasized nursing interventions. The nursing care is structured to integrate the five steps of the nursing process, centered around appropriate nursing diagnoses accepted by the North American Nursing Diagnosis Association (NANDA). The material can be used to develop individualized care plans quickly and accurately, and it meets the standards of nursing care required by the Joint Commission on the Accreditation of Hospitals (JCAH). By facilitating the development of individualized and authoritative care plans, this book can actually save you time to spend on direct patient care.

The format for Chapter 12, Nosocomial Infections, is different. The intent of this chapter is to provide nurses with recent information to prevent these hospital-acquired infections. Chapter 13, Therapeutic Procedures, presents the latest recommendations from the Centers for Disease Control on immunizations and isolation procedures.

In response to requests from scores of nurses participating in our research, a distinctive feature of this book is its use in patient teaching. Background information on diseases and medical interventions enables nurses to answer with authority questions patients often ask. The illustrations in the book, particularly those in the Color Atlas and the chapter on Diagnostic Procedures, are specif-

ically designed to support patient teaching. Chapter 14 consists of 13 Patient Teaching Guides written at a ninth-grade level so they can be copied, distributed to patients and their families, and used for self-care after discharge. Patient teaching sections in each care plan provide nurses with checklists of concepts to teach, promoting this increasingly vital aspect of nursing care.

The book concludes with a complete guide to antinfective drugs. The inside front cover contains frequently used information such as Universal Precautions, Immunization Schedules, and important reference phone numbers. Inside the back cover is a complete presentation on the nursing diagnosis for hyperthermia.

This book is intended for nurses practicing in both inpatient and outpatient care settings. We expect it to be a helpful reference for hospital medical-surgical, emergency room, and infection control nurses, and for nurses in ambulatory care clinics, school and college health programs, occupational health, home health, and public health care. We also anticipate that the book will be a valuable adjunct to medical-surgical and community health nursing texts for students learning nursing in a variety of settings.

We hope this book contributes to the advancement of professional nursing and the quality of patient care by serving to provide professional literature for nurses to call their own.

Contents

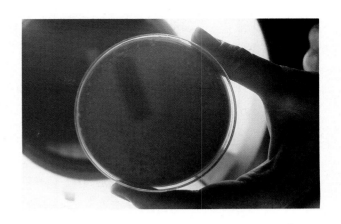

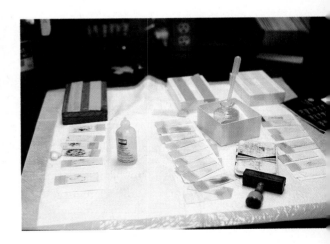

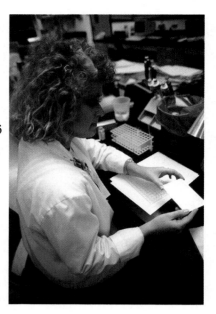
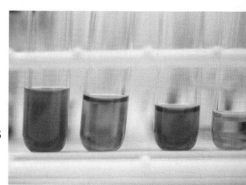

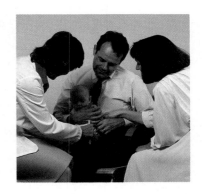

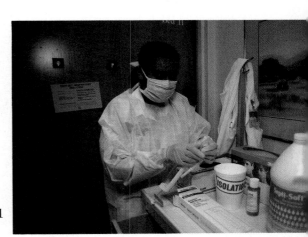

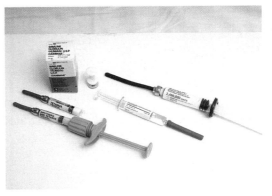

Color Plates

COLOR PLATE 1 Infectious hepatitis—closeup of rash. (Courtesy Dr. Thomas E. Sellers, Emory University, Atlanta, Georgia.)

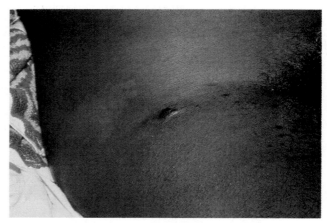

COLOR PLATE 2 Kaposi's sarcoma in groin of Haitian male with AIDS.

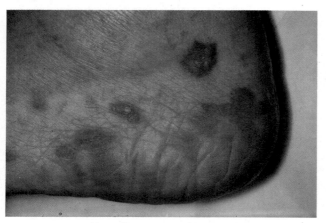

COLOR PLATE 3 Kaposi's sarcoma of heel and lateral foot.

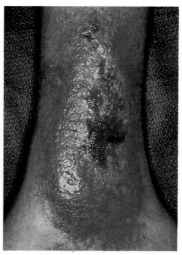

COLOR PLATE 4 Kaposi's sarcoma of distal leg and ankle.

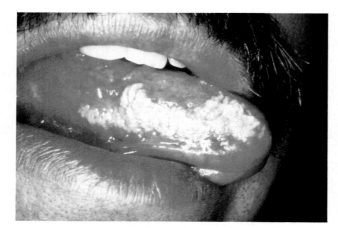

COLOR PLATE 5 Hairy leukoplakia on tongue of person with AIDS. (Courtesy J.S. Greenspan, B.D.S., University of California, San Francisco.)

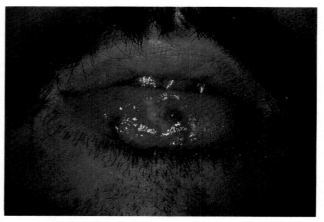

COLOR PLATE 6 Chronic mucocutaneous herpes simplex lesion in person with AIDS. (Courtesy Sol Silverman, Jr., D.D.S., University of California, San Francisco.)

Color plates courtesy The Centers for Disease Control, 1990.

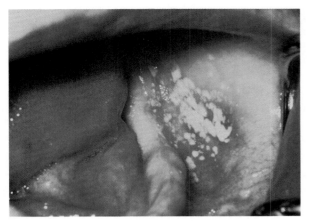

COLOR PLATE 7 Acute oral candidiasis in person with AIDS. (Courtesy Sol Silverman, Jr., D.D.S., University of California, San Francisco.)

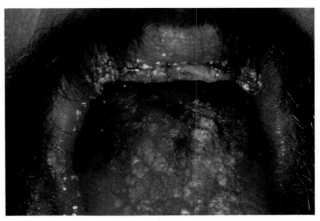

COLOR PLATE 8 Chronic oral candidiasis in person with AIDS. (Courtesy John Molinare, Ph.D., University of Detroit, Detroit, Michigan.)

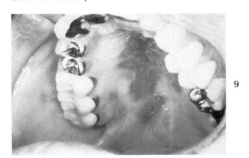

9

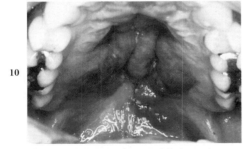

10

COLOR PLATES 9–10 Oral Kaposi's sarcoma. 9, Moderately advanced. 10, Advanced lesion. (Courtesy Sol Silverman, Jr., D.D.S., University of California, San Francisco.)

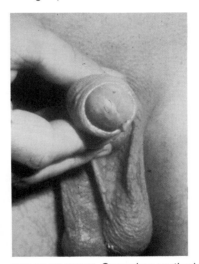

COLOR PLATE 11 Gonorrhea urethral discharge.

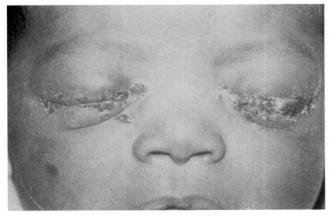

COLOR PLATE 12 Gonorrhea ophthalmia.

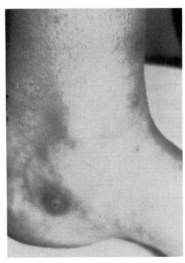

COLOR PLATE 13 Skin lesion of disseminated gonorrhea.

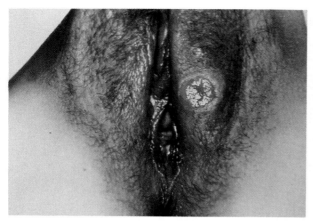

COLOR PLATE 14 Primary syphilis—chancre on labia.

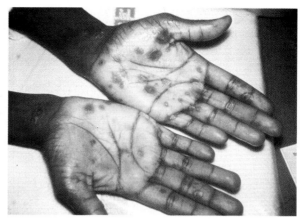

COLOR PLATE 15 Secondary syphilis—rash on hands.

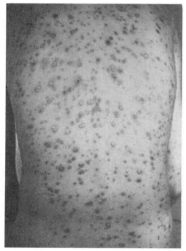

COLOR PLATE 16 Secondary syphilis—rash on back.

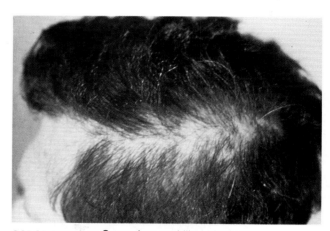

COLOR PLATE 17 Secondary syphilis—alopecia.

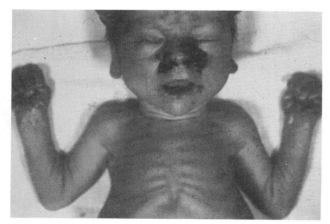

COLOR PLATE 18 Congenital syphilis.

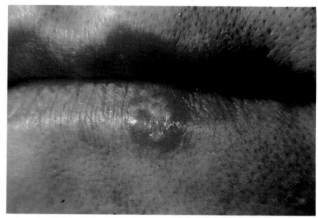

COLOR PLATE 19 Herpes simplex lesion of lowerlip— second day after onset.

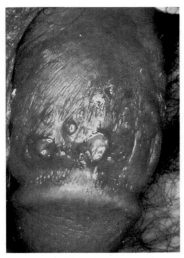

COLOR PLATE 20 Herpes corona.

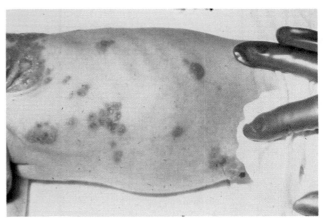

COLOR PLATE 21 Herpes simplex neonatorum.

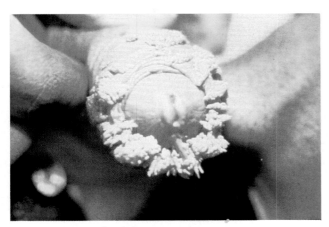

COLOR PLATE 22 Genital warts: male.

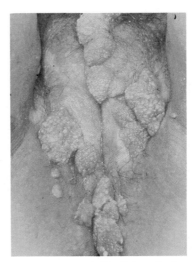

COLOR PLATE 23 Genital warts: female in lithotomy position.

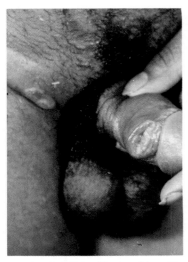

COLOR PLATE 24 Chancroid: male.

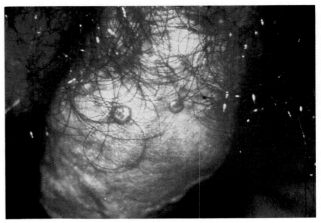

COLOR PLATE 25 Molluscum contagiosum: male.

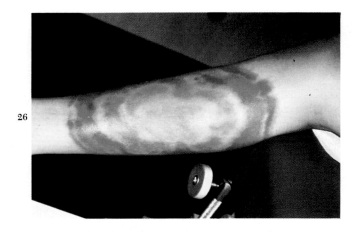

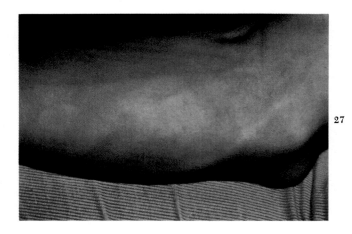

26

27

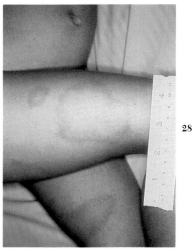

28

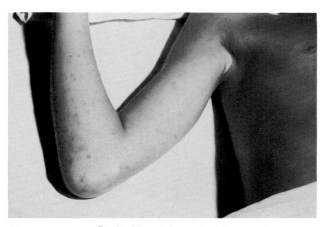

COLOR PLATES 26–28 Examples of erythema chronicum migrans of lyme disease. (Courtesy Dr. Allen C. Steere, et al.: An of Intern Med 86(6): 685–698, June 1977.)

COLOR PLATE 29 Rocky Mountain spotted fever rash on arm.

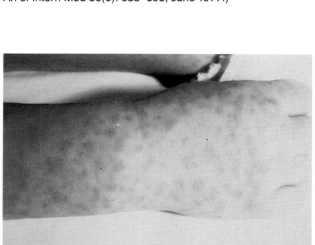

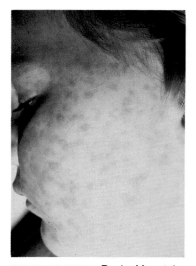

COLOR PLATE 30 Rocky Mountain spotted fever rash on wrist and hand.

COLOR PLATE 31 Rocky Mountain spotted fever rash on side of face 9 days after onset.

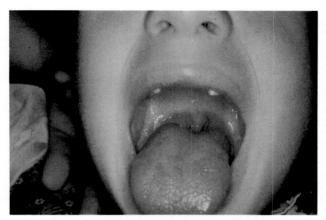

COLOR PLATE 32 Streptococcal throat with erythema and edema.

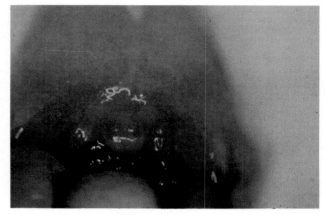

COLOR PLATE 33 Streptococcal throat with severe erythema and exudate beginning to form.

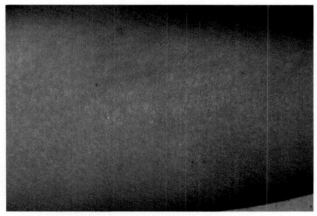

COLOR PLATE 34 Scarlet fever rash on forearm.

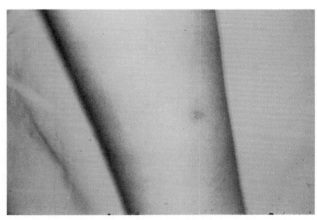

COLOR PLATE 35 Chickenpox vesicle on leg.

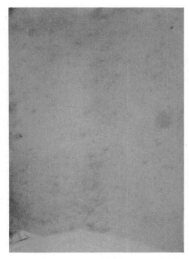

COLOR PLATE 36 Chickenpox lesions in various stages of development on chest.

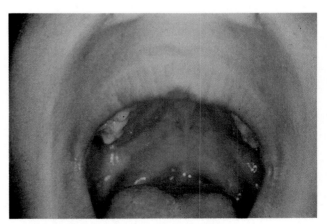

COLOR PLATE 37 Chickenpox in oral cavity.

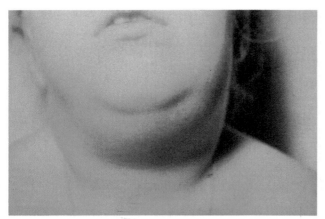

COLOR PLATE 38 Submaxillary mumps in infant.

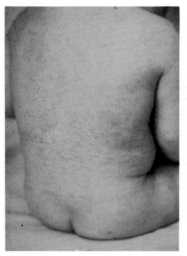

COLOR PLATE 39 Acquired rubella (German measles) in 11-month-old infant.

COLOR PLATE 40 Rubella (German measles) rash on abdomen (discrete, maculopapular erythematous rash).

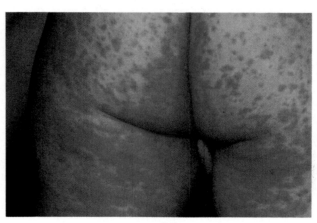

COLOR PLATE 41 Rubeola (measles) rash on third day.

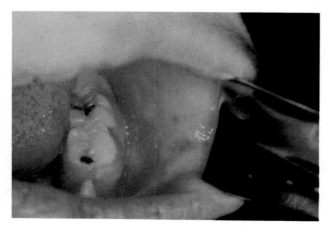

COLOR PLATE 42 Koplik spots on buccal mucosa 3 days before eruption of rubeola (measles) rash.

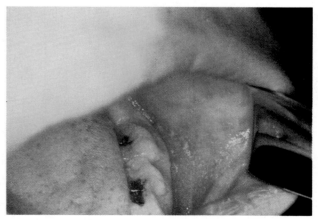

COLOR PLATE 43 Koplik spots after eruption of rubeola (measles) rash.

CHAPTER 1

Color Atlas of Infectious Disease Pathophysiology

Of all life-forms on earth, microorganisms compose the largest population. They are everywhere, living on and in water, soil, plants, animals, and even minerals—and, of course, humans. As a group, microbes are remarkably adaptable. That we are unaware of these invisible life-forms, at least most of the time, is a testament to their success. Many have evolved a friendly, mutually beneficial relationship with humans by performing a needed service in exchange for nutritional support.

Nonetheless, numerous organisms are pathogenic to humans. Infectious diseases rank as the fifth most common cause of death in the United States. They are an important complication of other disorders and cause a significant amount of morbidity even in healthy populations.

A susceptible host, an infectious agent, and an environment that permits transmission of the agent are not enough to produce an infectious disease. The infectious agent must also elicit symptoms of disease in the host, either from the action of the pathogen or its products on body cells or from physiologic responses elicited to eradicate the agent (Figure 1-1).

Each step in the infection process has more than one possible outcome. *Contamination*, the presence of an infectious agent on a body surface or object, is only a first step. *Infection* is implantation and successful reproduction of an infectious agent in a living host, but if no physiologic response occurs, then the agent has merely *colonized* the host. A colonized host who also sheds the agent, transmitting it to others, is a *carrier* but is not necessarily ill. A physiologic response that occurs without producing clinical symptoms is termed *subclinical infection*. Only if tissue injury or physiologic response produces clinical symptoms of illness is an *infectious disease* present.

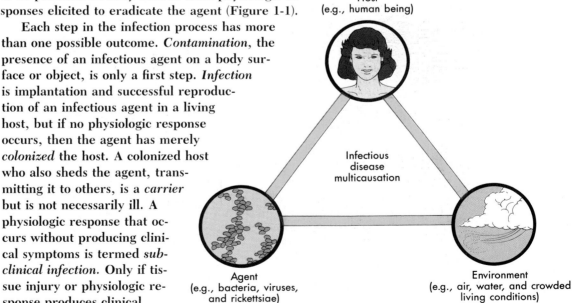

Host
(e.g., human being)

Infectious
disease
multicausation

Agent
(e.g., bacteria, viruses,
and rickettsiae)

Environment
(e.g., air, water, and crowded
living conditions)

FIGURE 1-1
Multicausation of infectious disease: agent, host, and environmental conditions interact to produce infectious disease in the host.

PATHOGENIC AGENTS

Pathogens are parasites that create pathologic process in their human host. Because they cannot synthesize their own amino acids, they must rely on a host to supply their nutritional requirements. Some pathogens are metabolically structured so that they can survive outside a host. By contrast, viruses depend on a host for all sustenance because they lack the ability to perform any metabolic function on their own and can only survive in the human cell.

Clearly, pathogens are a remarkably successful lifeform. One key to their success is viability, an organism's ability to survive in an adverse environment. This quality is determined by the morphology and chemical composition of the agent. The more viable the pathogen, the better able it is to resist an adverse environment. Many organisms are adaptable enough to evade physical, chemical, and thermal insults. For example, tetanus bacilli form spores that enable the bacilli to survive until they reach more welcoming environments. Genetic mutation creates antibiotic-resistant strains of bacteria and viruses that can parasitize previously immune hosts.

The Variability of Pathogenicity

The likelihood of a pathogen causing infectious disease is influenced by the organism's mode of action, infectivity, pathogenicity, virulence, antigenicity and toxigenicity.

Mode of action

Pathogens have various modes of action for invading and reproducing in a host. They may directly damage cells by causing hyperplasia, necrosis, and cell death. Intracellular pathogens, such as viruses, interfere with cellular metabolism, rendering the host cell dysfunctional by the accumulation of pathogens and their products inside the cell (inclusion bodies). Another mode of action is the production of toxins that cause local or systemic reactions (Figure 1-2).

Infectivity

Infectivity of the agent is its ability to invade and multiply in the host. It is affected by host defenses and pathogen-produced enzymes that facilitate invasiveness. Coagulase, an extracellular enzyme of some cells that causes coagulation, enables organisms, such as staphylococci, to clot plasma and form a sticky fibrin layer around themselves to protect against host defenses. Streptococci produce streptokinase to dissolve fibrin clots, allowing the organism to spread through host tissue. Hyaluronidase breaks down connective tissue and increases tissue permeability, enabling streptococci, pneumococci, and clostridia to spread throughout host tissues. Collagenase degrades collagen to facilitate deep invasion of *Clostridium perfringens* and other pathogens into tendons, cartilage, and bone.

Pathogens are graded according to their infectivity potential. For example, poliomyelitis virus is rated a highly infective agent, rubella virus has intermediate infectivity, and *Mycobacterium tuberculosis* has low infectivity.

Pathogenicity

The ability of an agent to produce disease depends on its speed of reproduction, extent of tissue damage, and production of a toxin. Agents can be graded according to pathogenicity. Examples of highly pathogenic agents are those that cause smallpox and rabies. Infection by them almost invariably results in disease. The rubella virus has intermediate pathogenicity, and the poliomyelitis virus has low pathogenicity.

Virulence

The potency, or virulence, of a pathogen determines the severity of disease it produces. Virulence is measured in terms of the number of microorganisms or micrograms of toxin required to kill a given host. Viru-

---

THE MANY RELATIONSHIPS BETWEEN HUMANS AND ORGANISMS

Symbiosis	Benefits only the human; no harm to the organism
Mutualism	Benefits the human and the organism
Commensalism	Benefits only the organism; no harm to the human
Pathogenicity	Benefits the organism; harms the human (**Opportunism** is the situation when benign organisms become pathogenic because of decreased human host resistance)

Some organisms that have a symbiotic or commensal relationship on one part of the body can become pathogenic when transferred to another area. For example, alpha-streptococci are part of the normal flora in the nasopharynx but become pathogenic when transferred to heart valves.

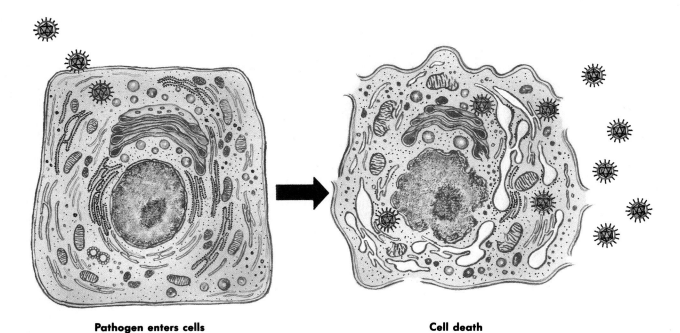

Pathogen enters cells   **Cell death**

FIGURE 1-2
Mode of action of pathogenic viruses. One factor influencing pathogenicity is an organism's mode of action. Viruses can replicate only within host cells. They interfere with cellular metabolism, leading to cell death.

lence can also be graded. The rabies virus is highly virulent, the poliomyelitis virus has intermediate virulence, the measles virus is of low virulence, and the common cold has very low virulence.

Antigenicity

The ability of pathogens to induce an immune response in the host varies considerably. Some have intrinsic antigens (e.g., proteins, polypeptides, or polysaccharides) that stimulate antibody production against the antigen. Others lack antigenic structures and may be able to evade destruction for a considerable length of time.

Toxigenicity

An important factor in determining a pathogen's virulence is toxigenicity. Agent products associated with toxigenicity are hemolysin, leucocidin, and toxins. Hemolysin destroys erythrocytes, and leucocidin destroys leukocytes. Both of these products are factors in the virulence of some streptococci and staphylococci.

Some bacteria secrete water-soluble antigenic exotoxins that are distributed rapidly by the blood, causing potentially severe systemic and neurologic manifestations. Diseases associated with exotoxins are tetanus, botulism, and diphtheria.

The cell walls of some bacteria are composed of endotoxins, which cause inflammation and local destruction of tissues. Endotoxins are weakly toxic, relatively stable, and not antigenic. Diseases associated with endotoxins include staphylococcal food poisoning and cholera.

CLASSIFICATION OF PATHOGENS

Pathogenic agents are classified according to morphology, chemical composition, growth requirements, and viability. Classifications are continually changing as new organisms are identified and additional distinguishing biochemical or morphologic characteristics of known organisms are recognized. The current classification scheme used includes protozoa, fungi, bacteria, rickettsiae, chlamydiae, mycoplasmata, viruses, and helminths.

PHYSIOLOGY OF THE HUMAN RESPONSE TO INFECTION

In the course of a single day, the average person is probably exposed to thousands of pathogenic organisms, yet most persons do not succumb to infectious disease. This is possible because the body is equipped with anatomic characteristics and physiologic processes that increase resistance to pathogens and fight the infectious process once it begins.

The first line of defense against infection is external and consists of mechanical barriers, chemical barriers, and the body's own population of microorganisms.

The two internal barriers come into play when the external line of defense is breeched. Operating as the second line of defense, the inflammatory response is aimed at preventing an invading pathogen from becoming established, reproducing, and invading other tissues. The third line of defense is the immune response, which is activated after the inflammatory response. Although inflammation and immune response are two events, they cannot always be easily separated because both events involve many of the same processes and cellular components.

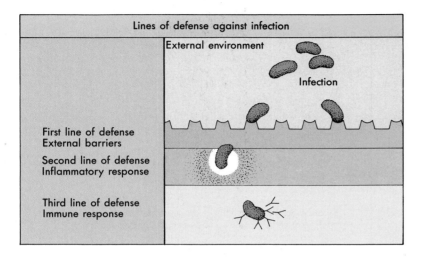

Lines of defense against infection

External environment

Infection

First line of defense
External barriers

Second line of defense
Inflammatory response

Third line of defense
Immune response

THE FIRST LINE OF DEFENSE: EXTERNAL BARRIERS

Every surface of the body that is exposed in any way to the environment is involved in first-line defense. The skin and mucous membranes of the digestive, respiratory, and genitourinary tract form a continuous, closed barrier between the internal organs and the environment (Figure 1-3). As long as they are intact, skin and mucous membranes are normally impervious to most pathogenic organisms. Body secretions provide an inhospitable environment by maintaining a pH level that discourages colonization or by "washing" the area to keep organisms from accumulating.

One of the most fascinating aspects of the body's first-line defense system is the normal microbial inhabitants (flora) that populate almost all of the body's surfaces. The process of colonization begins at birth. Operating on the principle of **microbial antagonism,** the presence of indigenous flora interferes with the establishment of pathogenic microorganisms in several ways. By occupying a surface, resident flora offer potential invaders stiff competition for both space and nutrients. Indigenous flora help maintain an optimal pH for their own growth, which is inhospitable to many pathogenic agents. Some of these benign organisms are known to secrete germicidal substances. There is evidence that indigenous flora also stimulate the development of the immune system.

The importance of microbial antagonism becomes evident when the normal flora is disturbed, as illustrated by the common occurrence of *Candida albicans* overgrowth following antibiotic therapy, resulting in diarrhea and vaginitis.

Some indigenous flora are themselves pathogenic under certain conditions. They can be responsible for infection when the immune system is impaired, the skin or mucous membranes are breeched, or the flora are displaced from their natural habitat to another area of the body. This latter event is explained by the fact that the normal flora are tissue specific—that is, a particular type of bacteria normally colonizes a particular type of tissue, adhering to specific receptors on epithelial cells. As a result, the normal composition of flora varies from one part of the body to another (Table 1-1). Displacement of indigenous flora to another area is a common cause of nosocomial (hospital-acquired) infection, such as urinary tract infection from enteric bacteria following catheterization.

THE SKIN

Penetration of the skin, with its stratified and cornified epithelium, is significantly more difficult for microorganisms than penetration of mucous membrane. With extremely rare exceptions, a break in the skin is necessary for pathogens to breech this mechanical barrier. Furthermore, the skin maintains a fairly acid pH, which inhibits the growth of most pathogenic bacteria. Microbes are continually sloughed from the epidermis with dead skin cells, and oil and sweat secreted from glands in the dermis wash microorganisms from the pores. Sebaceous secretions also contain bactericidal fatty acids.

THE NOSE

Inspired air travels across coarse nasal hairs and through the turbinates, which filter out larger particles and trap some pathogens. The sticky mucosal surface moves this material toward the throat for expectoration or swallowing, and the nasal passages can be cleared by sneezing. Nasal secretions contain some antimicrobial substances, such as IgA antibody and lysozyme.

THE LUNGS

The mucous membranes lining the upper airways clear inspired debris, including microorganisms, from the respiratory tract. Mucus-producing goblet cells located in the larger airways keep these passages replenished with mucus. Particles are trapped on the sticky mucosal surface, and cilia propel mucus toward

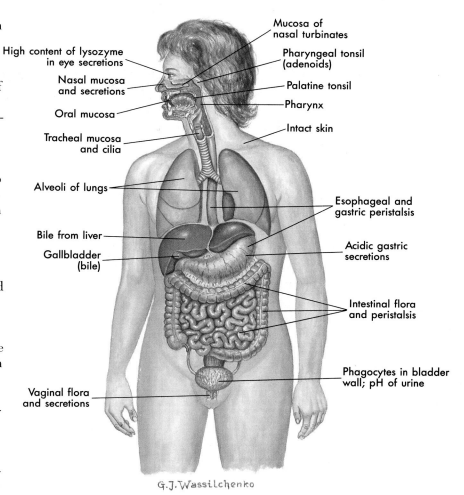

FIGURE 1-3
First line of defense—external barriers.

the throat at a rate of 10 to 20 mm/min. Coughing and sneezing expel particle-laden mucus from the respiratory tract.

The normal efficiency of the upper airways results in only the smallest particles reaching the lower respiratory tract. Microorganisms and other particles that remain in the alveoli are dispatched by alveolar macrophages. The pulmonary system is not inhabited by indigenous flora.

THE MOUTH AND PHARYNX

In addition to the mucous membrane lining these structures, lymph tissue of the tonsils and adenoids are located in the pharyngeal area. This permits a rapid lymphocytic response to pathogenic organisms entering the oral or respiratory routes.

THE DIGESTIVE SYSTEM

The stomach secretes extremely acid digestive enzymes, which neutralize or kill most bacteria. Bile de-

Table 1-1

NORMAL INDIGENOUS FLORA OF THE HUMAN BODY

Skin	Predominantly gram-positive cocci and rods.
	Staphylococcus epidermidis, corynebacteria, mycobacteria, and streptococci are primary inhabitants; *S. aureus* in some people; also yeasts (*Candida* and *Pityrosporum*) in some areas of skin. Numerous transient microorganisms may become temporary residents.
	In moist areas, gram-negative bacteria.
	Around sebaceous glands, *Propionibacteria* and brevibacteria.
	The mite *Demodex folliculorum* lives in hair follicles and sebaceous glands around the face.
Nose	Predominantly gram-positive cocci and rods, especially *S. epidermidis*.
	Some people are nasal carriers of pathogenic bacteria, including *S. aureus*, beta-hemolytic streptococci, and *Corynebacterium diphtheriae*.
Mouth	A complex population of bacteria that includes several species of streptococci, *Actinomyces*, lactobacilli, and *Haemophilus*.
	Anaerobic bacteria and spirochetes colonize the gingival crevices.
Pharynx	Similar to flora in mouth plus staphylococci, *Neisseria*, and diphtheroids.
	Some asymptomatic persons also harbor the pathogens pneumococcus, *H. influenzae*, *N. meningitidis*, and *C. diphtheriae*.
Distal intestine	Enterobacteria, streptococci, lactobacilli, anaerobic bacteria, and *C. albicans*.
Colon	*Bacteroides*, lactobacilli, clostridia, *Salmonella*, *Shigella*, *Klebsiella*, *Proteus*, *Pseudomonas*, enterococci and other streptococci, bacilli, and *Escherichia coli*.
Distal urethra	Typical bacteria found on the skin, especially *S. epidermidis* and diphtheroids. Also lactobacilli and nonpathogenic streptococci.
Vagina	Birth to 1 month: similar to adult.
	1 month to puberty: *S. epidermidis*, diphtheroids, *E. coli*, and streptococci.
	Puberty to menopause: *Lactobacillus acidophilus*, diphtheroids, staphylococci, streptococci, and a variety of anaerobes.
	Postmenopause: similar to prepubescence.

creases the surface tension of the cell wall in some bacteria, rendering the organisms more digestible. The esophagus and empty stomach have no resident flora, but microorganisms enter through food, saliva, and nasopharyngeal secretions. Within 1 hour of a meal, the stomach is again sterile.

Peristalsis discourages pathogenic colonization by preventing prolonged contact of fecal material with the mucous lining of the small intestine and colon. The sterile environment of the stomach extends to the upper portion of the intestinal tract, but near the terminal ileum the flora begins to resemble that of the colon.

The colon contains the largest concentration of bacteria of any area in the body. It is estimated that as much as 60% of feces, by weight, consists of bacteria and other microorganisms.

THE URINARY TRACT

Frequent flushing of the bladder and urinary tract through urination helps prevent microorganisms from colonizing the area. Urine contains urea nitrogen and ammonium, which are bacteriostatic to most pathogens. Prostatic fluid contains bactericidal substances that protect the male genitourinary tract. The bladder

wall is capable of mounting a phagocytic response within 30 minutes of pathogenic invasion. The distal portion of the urethra in both males and females is populated with bacteria found on the skin.

THE VAGINA

The microorganisms found in the vagina vary with age (Table 1-1). At birth the vagina is sterile, but within 24 hours glycogen is deposited in the vaginal mucosa under the influence of estrin, which is passively transferred from mother to infant. This establishes a pH of about 4.5, allowing flora to develop that resembles that of an adult. At about 1 month of age, glycogen secretion and the pH rises to about 7, changing the flora. At puberty, glycogen is again produced and the pH returns to about 4.5 until after menopause, when the vaginal flora again resembles that of prepubescence.

THE EYE

Tears have a high content of lysozyme, which is effective against most gram-positive bacteria. The continual flushing action of tears helps cleanse the eyes by transferring fluid through the lacrimal ducts and into the nasopharynx. No resident flora is present in the eye.

THE COMPONENTS OF INTERNAL DEFENSES

The second and third lines of defense (the inflammatory response and the immune system) share several components. These components include the lymphatic system, leukocytes, and a multitude of chemicals, proteins, and enzymes that facilitate the internal defense systems. An understanding of these components and their interactions aids in understanding inflammation and the immune response.

LYMPHATIC SYSTEM

The lymphatic system provides a network for components of the internal defenses to circulate throughout the body. It is designed to capture and destroy invading microorganisms. The lymphatic system functions in both the inflammatory response and immune reactions.

Every tissue supplied by blood vessels, except that of the brain and placenta, is invested with lymphatic vessels. The large lymphatic tissues are shown in Figure 1-4, but numerous smaller lymph nodes (varying from "pinhead" size to "lima bean" size) are grouped throughout the body. The lymphatic tissues are connected by a network of collecting ducts that parallel the vascular network, forming a closed but porous circle.

Lymph is a clear, opalescent or yellowish fluid containing a variety of white blood cells, particularly lymphocytes, and occasionally red blood cells. The fluid originates in the blood and enters the interstitial spaces, where it picks up microorganisms, cell debris, or other foreign material in the tissue. From here it passes into the profusion of microscopic lymph tubules that join to form ducts, which carry it to nearby lymph nodes.

Lymph nodes form two major functions—filtration and sensitization. Any foreign material entering a lymph node is filtered out. The "clean" lymph fluid exits the node and transfers proteins and fluids back into the circulatory system. Foreign material inside the lymph node generates one of the following events: (1) the material is destroyed by phagocytic cells inside the lymph node, or (2) a specific immune response is activated by sensitization of lymphocytes to the specific antigen of the foreign material. (See Activation of Lymphocytes in this section.)

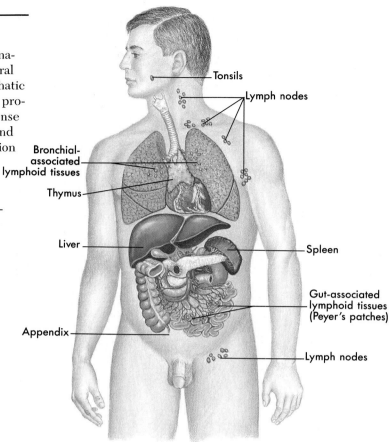

FIGURE 1-4
Components of the lymphatic system.

The thymus is critical to the maturation of T lymphocytes, a process that is influenced by thymic hormones. This gland reaches its greatest size during puberty, after which it gradually involutes as adipose tissue replaces thymic tissue. Acute disease or malnutrition can increase the involution process.

The spleen is the largest lymphatic organ. It produces leukocytes and filters venous blood. Tissue macrophages lining the splenic sinuses destroy circulating microorganisms and old red blood cells during the filtration process.

Lymphoid tissue can also be found in the tonsils and Peyer's patches. The tonsils are aggregations of lymphoid tissue, named according to their location. Those in the mouth and pharynx are termed **palatine, lingual,** and **pharyngeal** tonsils. The Peyer's patches are accumulations of the lymphoid tissue of the intestinal tract and the appendix.

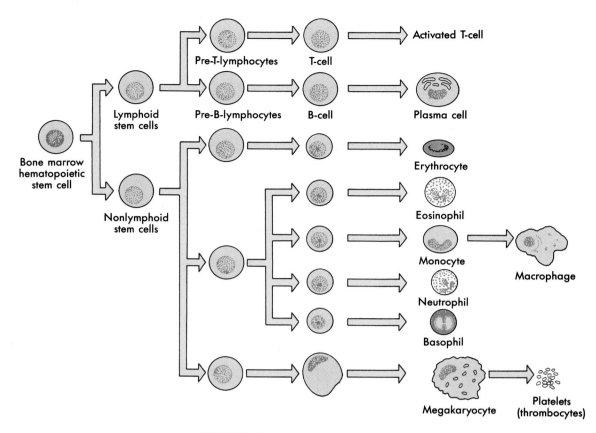

FIGURE 1-5
Lineage and differentiation of leukocytes.

LEUKOCYTES

Leukocytes, or white blood cells, are the blood components associated with the inflammatory and immune responses to the infectious process. All blood cells are created equal—that is, they originate from parent cells in bone marrow called **hematopoietic stem cells**—but by mechanisms that are not well understood, they undergo a process of differentiation, with some becoming erythrocytes (red blood cells) and others becoming leukocytes. The majority of leukocytes remain in an immature state in the bone marrow until they are needed to combat infection. Once activated to leave the bone marrow, leukocytes undergo a maturation process and further differentiate into five distinct types of cells—neutrophils, eosinophils, basophils, lymphocytes, and monocytes (Table 1-2):

1. Neutrophils ⎫
2. Eosinophils ⎬ Granulocytes
3. Basophils   ⎭
4. Lymphocytes ⎫
5. Monocytes   ⎬ Agranulocytes
                ⎭

The neutrophils and monocytes are involved in phagocytosis (part of the inflammatory response) and are fre-

quently referred to as phagocytes. Lymphocytes are predominantly involved in the immune process. The lineage and differentiation of leukocytes can be seen in Figure 1-5.

Neutrophils and Monocytes (Phagocytes)

Neutrophils and monocytes are the primary cells involved in inflammation and phagocytosis. They move through tissue by an amoeba-like action, chemically attracted to pathogens by chemotaxis and squeezing through blood vessel pores that are smaller than themselves by the process of diapedesis. Neutrophils are short-lived, having life spans of only about 12 to 14 hours, but they proliferate rapidly and are the first phagocytes to appear at a site of tissue injury. Most tissue-damaging processes, including inflammation, stimulate the production of neutrophils. Neutrophils are particularly effective against extracellular pyogenic organisms.

Mature monocytes are called macrophages. Macrophages are the second type of phagocytes to arrive via the circulation. Because they remain active for as long as 48 hours, macrophages are able to ingest more

Table 1-2

CHARACTERISTICS AND FUNCTIONS OF THE DIFFERENT LEUKOCYTES

Type of leukocyte	Percent of total; Function(s)	Characteristics
Polymorphonuclear granulocytes		Granules in the cytoplasm contain enzymes that digest organisms, debris, and other material. Nucleus may be single (band) or divided (segmented).
Neutrophils	50-75; Phagocytosis	First to arrive at site of injury; increase markedly during bacterial invasion, particularly in pneumococcal, streptococcal, and staphylococcal infection; remain active for 12-14 hrs.
		Contain opsonins that coat material before ingestion and release antibacterial chemicals and enzymes
Eosinophils	0-6; Weak phagocytosis; regulate hypersensitivity reactions	Same as neutrophils, plus contain enzymes that counteract inflammatory process in allergic reactions
		Increase in response to invasion by some protozoa and helminths; increased in allergic reactions
Basophils	0-1; Weak phagocytosis; release heparin and histamine from granules into surrounding tissue	Same as neutrophils, plus secrete heparin and histamine into surrounding tissue
Mononuclear agranulocytes		Have single nucleus; cytoplasm contains no granules
Lymphocytes	20-40; Active in immune responses	
B cells	Produce antibodies	Contact with antigen transforms them into plasma cells and memory cells
		Active for several days
T cells	Mediate immunologic responses	Contact with antigen transforms them into four different subsets. Helper and suppressor cells regulate the immune response; cytotoxic and delayed hypersensitivity cells engage directly in destroying cells.
		Active for 1 month to several years
Monocytes (macrophages)	2-10; Phagocytosis; stimulate maturation of T cells	Abundant cytoplasm and kidney-shaped nuclei
		A few tissue macrophages reach site of injury quickly, but circulating macrophages arrive after neutrophils; remain three to four times longer than neutrophils
		Maturation and division occur within injured tissue and increase metabolic activities in the area; active for 24-48 h
		Secrete interleukin-1, which activates T-cell response

pathogens than neutrophils. Macrophages are the predominant phagocyte seen in chronic inflammatory states. They also play an essential role as antigen-presenting cells in immune responses. After they digest pathogens, antigenic material appears on the surface of macrophages, activating lymphocytes with receptors for that antigen.

Neutrophils and macrophages may be circulating in the blood, as mentioned above, and in tissue, such as lymph nodes, spleen, liver sinuses (Kupffer cells),

lungs (alveolar macrophages), and other organs. This system of tissue phagocytes is called the **reticuloendothelial system** and operates in tandem with the lymphatic system. Tissue phagocytes mobilize as needed to destroy pathogens and can emigrate short distances to nearby tissue. These tissue phagocytes are longer-lived than circulating phagocytes and are more effective against intracellular bacteria, viruses, and protozoa.

The number of mature leukocytes in the blood at

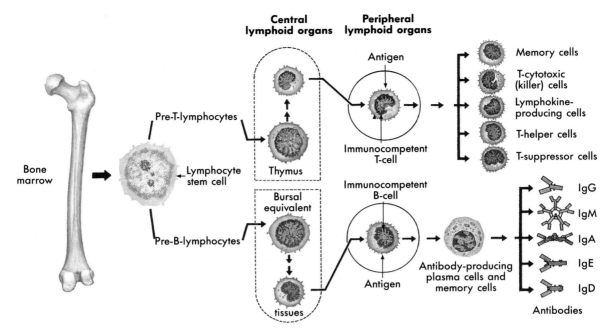

FIGURE 1-6
Maturation, differentiation, and activation of lymphocytes.

any one time is closely regulated with alterations in total number and type of leukocytes shifting with infection. These changes are discussed further in Chapter 3.

LYMPHOCYTES

Lymphocytes undergo a differentiation process that, as their name implies, is dependent on lymphoid tissue. The two classes of lymphocytes, T lymphocytes (also known as T cells) and B lymphocytes (also known as B cells), are the primary players in the immune response. Figure 1-6 demonstrates the maturation, differentiation, and activation of T and B lymphocytes.

Approximately 80% of the lymphocytes produced circulate to the thymus where, under the influence of thymic hormones, they proliferate and form mature T lymphocytes. The thymus is where the "education" process occurs, during which each T cell develops receptors for a specific antigen. As a result, each T cell can "recognize" and attach to a certain antigen.

The process of T-cell differentiation begins shortly before birth and continues for the first few months of life. Removal of the thymus after this time does not

interfere with T-cell immunity, because T cells clone themselves throughout life.

The remaining 20% of lymphocytes develop into B cells, which are responsible for producing antibodies. Similar to T cells, B cells are equipped with receptors that are antigen-specific. B-cell differentiation is thought to occur in bursal equivalent tissues of bone marrow, Peyer's patches (lymph tissue lining the small intestines), and in the liver during the prenatal and immediate postnatal periods. Also similar to T cells, B cells are renewed throughout life by cloning.

After they are formed, T and B cells circulate to lymph nodes, spleen, tonsils, and other lymph tissue. Since lymph tissue is positioned near the body's portals of entry, the lymphocytes are distributed to advantageous locations for intercepting antigens. The majority of T and B cells circulate continuously between the blood and lymphatic system, while others appear to reside in lymph tissue.

Activation of Lymphocytes

Until a T or B cell encounters in lymph tissue an antigen it recognizes, the lymphocyte is in a rather dormant state. At this point in the cycle the physical characteristics of the two cells are nearly identical, even under an electron microscope, although T and B cells do have different proteins on their cell membrane. Only after activation do T and B cells develop distinctive morphologic characteristics.

T cells are involved in both cell-mediated and humoral immunity (see page 17). Upon encountering an antigen it recognizes, the lymphocyte becomes activated and begins to proliferate wildly, producing identical cells that contain identical antigen receptors. Sensitized T cells develop into distinct subsets, each with a specific set of functions. T cell subsets are not structurally different from one another, but they carry different receptors, which forms the basis for immunologic assays. These subsets are classified as either effectors or regulators. Effector cells act directly on antigen, whereas regulatory cells direct other cells of the immune system, literally turning the immune response on and off (see box below).

B cells are involved in the humoral response (page 17). Activation of B cells produces two populations: antibody-secreting plasma cells and memory cells, which are reserved for future encounters with the same antigen and are the basis for developing acquired immunity. Plasma cells secrete antibodies into the blood at a rate of about 2,000 molecules per second. Antibodies bind to antigens, forming antigen-antibody complexes. Although not directly responsible for killing organisms, antibodies recruit complement, phagocytic cells, or cytotoxic T cells to destroy the antigens. Antibodies, which consist of large protein molecules called immunoglobulins, are discussed on page 17.

MEDIATORS

The internal defenses are orchestrated by a multitude of chemicals, proteins, and enzymes that, as a group, are termed *mediators*. Most of these substances are present throughout the body, remaining inactive until they are triggered by some event in the inflammatory process or by the immune system. Cell injury or death, for example, releases histamine, prostaglandins, and other mediators into the surrounding tissue. These substances initiate the vascular response, bringing into the area other mediators, such as complement system proteins, that normally circulate in the blood in an inactive form (see box on page 12).

Mediators have different properties, but most perform several functions. In many cases, one mediator activates other mediators. Table 1-3 summarizes the characteristics of the primary mediators. These substances are classified in the following manner:

- **Vasoactive substances**—cause small vessels to dilate and become more permeable
- **Leukocytosis promoters**—stimulate the release of leukocytes from bone marrow and the production of new leukocytes
- **Chemotactic substances or chemoattractants**—produce chemotaxis, which is the attraction of phagocytic cells either toward (positive chemotaxis) or away from (negative chemotaxis) the area
- **Leukotactic substances**—attract leukocytes to the area (leukotaxis)
- **Opsonins**—bind phagocytes to the invading microorganism, which promotes phagocytosis (opsonization)

T CELL SUBSETS

Effector cells

- Cytotoxic T cells (also known as killer T cells) are attracted to antigens, including microorganisms, cells that contain viruses, cancer cells, and transplanted cells. Cytotoxic T cells bind to the surface of an antigen, disrupt its cell membrane, and kill it directly with lymphokines. In addition, the release of lymphokines promotes phagocytosis.
- Delayed hypersensitivity T cells stimulate allergic reactions, anaphylaxis, and autoimmune reactions.

Regulator cells

- Helper T cells "turn on" the immune system by enhancing the response of B cells and cytotoxic T cells to antigens, stimulating the activity of all other T cells, and activating the macrophage system.
- Suppressor T cells "turn off" the action of helper and cytotoxic T cells, preventing them from causing excessive, potentially harmful immune reactions.

┌─────────────────── **COMPLEMENT SYSTEM** ───────────────────┐

Near the turn of the century, researchers recognized that blood plasma contained a substance that was required to "complete" the killing of bacteria, and the term **complement** was coined. We now recognize that complement is a complex of at least 20 serum enzymatic proteins that mediate the inflammatory reaction and amplify the specific immune response. These proteins circulate in the blood in an inactive state until they are activated by either immunologic stimuli (classical pathway) or nonimmunologic stimuli (alternate pathway). Once triggered, the complement proteins produce a cascade of reactions to increase vascular permeability, attract leukocytes, enhance phagocytosis, immobilize antigenic cells, and attack cell membranes.

- Classical pathway is activated by antigen-antibody reactions. IgG and IgM are complement-fixing antibodies that bind to an antigen, forming the initial connector molecule to which one of the complement proteins can attach. This initiates a systematic reaction referred to as the **complement cascade** that is eventually lethal to the invader. The reactions include activation of mast cells and basophils to release histamine; chemotaxis of neutrophils and macrophages; opsonization and phagocytosis by neutrophils and macrophages; lysis of the cell wall of some invaders; agglutination of some microorganisms; and neutralization of viruses.
- Alternate pathway is activated during inflammation by molecules in the cell membrane of yeasts and some bacteria.

└──┘

Table 1-3

PRIMARY MEDIATORS OF INFLAMMATION AND IMMUNE RESPONSE

Vasoactive amines Histamine Serotonin	Stored in tissue cells, basophils, and platelets; cause vasodilation and increased vascular permeability
Complement system	Complex of 20 or more enzymatic proteins found in the blood; increase vascular permeability; enhance phagocytosis as chemoattractants for leukocytes and opsonize antigens (see also the box above on Complement System)
Kinin (e.g., bradykinin)	A chemical produced in the blood that increases vascular permeability, causes vasodilation, and promotes chemotaxis
Prostaglandins (PG)	Enzymes produced by metabolic reaction of polyunsaturated fatty acids in most tissues; PGE and PGI are potent vasodilators and react with histamine and kinins to increase vascular permeability; stimulate hypothalmus to regulate temperature; stimulate pain receptors; may also have antiinflammatory actions and may modify immune function
Leukotrienes	Chemicals derived from same sources as PGs; found primarily in leukocytes; promote inflammation and hypersensitivity reactions; increase vascular permeability; chemoattractant for leukocytes; promotes adherence of leukocytes to endothelial cells; activates neutrophil enzymes
Platelet activating factor	A phospholipid found in neutrophils and macropages; stimulates chemotaxis, aggregation, and granule secretion of neutrophils and monocytes
Lymphokines	Proteins released primarily by T cells to stimulate other cells and neutralize toxins
Interleukin (IL)	IL-1 secreted by macrophages to activate helper T cells; stimulates the body's fever response; IL-2 secreted by activated helper T cells to stimulate cytotoxic T cells
Interferon	Produced by helper T cells; activates cytotoxic T cells to destroy intracellular pathogens; increases B cell production of antibodies
Tumor necrosis factor (TNF)	Bacterial endotoxin stimulates release of TNF from macrophages; activates neutrophils; stimulates production of prostaglandin E (PGE)
Platelet-derived growth factor (PDGF)	A chemoattractant
B-cell factors	Secreted by helper T cells; B-cell growth factor causes B cells to multiply; B-cell differentiation factor halts the multiplication of some B cells and prompts them to start producing antibodies
Proteinases (lysosomal enzymes)	Enzymes stored in lysosomes of leukocytes or produced in response to inflammation; they break down bacteria and proteins produced by the inflammatory process
Clotting system	Interacts with the complement system to produce several products important in the inflammatory response and tissue repair

THE SECOND LINE OF DEFENSE: THE INFLAMMATORY RESPONSE

Once a microorganism penetrates the first line of defense and invades cells, the inflammatory response is initiated. Inflammation is a local reaction to cell injury of any type, whether from physical, chemical, or thermal damage or microbial invasion. As a response to microbial injury, inflammation is aimed at preventing further invasion by walling off, destroying, or neutralizing the invading organism. Repair is also an integral part of inflammation, and in "clean" injuries, which do not involve microbes, repair is the primary beneficial result.

The early inflammatory response is protective, but it can continue for sustained periods of time in some infections. The production of new leukocytes (particularly phagocytic leukocytes) may be stimulated for weeks or months in some infections, as reflected in an elevated white blood cell count (particularly neutrophils and monocytes) for prolonged periods. However, sustained inflammation can become chronic and result in the destruction of healthy tissues. Extensive necrosis from persistent inflammation can actually increase tissue susceptibility to the infectious agent or provide an ideal setting for invasion by other pathogens.

The inflammatory response is limited to vascularized tissues, since the molecular components of inflammation are delivered via blood vessels. Inflammation develops in a series of interrelated steps that involve blood vessels, fluid and cellular blood components, the lymphatic system, and the surrounding connective tissue.

STAGES OF INFLAMMATORY RESPONSE

The complex mechanisms of the inflammatory response can be divided into three interdependent stages: cell response to injury, vascular response, and phagocytosis (Figure 1-7).

The cellular response to injury is the same regardless of the method of injury. A number of metabolic changes occur within the injured cell. The injured cell swells because it can no longer pump out sodium ions. Nearly all cells contain specialized sacs called *lysosomes* that contain a multitude of enzymes capable of digesting portions of the cell if its metabolic activity has been severely disrupted. The resulting cellular atrophy reduces metabolic demands on the cell. Cell death occurs if metabolism can no longer be maintained, and enzymes are released to dissolve the cellular contents and stimulate the inflammatory process in surrounding tissue.

The vascular response occurs shortly after injury. The arterioles, venules, and capillaries in the surrounding area dilate, producing a localized hyperemia.

This increases the filtration pressure of the blood and capillary permeability, causing fluid exudate to leak from the blood vessels into the interstitial spaces. Proteins, enzymes, and other chemical components in the exudate attract more fluid into the interstitial spaces, producing edema in an effort to wall off the inflamed area from uninvolved tissues.

Inflammatory exudate serves the important function of transporting phagocytic cells into the injured area. As fluid leaks from the blood, blood flow in the area slows, allowing leukocytes to collect (marginate) along the vascular endothelium. Leukocytes, particularly neutrophils and monocytes, emigrate through the endothelium to the injured tissue, attracted by chemicals released by the injured cells.

Phagocytosis is the process of engulfing, digesting, and destroying infectious agents and other material. This is done primarily by circulating macrophages, the majority of which are neutrophils and monocytes that are dispatched to an injured area in fluid exudate. Some macrophages reside in tissue and are found in lymph nodes, bone marrow, lungs (alveolar macrophages), spleen, liver (Kupffer cells), and other organs. Phagocytes also perform the essential "housekeeping" chore of cleaning up dead cells and other debris.

Intracellular phagocytosis occurs at the site of tissue invasion, but it also extends into lymphatic and blood circulation if infection becomes systemic. The intracellular activity of phagocytosis stimulates release of chemicals that induce lysis of the leukocytes. These dead leukocytes, together with dead organisms and fluid from the blood, make up the inflammatory exudate. Figure 1-7 illustrates phagocytosis.

PATTERNS OF INFLAMMATION

Both local and systemic symptoms of inflammation can occur. Heat, redness, swelling, and pain are local reactions to inflammation that may vary considerably in severity. The first three characteristics result from response of the vasculature to injury. Pain is produced partly from pressure of the exudate against nerve endings in the surrounding tissue, but prostaglandins and possibly other chemicals also play some role in causing pain.

Several types of inflammatory exudates can be produced locally (Table 1-4). Serous exudate, which typically occurs in early inflammation, contains only plasma and proteins. Mucinous or catarrhal exudate contains increased secretions from inflamed mucous membranes and may include both live and dead organisms. Fibrinous exudate forms on tissue, particularly mucous membranes, when large amounts of fibrinogen are extravasated into the tissue. Purulent exudate, such as pus, contains both live and dead leukocytes,

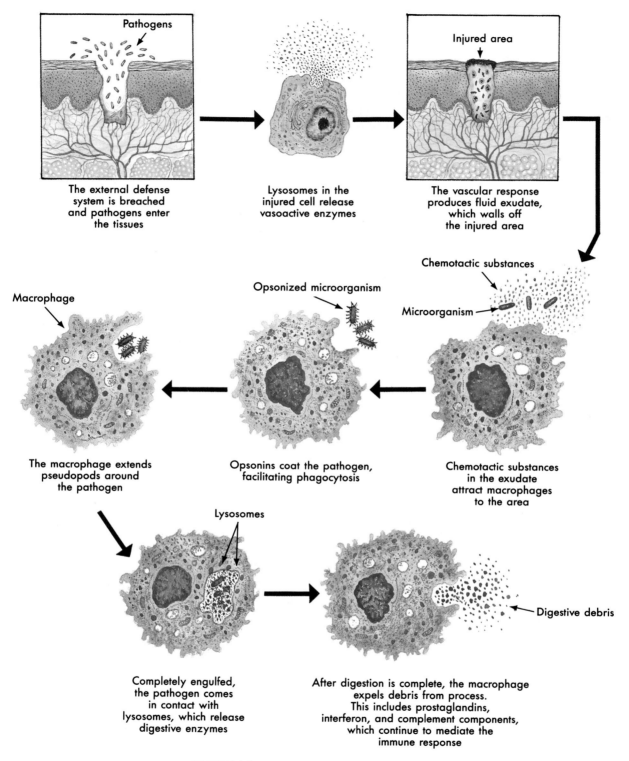

The external defense system is breached and pathogens enter the tissues

Lysosomes in the injured cell release vasoactive enzymes

The vascular response produces fluid exudate, which walls off the injured area

Pathogens

Injured area

Chemotactic substances

Microorganism

Opsonized microorganism

Macrophage

The macrophage extends pseudopods around the pathogen

Opsonins coat the pathogen, facilitating phagocytosis

Chemotactic substances in the exudate attract macrophages to the area

Lysosomes

Completely engulfed, the pathogen comes in contact with lysosomes, which release digestive enzymes

After digestion is complete, the macrophage expels debris from process. This includes prostaglandins, interferon, and complement components, which continue to mediate the immune response

Digestive debris

FIGURE 1-7
Second line of defense—inflammatory response.

live and dead microorganisms, serous exudate, and liquified digestive products of necrotic tissue. Some inflammatory conditions produce combinations of exudates. The characteristic fibrinopurulent exudate of diphtheria results from necrosis of the mucous membrane in the throat.

Inflammation and its exudates may remain localized, may permeate the tissue, or may spread throughout the body via the blood or lymph. An abscess is an example of a localized infection and inflammation with purulent exudate. Leukocytes form a wall around the organisms. The abscess deepens as more leukocytes are drawn into the area, more organisms are killed, and more necrotic tissue is dissolved. The exudate may eventually be autolyzed and resorbed by the body, in which case the inflammation and infection are resolved. Resolution may leave a cavity, ulcer, or scar tissue. Calcification around the exudate occurs in some instances, such as in tuberculosis walling off the live infectious agents inside the tissue. Rupture of the abscess and drainage into other tissues can spread the infection to other areas of the body.

Systemic symptoms can include fever and chills, diaphoresis, malaise, and nausea and vomiting. The inflammatory process also causes changes in blood components, such as an increased number of leukocytes or a change in the type of leukocytes.

Chronic inflammation may result from a low-grade inflammatory response that fails to elicit an acute response. Agents most often responsible for chronic inflammation are those that cannot penetrate deeply or spread rapidly, such as *M. tuberculosis*, the treponemata that cause syphilis, some viruses, fungi, and many helminths. Inadequate specific immune response or a hyperimmune response can also lead to chronic inflammation, such as occurs in autoimmune disorders.

Chronic inflammation is marked by tissue infiltration with macrophages, lymphocytes, and plasma cells rather than neutrophils. Exudates are not generally formed, although some types of chronic inflammatory disorders are characterized by certain types of exudates. Rheumatoid arthritis, for example, is accompanied by synovial effusions, an exudate into the joint. A proliferation of fibroblasts results in greater formation of scar tissue that sometimes replaces normal connective tissue or other tissue. Some chronic inflammations result in formation of granulomas, which are 1 to 2 mm lesions caused by the massing of macrophages surrounded by lymphocytes around an infectious agent. A dense membrane of connective tissue may encapsulate the lesion, as occurs in tuberculosis.

Several factors affect the outcome of the inflammatory process. Age, nutritional status, and general health greatly affect the individual's ability to mount an effective inflammatory response. Agent factors, such as virulence and size of inoculum, can overcome even an aggressive host defense and promote spread of the organism. In addition, some pathogens are effective intracellular parasites and are capable of surviving and multiplying in phagocytes. These include some viruses, *M. tuberculosis*, and *Rickettsia*. The immune response, the third line of defense, is activated to combat invaders that survive phagocytosis.

Table 1-4 ───────────────────────────────

INFLAMMATORY EXUDATES

Type of exudate	Characteristics
Serous	Clear; contains plasma and proteins
Mucinous (catarrhal)	Clear mucous membrane secretions; may contain live and dead microorganisms
Fibrinous	Contains fibrinogen extravasated into tissue
Purulent (pus)	Cloudy; contains leukocytes, live and dead microorganisms, serous exudate, and liquified necrotic tissue
Fibrinopurulent	Combination of characteristics of fibrinous and purulent
Hemorrhagic	Contains erythrocytes

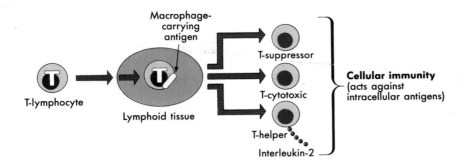

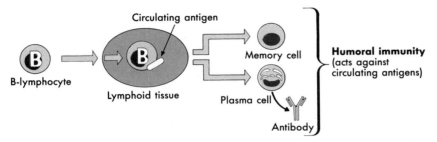

FIGURE 1-8
Cellular and humoral immunity. Cellular immunity results from activation of T lymphocytes by contact with intracellular organisms. Activated T cells differentiate and proliferate. Humoral (antibody mediated) immunity results from activating B lymphocytes.

THE THIRD LINE OF DEFENSE: THE IMMUNE RESPONSE

The first and second lines of defense are nonspecific—that is, they operate against all infectious agents in the same manner. In contrast, the immune system responds in a very specific manner to individual pathogens, as long as the organism has antigenic characteristics. Generally speaking, antigens are either proteins, large polysaccharides, or large lipoprotein complexes that stimulate an immune response. Not all microorganisms are antigenic, but some are bound by complement or other host-produced substances to form an antigen that elicits an immune response.

The immune system has several unique characteristics:

- Self-/nonself-recognition—It normally recognizes host cells as

nonantigenic and therefore responds only to foreign agents as antigens. In autoimmune diseases, there is a breakdown in this distinction, and the immune system attacks host cells as if they were antigens.
- Antibody production—It produces specific antibodies that target specific antigens for destruction, and it can produce new antibodies in response to new antigens.
- Memory—It remembers antigens that have invaded the body in the past, allowing a quicker response to subsequent invasion by the same antigen.
- Self-regulation—It monitors its own performance, turning itself on when antigens invade and turning itself off when infection is eradicated. This ability prevents destruction of healthy tissue.

An immune response is triggered after foreign materials have been cleared from an area of inflammation. After phagocytes digest the pathogens, antigenic material appears on their surface. Phagocytes, primarily macrophages, serve as antigen-presenting cells to introduce the pathogen to lymphocytes. Recognition of the antigen as "nonself" by receptors on lymphocytes in blood, lymph, or tissue exudate sets up a chain of responses to destroy or neutralize the antigen. Two types of immune responses can occur: cell-mediated immunity and/or humoral immunity (Figure 1-8). These processes begin with the differentiation of lymphocytes (Figure 1-6). These two types of responses overlap and interact considerably, but the distinction is useful in understanding how the immune system is activated.

CELL-MEDIATED IMMUNE RESPONSE

The cellular immune response is activated with the invasion of intracellular pathogens, such as viruses, mycobacteria, fungi, and protozoa, and it is a component of the host response to tumors and tissue transplants. Cell-mediated immunity, directed primarily by T cells, results from cell interaction with antigens expressed on phagocytes. T cell receptor binding to the antigen causes T cells to differentiate into subsets and proliferate. Helper T cells initiate the cell-mediated response by releasing interleukin-2, which stimulates the production of cytotoxic T cells. Cytotoxic T cells kill the antigen directly by releasing lymphokines, an event that also attracts more macrophages to the area. Suppressor T cells slow or completely halt the activity of other T cells.

Cell-mediated immunity is the basis for many skin tests, such as the tuberculin test. Cellular immunity cannot be transferred passively to another person.

HUMORAL IMMUNE RESPONSE

Humoral (antibody-mediated) immunity protects against many gram-positive and certain gram-negative bacteria. Antibody production also aids in neutralizing viruses, enhances phagocytosis, and activates the complement system. B cells, the antibody-producing lymphocytes, are responsible for humoral immunity.

Humoral immunity can be initiated in two ways. Some antigens are not recognized by T cells (T-independent antigens) and stimulate B cells directly. Most antigens, however, will bind to T cells (T-dependent antigens), and the helper T cells act to stimulate B cells. In either case, the stimulated B cells differentiate into antibody-producing plasma cells and memory B cells. Antibodies appear on the surface of plasma cells and bind to antigen. Once antigens are immobilized, cytotoxic T cells are activated and eradication of the pathogen begins. Suppressor T cells halt the humoral response after the infection is resolved.

The amount and type of antibody produced depend on the nature and amount of antigen present, the site of the antigen stimulus, and the number of previous exposures to the same antigen. The initial antibody production, the **primary response,** occurs the first time a particular antigen invades the body (from 1 to 7 days after initial exposure to the antigen). Depending on the nature of the antigen and the efficiency of antibody production, the response peaks in 1 to 10 weeks. Antibody titers can usually be detected within 10 days of exposure.

Memory B cells allow a more efficient humoral response on subsequent exposure to the same antigen (the **secondary response**). The memory cells generate more rapid, prolific, and sustained response, producing higher antibody titers that are usually detectable in a shorter period of time and for a longer duration.

The strength and persistence of the humoral immune response is determined by maintaining a correct balance between helper and suppressor T cells. Helper T cells must be present in sufficient numbers to stimulate B cell production of antibodies, and the correct proportion of T suppressor cells is needed to shut off the immune response. An imbalance can result in inadequate production of antibodies, leading to immune deficiency states, or the unchecked overstimulation of the immune response, resulting in autoimmune disorders. The normal helper to suppressor ratio is 2:1, whereas a 1:1 ratio is typical of acquired immune deficiency syndrome (AIDS).

The humoral immune response is more rapid than the cell-mediated response and is more frequently a factor in resistance to acute bacterial infections. Humoral immunity can be transmitted to another person, either by inoculation or by maternal transfer via the placenta or breast milk.

IMMUNOGLOBULINS

Immunoglobulins are the protein molecules that compose antibodies. There are five major classes of immunoglobulins that are able to combine in an endless number of ways to produce antibodies specific against a particular antigen. When the humoral immune response is initiated, more than one class may be activated. Table 1-5 summarizes the characteristics of the immunoglobulin classes.

Immunoglobulins perform four major functions:

1. Immunoglobulins directly attack antigens, destroying or neutralizing them through the processes of agglutination (clumping the antigens together to inactivate them), precipitating the toxins out of solution, neutralizing antigenic substances, and lysing the organism's cell wall.
2. Immunoglobulins activate the complement system (see Table 1-5 and the box on the Complement System, page 12).
3. Immunoglobulins activate anaphylaxis by releasing histamine in tissue and blood (see Table 1-5).
4. Immunoglobulins stimulate antibody-mediated hypersensitivity.

ACQUIRED IMMUNITY

Immunity refers to the presence of or acquisition of antibodies. Immunity can be acquired as a result of exposure to a specific antigenic agent or pathogen. Acquired immunity may be gained by natural means through inadvertent contact with an antigen (active) or antibodies (passive). Artificial immunity is intentionally induced through inoculation of antigen (active) or antibodies (passive) (Table 1-6). Active immunity, whether naturally or artificially induced, produces physiologically identical immune responses.

Table 1-5

IMMUNOGLOBULIN CLASSES

Immunoglobulin	Characteristics	Functions
IgG	Accounts for about 80-85% of antibodies in normal serum; most abundant in blood but also found in lymph, cerebrospinal, synovial, and peritoneal fluid and breast milk; the only immunoglobulin that crosses placenta and provides temporary immunity in neonate	Develops slowly during primary response, appearing about 1 wk or more after IgM, then reaches a peak in 1-3 wks or longer after IgM peaks; may persist for years; highest concentration during secondary immune response; activates complement system, involved in opsonization; attacks antigens directly
IgM	Accounts for about 5% of antibodies in normal serum	First antibody to form during viral or bacterial infection; usually peaks 1-2 wks after clinical symptoms appear; highest concentration during primary response; is increased in chronic infections; binds with viral and bacterial antigens in the circulation, which activates the complement cascade
IgA	Accounts for about 15% of antibodies in normal serum; found in blood and secretions (tears, saliva, colostrum, respiratory tract, and stomach and accessory organs)	Secretory antibody; increased in chronic infections and chronic inflammation
IgE	Accounts for <1% of antibodies in normal serum; found also in tissues	Sensitizing antibody; triggers release of histamine; involved with certain allergic disorders, especially atopic diseases; increased in parasitic diseases
IgD	Accounts for <1% of antibodies in normal serum	Function unclear, but increases in chronic infection

Table 1-6

TYPES OF ACQUIRED IMMUNITY

Type of immunity	How acquired	Length of resistance
Natural		
Active	Natural contact and infection with the antigen	May be temporary or permanent
Passive	Natural contact with antibody transplacentally or through colostrum and breast milk	Temporary
Artificial		
Active	Inoculation of antigen	May be temporary or permanent
Passive	Inoculation of antibody or antitoxin	Temporary

MANIFESTATIONS OF INFECTIOUS DISEASE

STAGES OF INFECTION

The progression from infection to infectious disease follows definable stages that arise in a predictable order, as demonstrated in Figure 1-9. The duration of each stage and the potential outcomes vary considerably, depending on the infecting agent and host factors.

The disease stage is extremely variable, since it may be asymptomatic or manifested clinically. It sometimes extends longer than the period of communicability. Complete resolution may be simultaneous with or may precede complete eradication of the agent. Some infections revert to latent disease characterized by intermittent infectious episodes, as occurs in malaria. With other infections, the host may become an asymptomatic carrier, continuing to harbor and shed the agent.

The communicability stage is also variable and is often the main determining factor for how easily a disease is transmitted. A number of infections are transmissible as long as the agent persists in the body. Such is the case with hepatitis B. Some viruses, such as mumps, are more communicable during the incubation period than during the disease stage. The communicable state can also be intermittent in diseases, such as tuberculosis, leprosy, syphilis, and gonorrhea, and infections characterized by recurrent disease states, such as malaria.

FEVER: THE HALLMARK OF INFECTIOUS DISEASE

Signs and symptoms of infectious disease vary, depending on the pathogen and the organ system affected. Manifestations can arise directly from the infecting organism or its products, but in most diseases the majority of symptoms results from host responses. Infectious diseases typically begin with the general symptoms of malaise, fatigue, weakness, and loss of concentration. Generalized aching and anorexia are common complaints. However, the hallmark of most infectious diseases is fever.

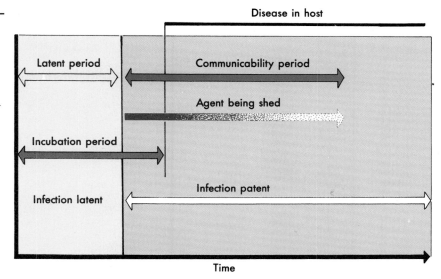

FIGURE 1-9

Stages of infection. Infection in the host proceeds in identifiable stages; the length of each stage varies with the pathogenic agent and host factors. The **latent period** begins with pathogenic invasion of the body and ends when the agent can be shed (communicability period). The **incubation period** begins with invasion of the agent, during which the organism reproduces, and ends when the disease process begins. The **communicability period** begins when the latent period ends and continues as long as the agent is present. The **disease period** follows the incubation period and ends at variable times. This stage may be subclinical or produce overt symptoms, and it may resolve completely or become latent.

Fever is not a failure of the body to regulate temperature; rather the body temperature is regulated at a higher level than normal. Body temperature is regulated by nervous system feedback to the hypothalamus, which functions as a central thermostat.

Changes in regulation of the thermostat are stimulated by pyrogens that are released by the body or by the pathogens. Heat-sensitive neurons located on the skin, in the spinal cord, and in the abdomen monitor environmental and metabolic conditions and transmit signals to the hypothalmus. Based on the information received from these neurons, efferent signals from the hypothalmus are transmitted throughout the body to control heat loss, heat conservation, and heat production. Fever is produced by heat conservation and increased heat production. Body temperature returns to normal via heat-loss mechanisms.

Heat conservation is promoted by vasoconstriction and abolition of sweating. Heat production is increased by stimulating tone and shivering in skeletal muscles; by releasing epinephrine and norepinephrine to increase cellular metabolism (a more common means of heat production in infants than in adults); and by the release of thyroxine from the thyroid gland to increase cell metabolism. This latter mechanism results in a slower response than the other two methods of in-

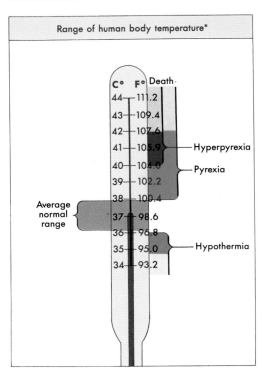

Range of human body temperature*

FIGURE 1-10
The range of human body temperature (measured orally).

creasing heat production. Heat loss occurs from evaporation of sweat and peripheral vasodilation.

During infection helper T cells and macrophages secrete interleukin-1, which, in addition to its activities as a messenger protein, is a pyrogen. Some bacteria also produce pyrogenic endotoxins. Pyrogens cause the "set point" of the hypothalamus to rise, increasing the metabolic rate of cells to assist rapid generation of lymphocytes and phagocytic cells. Thus fever has a

beneficial effect—up to a point. For each degree Fahrenheit of temperature elevation, body metabolism increases 7%, and extreme elevations can damage cells irreversibly. Temperatures of 104° F (40° C) can cause delirium and convulsions, particularly in children, and fever above 106° F (41.1° C) can irreparably impair the hypothalamic control center.

Physiologic responses to fever occur in four stages:

- **Direct transmission** with an infected person or animal occurs by direct body contact (e.g., touching, kissing, or sexual contact) and by transfer of secretions through sneezing or coughing. Diseases that are transmitted only by direct contact are sometimes called **contagious**.
- **Indirect transmission** occurs through an intermediate animal host (e.g., a rabid dog), a vector (e.g., a mosquito carrying malaria), or a contaminated object (e.g., a needle or food).

1. First stage (prodromal period)—The hypothalamus has sent signals to begin heat conservation and nonspecific symptoms of discomfort (e.g., malaise) appear before temperature change occurs.
2. Second stage—Body temperature rises toward a higher thermostat setting, producing chills.
3. Third stage—Flushing occurs when the temperature has reached the new set point.
4. Fourth stage—Body temperature begins to return toward normal (defervescence), causing sweating.

Fever patterns can vary considerably and do not necessarily reflect disease severity (Figure 1-10). Fever may be continual or intermittent, extremely high or low grade, or abrupt or gradual in onset.

TRANSMISSION OF INFECTION

The ability of a pathogen to produce infectious disease requires an intact chain of transmission that includes the pathogen, a reservoir, a portal of exit from the reservoir, an environment conducive to transmission of the pathogen, a portal of entry to a new host, and the susceptibility of the new host to the infectious disease (Figure 1-11).

RESERVOIR

The environment in which a pathogen lives and multiplies may be a person, animal, arthropod, plant, soil, water, food, or other organic substance or a combination of these reservoirs. The agent (pathogen) depends on the reservoir for its reproduction and consequent survival. Humans are the only reservoir for some

pathogens, whereas other agents require an intermediate animal(s) or an inanimate reservoir. The human reservoir may be clinically ill, have a subclinical infection, or be a carrier.

PORTAL OF EXIT

In exiting an animal or human reservoir, the pathogen usually escapes from a portal nearest its breeding site. Portals of exit include the genitourinary tract, intestinal tract, oral cavity, respiratory tract, open lesions, or any wound through which blood escapes. A pathogen may escape through more than one portal of exit.

The period of time a pathogen can escape coincides with the period of communicability, which varies with each disease. Generally there is an inverse relationship between length of the communicable period and the infectivity of the organism. Highly infectious pathogens, such as the orthomyxoviruses, which cause influenza, have a short duration of escape and high communicability, whereas the less infective *M. tuberculosis* has a long duration of escape and lower communicability.

TRANSMISSION

The portal of exit determines the mode of transmission and, as with exit points, may have a single or multiple route of transmission. In general, most pathogens are transmitted either directly or indirectly. Direct transmission occurs when there is actual physical contact between the source and the victim, as occurs with diseases transmitted sexually or orally, by fecal contamination, or by airborne mucous droplets. Indirect transmission requires that organisms survive on animate or inanimate vehicles for a time without a human host. Inanimate vehicles include air, food, water, soil, fomites, or biologic materials. An inanimate vehicle that has the potential for infecting many persons is called a **common vehicle.**

PORTAL OF ENTRY

Portal of entry into a new host often corresponds with the portal of exit from a human reservoir. Entry may be by ingestion, inhalation, or percutaneous injection and through the mucous membranes or across the placenta. The duration of exposure to the pathogen and the number of organisms required to start the infectious process vary with each disease.

HOST SUSCEPTIBILITY

Earlier in the chapter, we discussed the defense systems against infectious disease. Host susceptibility is also influenced by general human characteristics, such as age, sex, ethnic group, and heredity; cultural behaviors regarding eating and personal hygiene; geographic and environmental conditions; and general

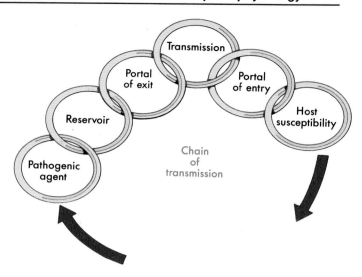

FIGURE 1-11
Chain of transmission for infection. The chain must be intact for an infection to be transmitted to another host. Transmission can be controlled by breaking any link in the chain.

health status, including nutrition, hormonal balance, and the presence of concurrent disease. These factors contribute to the host's susceptibility to exposure to specific pathogens and the host response.

CONTROL OF TRANSMISSION

Control of infectious disease relies on breaking the chain of transmission at one or more links. Control measures may be directed at killing or altering the virulence of the pathogen, destroying nonhuman reservoirs and vectors, isolating infected persons, using precautions with infected body fluids and contaminated objects, and improving host resistance. Effective control is also based on monitoring disease occurrence to facilitate early intervention. Many infectious diseases must be reported to the local health department (see inside front cover).

SPECTRUM OF DISEASE OCCURRENCE

Characteristics of the organism and mode of transmission are the two most important factors in how often a particular infectious disease occurs and how many people are affected.
- **Sporadic disease** is the occasional, irregular appearance of cases in a population over a given period of time.
- **Endemic disease** occurs at a constant rate, affecting about the same number of people in a population over a given period of time.
- **Epidemic disease** is a definite increase over its expected endemic pattern.
- **Pandemic disease** is an epidemic occurring over a very wide area and usually affecting a large proportion of the population.
     Some diseases also demonstrate predictable seasonal, yearly, or geographic variation in occurrence.

Assessment

Infectious agents cause a wide range of diseases, from mild, self-limiting infections to severe, life-threatening illness and from localized to systemic infections. Symptoms vary from highly specific, such as occurs with an infected wound, to a generalized feeling of illness. Although susceptibility to infection increases with poor nutrition, chronic disease, immunosuppression, fatigue, and stress, healthy individuals are also victims of pathogenic agents.

Many infectious diseases follow a reasonably predictable risk pattern in which they occur more commonly in certain individuals. Age is a factor in some diseases, such as chickenpox, which most often affects children. Some infections, such as tuberculous infections, have a higher prevalence in lower socioeconomic groups because of crowded conditions, poor sanitation, and poor nutrition. Certain behaviors—for example, IV drug use—place individuals at risk for blood-borne infectious agents, such as HIV and hepatitis B. However, with very few exceptions, there can be considerable crossover to low-risk individuals. Chickenpox can and does affect adults, tuberculosis can and does affect individuals of all socioeconomic groups, and HIV and hepatitis B are transmitted by maternal transfer and by blood products.

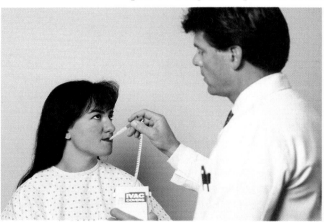

For all these reasons, the nurse often faces a challenge in assessing patients with infections and those who have been exposed to infectious agents. Infections encompass the entire spectrum of illness and strike individuals from all socioeconomic and cultural backgrounds. Because not all patients will fit the expected profile associated with a particular infection, it is important for the nurse to keep an open mind and avoid making assumptions.

It is equally important to provide a confidential atmosphere and project a nonjudgmental attitude. Although it is obvious that a diagnosis of a sexually transmitted disease (STD) can cause great embarrassment to the patient, it may be less obvious that some patients may find other types of infection equally embarrassing. For example, some patients associate food poisoning with carelessness or skin infections with lack of cleanliness. A child's parasitic infestation may arouse feelings of guilt in a parent.

Finally, the nurse must consider the potential for transmission to others. This requires an understanding of the mode of transmission of the pathogenic agents and the degree of infectivity. Gloves must be worn when handling body fluids or secretions and while examining the nasopharyngeal area, genitourinary area, or skin lesions. In addition, persons who have close contact with patient and are therefore at risk should be identified during the assessment process, and appropriate instructions should be given to the patient regarding his or her responsibility in informing these contacts that they are at risk. During assessment, patient teaching about transmission may be necessary even before a definite diagnosis has been established if the transmission chain is to be broken. For example, a patient who has a probable STD needs to understand the importance of protecting sexual partners against infection.

Because infectious diseases can involve any system in the body, the nurse will direct the physical assessment based on the patient's description of his or her symptoms, other relevant history (such as coexistent ;ease), and objective signs and symptoms.

HISTORY

The nursing interview serves three primary purposes: to obtain details about the patient's chief complaint, to investigate the patient's history for factors that may contribute to infection and influence the outcome of treatment, and to observe the patient for clues to his or her health status and emotional state. The interview provides an opportunity for the nurse to establish rapport with the patient. By demonstrating interest and concern, the nurse can often elicit information that is helpful in arriving at a diagnosis more quickly.

The exact nature of the complaint will determine the line of questioning, but the questions should be direct, specific, and worded in a way to avoid suggesting answers. Following is a guideline for eliciting information about the patient's medical history and other factors that may relate to infection.

HEALTH HISTORY

Patient history: factors relating to infectious diseases
Potential exposure to infectious agents

Contact with infected persons
Possible ingestion of contaminated food or water
    Close contacts have same symptoms
    Ingested raw seafood or undercooked meat
    Poor sanitation in the home (e.g., lack of refrigeration or poor disposal of sewage)
    Drinking untreated water
Animal (domestic or wild) bites
    Insect bites
    Surgery or other invasive medical procedures
    High-risk sexual practices or multiple sexual partners
    Dental procedures
    IV drug use
    Foreign travel

Risk factors that alter host resistance to infectious agents

Recent injury
Exposure to environmental irritants (e.g., chemicals and pollens)
Living and working conditions
Smoking—amount per day, number of years
Alcohol—amount per day or week, number of years
Dehydration or altered food intake

Medical history related to increased risk of infection

Metabolic and immune disorders
    Diabetes mellitus
    Renal disease
    Arthritis
    Autoimmune disease

Immune deficiency disease
Cancer and cancer therapy
Antibiotic therapy

Previous infections

Childhood infectious diseases—rubeola, rubella, mumps, pertussis, scarlet fever, chickenpox, and strep throat
Encephalitis or meningitis
Tuberculosis
Gastrointestinal infections and parasites
Hepatitis
Rheumatic fever
Hematolymphatic infections
HIV infection
Sexually transmitted disease
Hospital-acquired infections
Vector-transmitted infections

Immunization history

Tetanus, diphtheria, pertussis
Mumps
Rubella
Rubeola
Polio
Tuberculosis skin test or BCG vaccine
Influenza
Haemophilus influenzae B

Present complaint: guidelines for interviewing patients with possible infectious diseases

Reason for visit—The patient's statement, in his or her own words, for seeking medical attention

HEALTH HISTORY

Body system(s) affected by symptoms

Skin
Eyes, ears, and nose
Throat and mouth
Lungs
Gastrointestinal tract
Genitourinary tract
Musculoskeletal system
Central nervous system
Generalized

Skin

Inflammation
Rashes or lesions
Wounds or bites
Pruritis or pain

Eyes

Discharge
Pruritis
Lacrimation
Pain
Periorbital edema
Photophobia
Vision changes

Ears

Pain
Ringing
Hearing loss
Vertigo
Discharge

Nose

Discharge
Sinus pain
Postnasal drip
Sneezing
Lesions around nares

Mouth and throat

Soreness
Lesions of tongue, mouth, or lips
Hoarseness
Laryngitis
Swallowing difficulty

Lungs

Pain
Cough
Sputum production
Shortness of breath

Gastrointestinal

Nausea/vomiting
Diarrhea

Jaundice
Pain
Changes in eating and elimination patterns

Urinary

Pain or burning on urination
Urinary urgency
Suprapubic pain
Flank pain
Pyuria or hematuria

Genital—women

Lesions
Discharge
Odor
Genital pain, burning, itching, or swelling
Pelvic pain
Pain with intercourse
Unusual bleeding

Genital—men

Lesions
Discharge
Anal pain, itching, or burning; lesions; discharge

Musculoskeletal

Joint or bone pain
Swelling
Limited movement
Redness
Stiffness
Myalgia or arthralgia
Recent streptococcal infection

Central nervous system

Headache
Stiff neck
Alteration in consciousness

General symptoms

Fatigue
Weakness
Listlessness
Inability to concentrate
Fever
Anorexia
Weight loss
Enlarged lymph nodes

Previous efforts to treat

Over-the-counter drugs
Prescription drugs
Previously sought medical treatment
Other

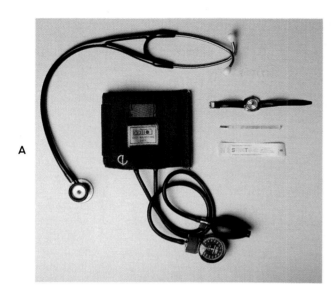

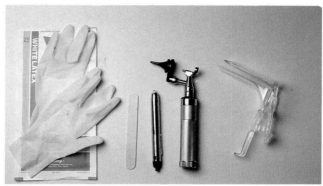

FIGURE 2-1
A, Complete vital signs are monitored to detect fever and systemic responses to fever. **B,** Examination, when infection is suspected, will be directed to the organs or systems that manifest symptoms. Gloves should be worn when examining mucous membranes of eyes, ears, nose, throat, and genital areas and any lesions anywhere.

GENERAL ASSESSMENT

Many infectious diseases produce signs and symptoms that are obvious to both patient and examiner, such as an infected wound. In such cases, the patient often makes the diagnosis before seeking treatment, and the examiner confirms the diagnosis through a brief evaluation, which includes a general assessment and examination of the symptomatic site. Infections that produce generalized or equivocal systemic symptoms may require a complete examination to establish a probable diagnosis that must often be confirmed by diagnostic tests.

Before starting the assessment, determine whether cultures or examination of specimens will be necessary and have the appropriate sterile container on hand. If you are unsure of the proper container, consult your-

procedures manual or laboratory personnel. Chapter 3 details the techniques for obtaining the various specimens.

The equipment needed will depend on how detailed an assessment is necessary and which systems will be examined. To perform a general assessment the following

> **The cardinal symptoms of infection** are fever, localized inflammation, and subjective findings (such as malaise, fatigue, pain, nausea).

equipment is needed: a thermometer, sphygmomanometer with appropriate-size cuff, stethoscope, and watch with a second hand (Figure 2-1).

ASSESSMENT OF PATIENT BEHAVIOR

Nursing Assessment: Observe patient's behavior and appearance. Listen to patient's nonspecific complaints.

Many symptoms of infection manifest as subjective complaints that are not easily confirmed by objective assessment. Through observing the patient's behavior and appearance, the nurse can often validate these complaints. Slowed movement, using objects for sup-

port, slumped posture, faint speech, or careless grooming may indicate malaise, listlessness, fatigue, and weakness. Other frequently cited nonspecific complaints are myalgia, arthralgia, and headache, which may be reflected in the patient's facial expression, as well as other signs of distress, such as acute pain and shortness of breath. Loss of concentration and anorexia are other common complaints.

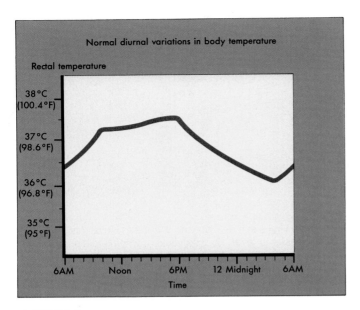

FIGURE 2-2
Normal diurnal variations in body temperature. Normal body temperature varies during a 24-hour period to correspond with changes in metabolism.

MONITORING TEMPERATURE AND OTHER VITAL SIGNS

Nursing assessment: Monitor temperature, pulse, respirations, and blood pressure every 4 hours to detect fever and systemic responses to fever. Monitor for flushing and diaphoresis associated with fever.

Most infectious diseases produce fever, and fever is sometimes the only clinical manifestation of an infectious process. Fever, however, is a nonspecific response that is also associated with a number of noninfectious events, including drug reactions, traumatic injuries, vascular disease, malignancies, and immunologic disorders.

The "normal" body temperature is 98.6° F (37° C) measured orally, although individual variations range from about 97°F to 99.6°F (36.1°C to 37.5°C). In addition, everyone experiences a diurnal variation in body temperature, with the highest readings occurring in late afternoon or early evening and the lowest readings occurring during early morning hours from 3 to 5 AM. Figure 2-2 demonstrates temperature variations in a typical 24-hour period.

Fever is defined clinically as an oral temperature over 100° F (37.8° C) or a rectal temperature over 100.8° F (38.2° C). Infectious disorders rarely cause the body temperature to exceed 106° F (41° C) except for central nervous system infections. Temperatures above this are usually the result of overheating in a hot environment.

It should be remembered, however, that the very young and the elderly often have quite different fever responses. Young children can spike temperatures to 105° F (40.5° C) with trivial infections, although children under 3 years sometimes have only minor temperature elevations with infections that normally produce marked elevation in older children and adults. Patients over 65 years may have serious infections with no or only slight fever, or they may even be hypothermic.

Several fever patterns have been recognized. The most common pattern seen in infections is *remittent fever*, in which the temperature waxes and wanes 2 or 3 degrees without returning to normal. A *sustained fever* demonstrates little variation over a 24-hour period and is common in streptococcal pneumonia. *Intermittent fever* is a predictable cycle of fever alternating with normal temperatures, usually with the highest point occurring in the evening and normal temperatures during the day. A low-level fever that persists sometimes for years is a *habitual fever*. *Relapsing fevers* recur after apparent recovery.

Both the onset and the resolution of fever may be sudden or gradual. Some infections follow a "saddle-back" curve characterized by a high fever initially, followed by a few days of remission, and then a second period of high temperature elevation.

As the body's temperature increases, there is usually an increased heart rate of about 10 bpm for every degree Fahrenheit. The respiratory rate also increases. Blood pressure is typically in the normal range, although hypotension may develop in severe infections.

Chills occur as the body temperature rises and sometimes precedes fever. The patient's extremities may be cool and pale during this phase. Fever of 101° F or more can give the patient a flushed look, with the skin warm to the touch. Sweating occurs with high fevers and with defervescence.

EXAMINATION OF LYMPH NODES

Nursing Assessment: Inspect and palpate lymph nodes in the region where localized infection is suspected. Examine all lymph nodes for systemic infection.

Inspect the lymph nodes in the head, neck, axilla, and inguinal areas for erythema, swelling, tenderness, or red streaks. Pay particular attention to sites of injury or obvious infection that may have erythematous streaks indicating lymphangitis originating from these areas.

Palpate the lymph nodes (Figures 2-3 and 2-4), using a firm but gentle touch and moving skin over the area to be palpated to detect swelling, heat, or tenderness. Note texture and movement of any nodules. Detection of superficial nodes less than 1 cm in diameter is a common finding in healthy adults. Lymph tissue may be up to 3 cm in healthy children age 6 to 12.

Tender, warm lymph node enlargement is a common finding in a variety of infections. The nodes may be either fixed or matted. In children enlarged postauricular nodes often accompany otitis media.

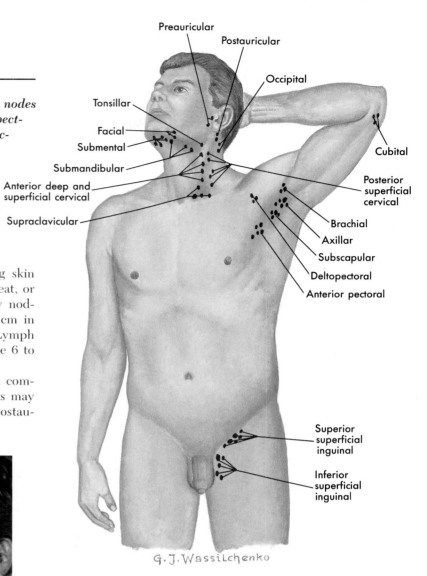

FIGURE 2-3
Location of palpable lymph nodes.

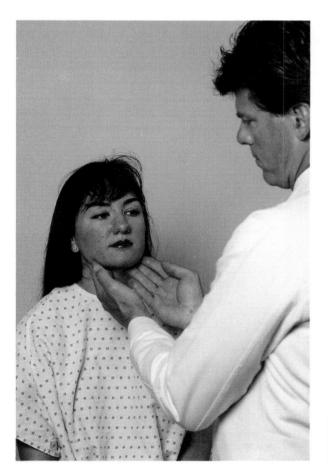

FIGURE 2-4
Palpate lymph nodes by moving skin over area to be palpated. Feel for swelling, heat, tenderness, texture, and movement of any nodules.

EXAMINATION OF SKIN

Nursing Assessment: Note the presence of erythema, edema, heat, excessive moisture or dryness, or lesions.

Skin lesions are a common sign of numerous viral, bacterial, and fungal infections. Lesions may be a manifestation of systemic infection, such as occurs in chickenpox, or the infection may be a local process. In evaluating patients with skin lesions, be cautious in touching the skin because pain or pruritis may be present.

In assessing skin lesions, note the type and characteristics (e.g., size, shape, color, texture, and elevation or depression), location and distribution, pattern of arrangement (e.g., annular, grouped, linear, arciform, or diffuse), and any exudate (e.g., amount, color, and consistency) (Figure 2-5). Skin lesions typically associated with infection are described below (not all of those listed result from an infectious process).

Parasitic infestations can produce unusual patterns of inflammation. Fine, dark, wavy lines up to 1 cm long and ending with a tiny papule indicate scabies. Hookworm produces a narrow winding trail of inflammation appearing most commonly on the feet, legs, buttocks, or back.

Using a magnifying glass, inspect the scalp and other areas of the body covered by hair for signs of lice. Nits are small, oval, greyish-white ova that adhere to the hair shaft. Lice infestation is sometimes accompanied by a nonspecific dermatitis, and secondary bacterial infection may occur in excoriated areas.

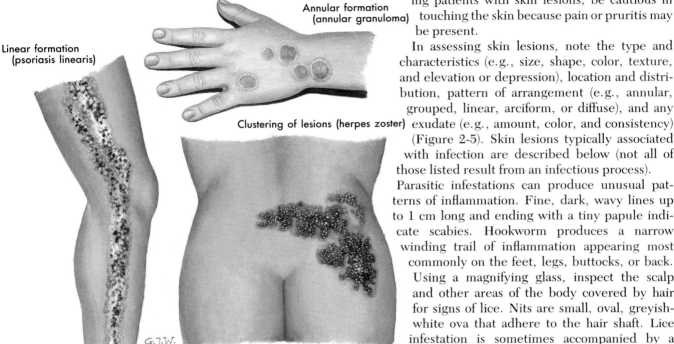

Linear formation
(psoriasis linearis)

Annular formation
(annular granuloma)

Clustering of lesions (herpes zoster)

G.J.W.

FIGURE 2-5
Patterns of skin lesions.

—SKIN LESIONS—

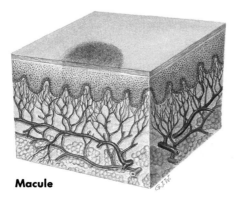

Macule

Flat; nonpalpable; circumscribed; less than 1 cm in diameter; brown, red, purple, white, or tan

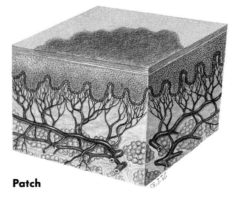

Patch

Flat; nonpalpable; irregular in shape; macule that is greater than 1 cm in diameter

—SKIN LESIONS—

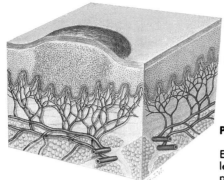

Papule

Elevated; palpable; firm; circumscribed; less than 1 cm in diameter; brown, red, pink, tan, or bluish red

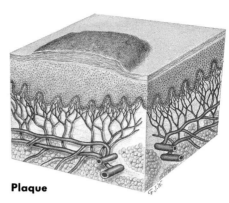

Plaque

Elevated; flat topped; firm; rough; superficial papule greater than 1 cm in diameter; may be coalesced papules

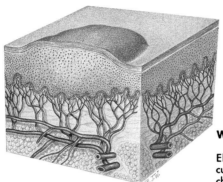

Wheal

Elevated; irregular-shaped area of cutaneous edema; solid, transient, changing; variable diameter; pale pink

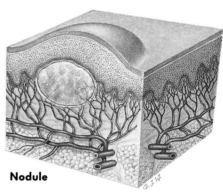

Nodule

Elevated; firm; circumscribed; palpable; deeper in dermis than papule; 1 to 2 cm in diameter

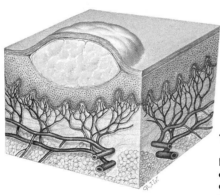

Tumor

Elevated; solid; may or may not be clearly demarcated; greater than 2 cm in diameter; may or may not vary from skin color

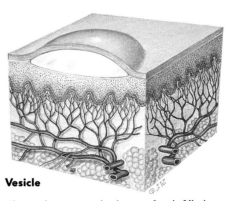

Vesicle

Elevated; circumscribed; superficial; filled with serous fluid; less than 1 cm in diameter

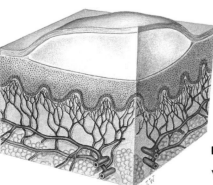

Bulla

Vesicle greater than 1 cm in diameter

—SKIN LESIONS—

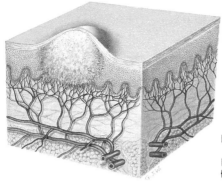

Pustule

Elevated; superficial; similar to vesicle but filled with purulent fluid

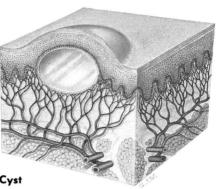

Cyst

Elevated; circumscribed; palpable; encapsulated; filled with fluid or semisolid material

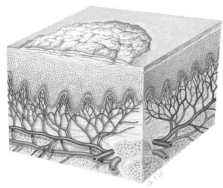

Scale

Heaped-up keratinized cells; flaky exfoliation; irregular; thick or thin; dry or oily; varied size; silver, white, or tan

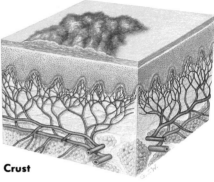

Crust

Dried serum, blood or purulent exudate; slightly elevated; size varies; brown red, black, tan, or straw

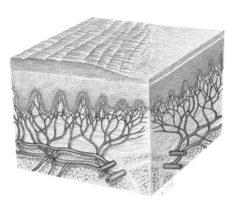

Lichenification

Rough, thickened epidermis; accentuated skin markings caused by rubbing or irritation; often involves flexor aspect of extremity

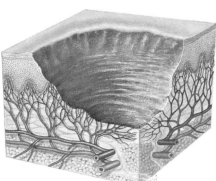

Ulcer

Loss of epidermis and dermis; concave; varies in size; exudative; red or reddish blue

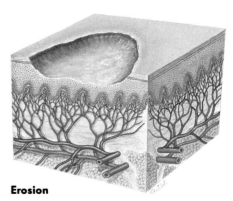

Erosion

Loss of all or part of epidermis; depressed; moist; glistening; follows rupture of vesicle or bulla; larger than fissure

REVIEW OF SYSTEMS

Infectious diseases may occur in any organ system, so if infectious disease is suspected, an examination in all or some organ systems may be necessary. The outline below provides a screening examination for each of these areas:

Skin: Inspect exposed and unexposed skin for color (e.g., erythema associated with inflammation; jaundice with hepatitis), hair distribution, lesions, and parasites; palpate for moisture, temperature, texture, turgor, and mobility to detect signs of fever and dehydration associated with fluid loss; palpate for consistency of lesions; collect specimen of any lesion exudate for lab analysis

Eyes: Inspect periorbital area for edema; inspect eyelid margins for exudate or excessive lacrimation, flakiness, redness, swelling, or lesions; inspect conjunctiva for erythema or cobblestone appearance, indicating conjunctivitis and for jaundice associated with hepatitis; inspect eye movement for excessive blinking, indicating photophobia; collect discharge for lab analysis

Ears: Inspect and palpate the auricles for tenderness, swelling, presence of nodules, or pain; perform otoscopic examination—inspect external canal for redness, exudate, or scaling, and inspect tympanic membrane for bulging, redness, retraction, bubbling, rupture, or exudate; collect any discharge or exudate for lab analysis

Nose and sinus: Inspect nasal passages for discharge (e.g., watery, mucous, purulent, crusty, or bloody); inspect frontal and maxillary sinus areas for swelling; palpate sinuses for pain; collect nasal secretions for lab analysis

Mouth and throat: Inspect lips for lesions and unusual color; inspect buccal mucosa and gums for lesions, edema, and inflammation; inspect pharynx and tonsils for edema, inflammation, lesions, or exudate; collect lesion or pharyngeal exudate for lab analysis

Thorax: Inspect respiratory rate and depth for tachypnea; palpate thoracic expansion from posterior and anterior positions (limitation in expansion may indicate inflammation and pain); palpate the chest wall for tactile fremitus (e.g., increased with pneumonia; normal in bronchitis); percuss the chest wall systematically from side to side and compare tones (e.g., dull over areas of consolidation of pneumonia; resonant with bronchitis); auscultate breath sounds (e.g., bronchial sounds and crackles with consolidation; prolonged expiration, wheezes or crackles may indicate bronchitis); evaluate characteristics of cough; collect sputum specimen

Heart: Auscultate for abnormal heart sounds—such as holosystolic murmur (at apex) (indicates mitral regurgitation) or diastolic murmur (indicates mitral stenosis)—both associated with rheumatic valvulitis; inspiratory pericardial friction rub associated with pericarditis; ventricular gallop (S_3) associated with endocarditis and myocarditis

Abdomen: Auscultate abdomen with diaphragm of stethoscope to detect increased bowel sounds associated with gastroenteritis; auscultate over liver and spleen for friction rubs associated with edema; palpate and percuss abdomen to identify organ enlargement and areas of tenderness; palpate for splenic enlargement; collect vomitus and stool specimens for laboratory analysis and culture

Peripheral vascular: Inspect extremities for color and edema; palpate peripheral pulse: absent or diminished may be associated with arteritis; palpate for heat associated with inflammation; test for Homan's sign (Have the patient bend the knee while you sharply dorsiflex the foot; calf pain indicates a positive Homan's sign associated with thrombophlebitis)

Musculoskeletal: Inspect muscles and joints for swelling, erythema; palpate for heat and tenderness; assess for weakened muscle strength, which may be associated with myelitis; evaluate movement and gait for signs of pain

Central nervous system: Assess for decreased level of consciousness or for confusion indicating CNS infection; assess changes in behavior or emotional responses; assess flexion of neck for nuchal rigidity associated with meningitis

Genitourinary: Percuss costovertebral angle (flank area of back) for kidney tenderness; collect urine specimen for lab analysis; inspect external genitalia for signs of lice or nits, edema, erythema, lesions, or discharge; with gloved hands, palpate any lesions for consistency or tenderness
  Female: Using a speculum, inspect cervix and vaginal walls for edema, erythema, lesions, and exudate; obtain specimen of exudate for lab analysis
  Male: Inspect testes for asymmetric enlargement; palpate scrotum for tenderness; obtain specimen of urethral discharge for lab analysis

Rectal: Inspect perianal area for inflammation, lesions, exudates, and signs of parasites (e.g., lice and nits); palpate rectal area for tenderness; insert gloved finger into anal opening to palpate for lesions and tenderness; collect exudate and/or fecal specimen for lab analysis

Diagnostic Procedures

Chapter 3 is organized into two sections. The first part (pages 32-45) describes procedures for collecting and handling specimens. The second part (pages 45 to 51) describes diagnostic tests. These include skin tests, microscopic examination, cultures, immunologic tests, and antibiotic sensitivity tests.

COLLECTING AND HANDLING SPECIMENS

If pathologic agents responsible for infectious diseases are to be correctly identified, specimens must be collected and handled very carefully. Failure to use proper techniques to obtain a specimen can result in contamination with normal flora, which leads to inaccurate laboratory results. Incorrect handling of the specimen after it is collected may result in killing the organisms before culturing or in spurious overgrowth of the organism in the culture. It is essential that you become familiar with your institution's laboratory procedures for handling and transporting specimens. If in doubt, ask questions.

The danger inherent in handling specimens (or any body fluids of infected patients) cannot be overemphasized. To protect yourself, your colleagues, and other patients, you must be compulsive about practicing measures that prevent contamination and spread of infection.

Although procedures differ according to the type of specimen, the following general principles apply to the collection and handling of all fluids and tissues.

OBTAINING ADEQUATE SPECIMENS

- Prevent embarrassment by assuring complete privacy and confidentiality for the patient. This will help the patient relax and facilitate collection of a good specimen.
- Obtain the specimen during the acute stage of infection and before initiating antibiotic therapy, if possible.
- The specimen must be representative of the infectious process. Secretions or excretions from unin-

volved areas should be avoided during collection.
- Obtain an adequate amount of the specimen necessary for tests. Check with your laboratory if you are not sure.
- Use the proper collection instruments and containers and place the specimen in a sterile or clean container, as indicated.
- Label the container to identify the patient, source of the specimen (e.g., sputum, urine, or venous blood), date, time collected, test(s) to be performed, and organism suspected (Figure 3-1).
- For specimens that must be inoculated directly into culture or transport medium, do not open the container until you have obtained the specimen. This prevents environmental organisms from contaminating the medium.
- If the specimen or collection materials are accidentally contaminated by contact with other secretions, the patient's skin, or nonsterile objects, discard the specimen and obtain another.

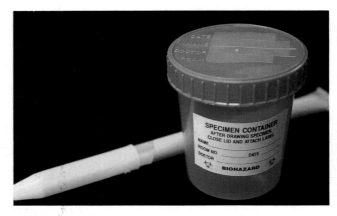

FIGURE 3-1
Properly label the specimen container.

- When the patient will collect his or her own specimen, give complete verbal and written instructions. (Chapter 14 provides patient teaching materials that can be photocopied and given to the patient.)
- Maintain the recommended temperature of the specimen, and deliver it to the laboratory as soon as possible to maintain viability of the pathogen.

PROTECTING YOURSELF AND OTHERS

- Always wash your hands before and after collecting specimens or handling body fluids.
- Always wear gloves while collecting and handling specimens. Sterile gloves are necessary for some procedures.
- Wrap securely and properly dispose of contaminated equipment, gloves, linens, and other contaminated objects.
- Protect yourself against needle-stick injury. Do not recap needles. Dispose of needles in a "sharps" container (Figure 3-2).
- Clean up any spilled specimen.
- Take care not to contaminate the outside of the container with the specimen. If contamination occurs, transfer specimen to another or place contaminated container inside another container or plastic bag.

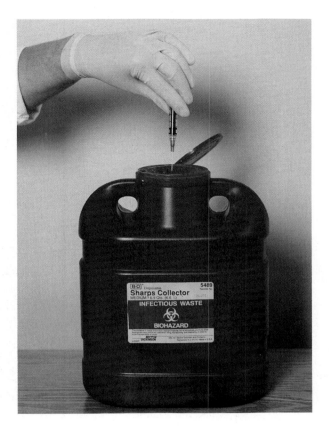

FIGURE 3-2
Dispose of needles properly.

BLOOD SPECIMENS

Blood is normally sterile, although mild, transient, asymptomatic bacteremia is common. However, septicemia is a serious, life-threatening event necessitating rapid identification of the causative organism. Organisms may be isolated and identified in the laboratory through cultures, microscopic examination, or a variety of serologic tests. Samples obtained by venipuncture are preferred over sampling from intravenous catheters.

It is preferable that blood samples for cultures be obtained before antibiotic therapy is started because otherwise culturing may be ineffective. This is not always possible because patients may have already received antibiotics. If so, note this on the specimen sent to the laboratory.

Serial blood cultures are usually necessary. Ideally, three blood samples are obtained over a 24-hour period. When this isn't possible because of need to initiate therapy, three samples can be obtained 30 minutes apart, or three specimens from three different sites can be drawn concurrently. In addition, blood samples for cultures may need to be obtained daily to monitor the patient's response to therapy until clinical improvement is demonstrated.

Most organisms will grow within 3 days, but some require 7 days for adequate growth. In rare cases, cultures are maintained up to 28 days if unusually fastidious organisms or anaerobic bacteria are suspected.

In addition, Gram's stains are performed immediately to provide a general guide for initiating antimicrobial therapy before culture results are available.

CONTRAINDICATIONS

Patients with coagulation disorders require special precaution. In addition, venipuncture is contraindicated at sites where there are lesions or infection.

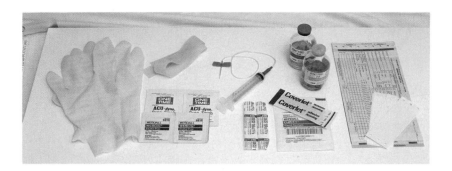

FIGURE 3-3
Equipment for blood collection.

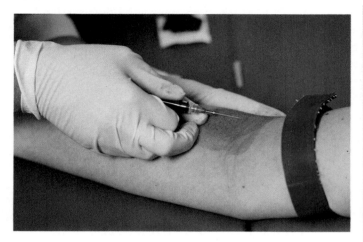

FIGURE 3-4
Performing venipuncture.

SPECIMEN PREPARATION

Special media are used for blood cultures, and the correct procedure for preparing the culture bottles or tubes will depend on laboratory protocols at your institution and the type of pathogen suspected. In general, these basic guidelines for preparing blood specimens should be followed:

- Broth cultures require a blood/broth ratio of 1:5 or 1:10, according to instructions. Thus a 1:5 dilution requires that 10 ml of blood are added to a 50-ml bottle.
- For special resins inject the blood into the specimen container and invert the bottle to mix.
- Lysis-centrifugation technique involves drawing blood directly into a special processing tube that is sent to the laboratory. This requires no further preparation.

COLLECTION PROCEDURES

Aseptic technique is essential to avoid contaminating the specimen with microorganisms residing on the skin. The following procedure should be followed carefully:

1. Assemble this equipment (Figure 3-3): culture tubes with the appropriate media, 10- or 20-ml syringes (one for each venipuncture), 21-gauge needle (two for each venipuncture), butterfly needles if they will be used, sterile gloves, antiseptic solution (2% iodine or povidone), alcohol swabs; tourniquet, and labels for identification.
2. After washing your hands, clean the venipuncture area with an alcohol sponge to remove superficial dirt and body oil.
3. Using a sponge saturated with an antiseptic solution, clean the venipuncture site in a widening circle, working from clean to dirty. The cleaned area should be about 5 cm (2 inches) in diameter.
4. Wait about 1 minute for the solution to dry and then wipe off the excess antiseptic with an alcohol swab. (Note: if an iodophor compound has been used as the antiseptic, do not remove with alcohol; allow the iodophor solution to dry completely on the skin before venipuncture.)
5. Apply the tourniquet.
6. Put on sterile gloves before palpating the vein.
7. Perform the venipuncture and draw 10 to 20 ml of blood into the syringe (between 2 and 6 ml for small children, depending on their size) (Figure 3-4).
8. Remove the needle and recap, using either the one-handed technique or a hemostat to avoid needle-stick injury.
9. Apply pressure to the puncture site, using sterile gauze, and cover with a small bandage.
10. Still maintaining aseptic technique, insert a sterile needle into the syringe.

11. Clean the diaphragm tops of the culture bottles with alcohol or iodine and inject the specified amount of blood (usually 3 to 6 ml) into each of the tubes containing culture media.
12. If concurrent specimens are required, repeat these steps at other venipuncture sites.
13. Label each tube with the following information: the patient's name, exact time the blood was drawn, site from which it was obtained or whether it was taken from an IV catheter, and any antibiotics the patient has received within the past 10 days. Keep the culture tubes at room temperature and transport immediately to the laboratory.

PATIENT TEACHING

Explain the procedure and its purpose. Let the patient know that the needle will "stick." After the needle is withdrawn, patients who are not too ill can hold the pressure gauze in place for a minute to stop the bleeding and prevent a hematoma. Explain to the patient that a hematoma may occur. Culture results are usually available in about 3 days.

URINE SPECIMENS

Urine in the bladder is normally sterile. However, microorganisms do inhabit the distal portion of the urinary tract. Catheterization is the most direct method of obtaining a urine sample, but this should be avoided if at all possible because of the risk of urinary tract infection. Urine is an excellent growth medium. For this reason, 24-hour collections, samples from a drainage bag, and specimens that have been at room temperature for longer than 30 minutes are of no use for microbiologic analysis. The best method of obtaining a urine sample for detecting infection is the clean-catch midstream collection.

Urine specimens that contain bacteria of less than 10,000/ml of urine are considered free of infection. Bacterial levels of 10,000 to 100,000/ml urine are inconclusive and usually require a second specimen. Bacterial counts greater than 100,000/ml urine indicate definite urinary tract infection.

COLLECTION PROCEDURES

Clean-catch midstream collection

The procedure below must be carefully followed so that only a midstream voiding is collected and contamination does not occur. A midstream collection allows microorganisms in the distal tract to be flushed out at the beginning of the stream. In addition, closing of the urinary sphincter at the end of voiding can dislodge a misleadingly large amount of bacteria, and in men, cause ejection of bacteria from the prostate. Also, contamination of the urine by external structures results in misleadingly higher bacterial counts. Depending on the situation, the nurse or the patient may be collecting the specimen, using the following procedure:

1. Clean the external genitalia with three pads—either sealed sterile Peri-wipes or 2 × 2 gauze pads soaked in povidone-iodine solution.
2. Remove the plastic wrap from a sterile specimen cup, taking care not to touch the rim or inside of the cup.
3. **For men** (Figure 3-5, *A*): Retract the foreskin, if uncircumcised, and wash the glans penis with soap and water. Wipe the urethral meatus with the pads, making only one wipe with each pad.
   For women (Figure 3-6, *A*): Wash the vulva, labial folds, and around the urinary meatus with soap and water, and rinse. Separate the labia minora with the fingers of one hand, making sure to keep them separated throughout the procedure. Using the first pad, wipe once down one side of the urinary meatus; repeat on the other side with the second pad; with the third pad wipe once directly over the urinary meatus.
4. Have the patient start voiding and then stop.
5. Position the cup to catch the stream, and ask the patient to restart the urine, (Figures 3-5, *B* and 3-6, *B*) making sure that the urine stream does not touch external structures.
6. When 5 ml have been collected (15 to 30 ml if a urinalysis will also be performed), have the patient stop voiding and remove the cup.
7. Carefully label the specimen container.
8. Transfer to the laboratory within 30 minutes. If this is not possible, the specimen can be refrigerated at 4° C (39.2° F) for up to 5 hours.

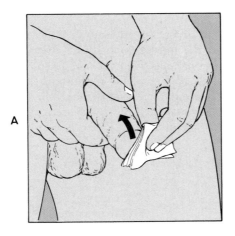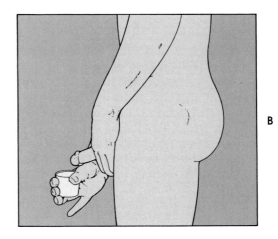

FIGURE 3-5
Clean-catch urine collection for men. **A,** Preparation and **B,** collection. (See text for instructions.)

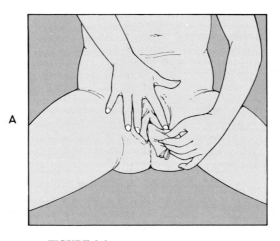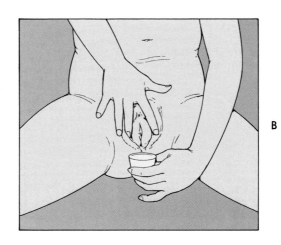

FIGURE 3-6
Clean-catch urine collection for women. **A,** Preparation and **B,** collection. (See text for instructions.)

9. Record on the patient's chart the appearance of the specimen (e.g., straw-colored, cloudy, or dark or if containing sediment).

Indwelling catheters

1. Clamp the collection tube about 30 minutes before taking the sample to allow the bladder to fill.
2. Wipe the catheter sampling port with alcohol and insert a sterile needle into the port at a 90° angle.
3. Unclamp the catheter and draw 5 ml (15 to 30 ml if a urinalysis will also be performed) into the syringe as the urine leaves the bladder.
4. Transfer the specimen to a sterile container la-

beled with the patient's name and time of collection; make sure to note that the specimen was obtained via an indwelling catheter.

5. See 8 and 9 under clean-catch Midstream Collection.

PATIENT TEACHING

Explain the procedure and its purpose. If the patient is to self-collect a specimen by the clean-catch midstream method, provide a photocopy of the Patient Teaching Guide on page 301. For patients with indwelling catheters, explain that you are clamping the drainage tube for about 30 minutes to allow urine to collect in the bladder but that this should cause no discomfort.

FECAL SPECIMENS

Fecal specimens are obtained to culture organisms that are not part of the normal bowel flora. Microscopic examination of the specimen is performed to identify ova and parasites, to detect an increased number of white cells (indicating pathogenic invasion of the intestinal wall), and to detect red blood cells (indicating gastrointestinal bleeding). Some viruses can be identified by either electron microscopy or immunoassay.

Normally, stools contain only normal flora in the expected proportions: over 95% consists of anaerobes (e.g., nonspore-forming bacilli, clostridia, and streptococci) and the remaining consists of gram-negative aerobes (e.g., mostly *Escherichia coli*, other Enterobacteriaceae, and some *Pseudomonas*), gram-positive cocci, and yeasts. The finding of an unusually high population of normal flora is pathogenic, and additional tests may be performed to identify toxin production. Organisms such as *Clostridium difficile* and *E. coli* are examples of normal flora that can become pathogenic under certain circumstances. Stools that are watery and contain blood or mucus are abnormal.

COLLECTION PROCEDURES

The stool specimen should not contain urine or water from the toilet bowl. The patient may defecate into a clean bedpan or onto a plastic bag or newspaper taped under the toilet seat (Figure 3-7). With proper instructions, ambulatory patients can easily collect their own fecal specimen in the same manner as described below. Fecal specimens may also be obtained directly from the rectum using a sterile swab, if necessary, for unconscious patients or for infants and young children.

Fecal collection

1. If the specimen will be tested for viruses, check with the laboratory for the proper procedure.
2. Assemble this equipment: a waxed or plastic cup with a lid, label for identification, clean gloves, a tongue blade, and either a clean, dry bedpan *or* plastic or newspaper taped securely under the toilet seat.
3. Instruct the patient to defecate without voiding.
4. Wearing gloves, collect the stool specimen with the tongue blade. If the stool is formed, a walnut-sized specimen is sufficient. If the stool is liquid, 15 to 20 ml is collected.
5. Place the specimen in the cup, being careful not to contaminate the outside of the container.
6. Wrap the tongue blade and gloves and discard properly.
7. Place the lid on the container and label it with

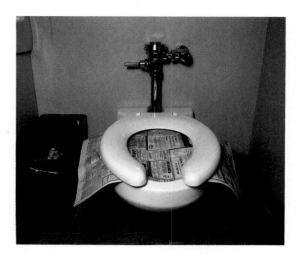

FIGURE 3-7
A stool specimen can be obtained directly from newspaper taped under a toilet seat.

the patient's name, time of collection, and suspected diagnosis and note if the patient has received antibiotics.
8. Wash your hands.
9. Transport the specimen to the laboratory immediately. (If the fecal specimen will not be tested for parasites, transport may be delayed. However, check with the laboratory for instructions about storing the specimen.)

Rectal swab

1. Assemble this equipment: sterile swab, gloves, and a wax or plastic cup with a tight fitting lid (label for identification).
2. Place the patient in the left lateral recumbent position, knees bent toward the chest.
3. Separate the buttocks and ask the patient to bear down to relax the external sphincter. Insert the sterile swab into the rectum just inside anal opening (Figure 3-16).
4. Keeping the buttocks separated, withdraw the swab and deposit the fecal material in the cup. If more material is needed, repeat the procedure with another sterile swab.
5. Discard gloves and swab.
6. See 8 and 9 under Fecal Collection.

PATIENT TEACHING

Explain the procedure and its purpose. If the patient is to collect the specimen without supervision, explain each step in detail, including the importance of not contaminating the fecal material with urine or toilet paper.

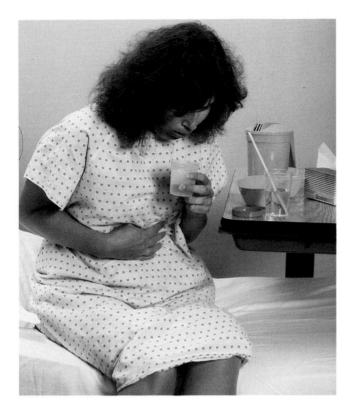

FIGURE 3-8
Collection of sputum specimen. The specimen should be representative of pulmonary secretions—not saliva.

SPUTUM SPECIMENS

All too often, sputum samples sent for culturing are little more than saliva and oropharyngeal secretions, rather than specimens from the lower respiratory tract. Failure to follow the proper techniques for obtaining sputum can result in delayed diagnosis. Most laboratories will perform a Gram's stain on a sputum specimen to determine whether it does indeed represent lung secretions. If the majority of cells are from squamous epithelium, the sample is primarily oropharyngeal secretions, and another specimen will be requested. Specimens from the lower respiratory tract of patients with pulmonary infections contain mostly white blood cells and will be cultured.

The most common method used for sputum collection is expectoration. Other less frequently used methods include bronchial aspiration, tracheal cannulation, and translaryngeal aspiration. With the exception of translaryngeal aspiration, all collection techniques are subject to some contamination with oropharyngeal secretions. Following the expectoration procedure carefully, however, reduces the amount of contamination

and should produce a specimen that is representative of pulmonary secretions. This method is also without complications.

COLLECTION PROCEDURES

Expectoration

Expectorated sputum can be obtained from a cooperative patient with a productive cough. The specimen should be collected first thing in the morning because pooling of lung secretions during sleep results in a larger quantity of sputum that contains a maximum number of pathogens.

1. Assemble this equipment: a wide-mouthed container with identification label, gloves, tissues, water, and mouthwash.
2. Have the patient blow his or her nose to expell excess nasopharyngeal secretions. The patient should then brush and rinse with mouthwash to reduce the number of oral organisms.
3. Have the patient take a deep breath and cough deeply to bring up sputum. If possible, have the patient hold the container and expectorate directly into it (Figure 3-8).
4. If this fails to produce sputum, there are several techniques you can use to loosen thickened secretions. An **aerosol nebulizer** increases the moisture content in the lungs, or **intermittent positive-pressure breathing** with an aerosol may be prescribed. **Chest physiotherapy** also loosens secretions from the airways.
5. While wearing gloves, cap the container, taking care that the outside is not contaminated with sputum.
6. Label the container "sputum specimen," with the patient's name, time of collection, and whether antibiotics have been given. Transport immediately to the laboratory.

NURSING CARE

Describe the procedure and its purpose to the patient. For collection by expectoration, encourage the patient to drink fluids the evening before collection. For bronchoscopy and for translaryngeal aspiration, informed written consent must be obtained, and sedatives are administered as ordered.

After expectoration, provide good mouth care and encourage liquids.

PATIENT TEACHING

For collection by expectoration, explain the procedure carefully to ensure the patient understands that sputum, not saliva, is needed.

THROAT, EYE, EAR, AND NOSE SPECIMENS

Secretions and excretions from mucous membranes will invariably contain normal flora as well as pathogens. Therefore the specimen obtained must be representative of the pathologic process rather than the surrounding skin.

Mucous membrane specimens should be collected with a sterile polyester swab, not a cotton swab. Preparation of the specimen will depend on the suspected diagnosis. The appropriate culture medium should be available, and if the specimen will be examined microscopically, you will need a slide with coverslip and the appropriate solution for wet-mount preparations.

COLLECTION PROCEDURES

Throat

1. Assemble this equipment: tongue blade, penlight, sterile polyester swab, gloves, slide and solutions, as indicated, appropriate culture medium, and labels for identification.
2. Put on gloves. Moisten the tongue blade with warm water. (A moist tongue blade does not stimulate the gag reflex as readily as a dry blade, although most patients will gag to some extent.)
3. With the patient's head tilted back, depress the patient's tongue and insert the sterile polyester swab. (Be careful not to touch the swab to the patient's lips, teeth, or buccal mucosa when entering and exiting the mouth.)
4. Swab both tonsils and the posterior pharynx, as shown in Figure 3-9. (Repeat with a second swab if culturing for *Corynebacterium diphtheriae*.)
5. Prepare the specimen for laboratory examination.
6. Discard gloves and swab properly. Wash hands thoroughly after the procedure.
7. Label the container as to body source of specimen, with the patient's name, date and time of collection, suspected diagnosis, and whether recent or current antibiotic therapy has been given. Transport the specimen to the laboratory immediately.

Eye

1. Assemble this equipment: sterile polyester swab, gloves, slide and solutions, as indicated, appropriate culture medium, and labels for identification.
2. Put on gloves. With the thumb of one hand, place gentle downward traction below the eye to expose the conjunctiva.

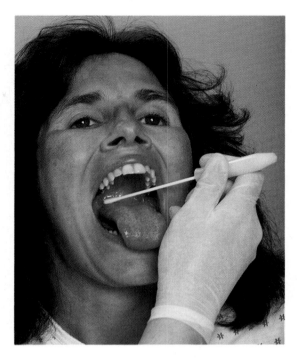

FIGURE 3-9
Collection of specimen from posterior pharynx.

3. Instruct the patient to look up. This will help avoid touching the cornea with the swab.
4. Gently place a sterile polyester swab against the conjunctiva, holding in place for about 10 seconds to allow the exudate to absorb into the swab.
5. See 5, 6, and 7 from Throat.

Ear

A specimen should be obtained when there is drainage from the middle ear from a ruptured tympanic membrane.

1. Assemble this equipment: sterile polyester swab, gloves, slide and solutions, as indicated, appropriate culture medium, and labels for identification.
2. Put on gloves. Have the patient tilt the head forward and slightly to the affected side. This will help move the exudate into the distal canal where it can be reached more easily.
3. Gently insert a sterile polyester swab just inside the external canal, holding in place for about 10 seconds to allow the swab to absorb the exudate.
4. See 5, 6, and 7 from Throat.

Nose

1. Assemble this equipment: penlight, sterile polyester swab, gloves, slide and solutions, as indi-

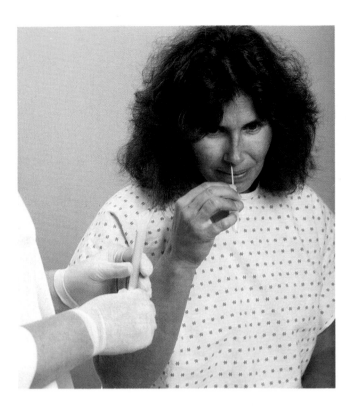

cated, appropriate culture medium, and labels for identification.

2. Put on gloves. While steadying the patient's head with one hand, insert a sterile polyester swab into the nose (until you reach the turbinates).

3. Rotate the swab gently against the septum and floor of the nares for about 10 seconds to allow the swab to absorb the exudate (Figure 3-10).

4. See 5, 6, and 7 from Throat.

PATIENT TEACHING

Describe the procedure and its purpose. Assure the patient that it will take only a few seconds to obtain the specimen.

FIGURE 3-10
Collection of nasal specimen may be performed by the nurse or by a cooperative patient.

CEREBROSPINAL FLUID SPECIMENS

When infection of the central nervous system is suspected, cerebrospinal fluid (CSF) analysis provides the only means of making a definitive diagnosis. CSF is usually obtained by lumbar puncture, which is usually performed between the third and fourth lumbar vertebrae. A cisternal puncture may be necessary if there is an infection or deformity in the lumbar area. Cisternal puncture is done with a short needle inserted below the occipital bone, just above the first cervical vertebrae. Both procedures are performed by the physician, usually at bedside.

In rare cases, ventricular puncture must be performed in patients for whom the standard procedures are contraindicated. This is a surgical procedure that requires drilling a hole through the skull and aspirating CSF directly from a lateral ventricle.

A minimum of three tubes of CSF are usually collected for laboratory analysis, one of which is for Gram's stains, culturing, and antibiotic sensitivity tests. Additional tests include electrolyte analysis, glucose testing, serologic tests, such as the VDRL for syphilis, and cytologic analysis for protein and unusual cells.

Spinal fluid is normally clear and contains 15 to 45 mg of protein/100 ml, 50 to 80 mg glucose/100 ml, 118 to 130 mEq chloride/L, less than 5 white blood cells (WBCs) and no organisms. Bacterial meningitis, brain abscess, or other infective process of the CNS produce a cloudy CSF containing increased numbers of WBCs, and glucose and chloride levels are often decreased.

CONTRAINDICATIONS

CSF puncture cannot be performed on the uncooperative patient, in patients with severe spine disorders, or if there is an infection at the puncture site. Increased intracranial pressure is a relative contraindication, requiring that the procedure be performed with extreme caution to avoid cerebellar herniation and compression of the medulla.

COMPLICATIONS

Headache following the procedure is extremely common. Puncture of a nerve root during the procedure may occur.

COLLECTION PROCEDURES

1. Obtain informed consent.
2. Administer sedative as ordered. Be sure the patient urinates immediately before the procedure.
3. Assemble lumbar or cisternal puncture tray,

sterile gloves and bandage, local anesthetic, antiseptic solution, and identification labels.

4. Assist the patient into a lateral recumbent position with the spine close to the edge of the bed or table (Figure 3-11). The patient's knees are drawn up against the abdomen and the chin is resting on the chest, curving the spine forward to provide maximum space between the vertebrae. Use pillows as needed to position the spine in a horizontal alignment. You or another nurse must help the patient maintain this position throughout the procedure by placing one arm around the patient's knees and the other arm around his or her neck (or head if a cisternal puncture is performed). (Note: Some physicians prefer performing the procedure with the patient sitting, chest and head bent forward on the thighs.) Quietly reassure the patient throughout the procedure.

5. Medical procedure: The puncture site is scrubbed and draped by the physician, and a local anesthetic is injected to anesthetize the skin. A spinal needle is injected at the midline, usually between L3 and L4 for lumbar puncture, or above C1 for a cisternal puncture. The stylet is removed by the physician, allowing spinal fluid to drip from the needle if it is correctly positioned. The initial CSF pressure is measured with a stopcock and manometer attached to the needle. This initial pressure should be recorded. CSF samples are then collected and placed into specimen tubes. The CSF pressure is again taken and recorded, and the needle is removed. The puncture site is cleaned with an antiseptic, and a bandage is applied.

6. Fill three or four sterile tubes, following specifications of the laboratory. Label each tube with the words "spinal fluid" and the patient's name, time of collection, and test to be performed. Notify the laboratory that CSF specimens are ready so that the personnel are prepared for immediate analysis, and immediately transport the specimens to the laboratory. Do not refrigerate unless the laboratory requests chilling for viral culture.

7. On the patient's chart, record the color and clarity of the specimen and the patient's reaction to the procedure.

NURSING CARE

During the procedure, observe the patient for any signs of adverse reaction and alert the physician immediately. An elevated pulse rate, pallor, and clammy skin may indicate shock.

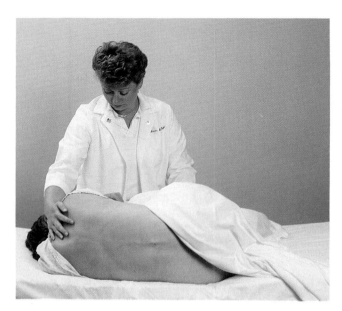

FIGURE 3-11
Positioning patient for lumbar puncture.

After the procedure, maintain the patient in bed as ordered by the physician. Most physicians require that the patient remain flat for 4 to 6 hours, but some allow the head to be elevated 30°. However, the patient may turn from side to side. Monitor the patient's neurologic status (including level of consciousness, mentation, and pupillary reactivity) and vital signs every 15 minutes for 4 hours and then hourly, if the patient remains stable. By 6 hours after the procedure, assess neurologic status every 4 hours or as ordered. Check the puncture site for swelling, erythema, and drainage once an hour for 4 hours and then every 4 hours for the next 24 hours. Encourage the patient to drink fluids. If headache occurs, administer analgesics as ordered.

PATIENT TEACHING

Before the procedure, describe the procedure and explain its purpose. Stress the importance of keeping completely still and breathing normally throughout the procedure. Provide assurance you will help the patient maintain the correct position. Explain that a local anesthetic will be injected first, which will sting, and that the spinal needle will cause some brief pain. Tell the patient to let you know if the pain continues or if any other unusual sensations occur during the procedure, such as pain radiating to either leg. Explain that headache after the procedure is common but staying in bed as ordered by the physician will help minimize this side effect.

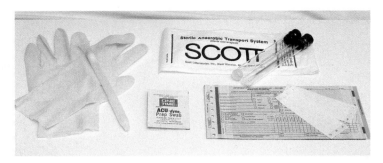

FIGURE 3-12
Equipment for collection of specimens from wound and decubiti.

WOUNDS AND DECUBITI SPECIMENS

A clean wound or ulcer contains essentially no pathogens. Signs of infection mandate microscopic examination and culturing of a specimen from the lesion to identify the responsible pathogen(s). Specimens for deep wounds and decubitus ulcers are cultured for both aerobic and anaerobic organisms. The technique for collecting specimens for anaerobic cultures must be precise because anaerobic organisms are destroyed quickly when exposed to oxygen and will fail to grow in culture.

COLLECTION PROCEDURES

Aerobic and anaerobic cultures

1. Assemble this equipment (Figure 3-12): A sterile 21-gauge needle and 10-ml syringe or sterile cotton swab, aerobic and anaerobic culture tubes, antiseptic solution, sterile gauze pads, gloves, and labels for identification.
2. Put on gloves and cleanse the area surrounding the wound with gauze pads soaked in the anti-septic solution to reduce contamination by normal flora nearby. Take care that no solution touches the wound, however, since this may affect culture growth.
3. **For aerobic cultures:** Express the wound (if necessary) by pressing on skin around the wound with sterile gauze pads to obtain an exudate. With a sterile cotton-tipped swab, collect as much exudate as possible. If the wound is deep, you may need to insert the swab into the wound and rotate gently to collect the specimen. Place the swab immediately in the aerobic culture tube and cap.
   For anaerobic cultures: Insert the needle into the wound and aspirate 1 to 5 ml of exudate or insert the swab deeply into the wound and gently rotate. Depending on instructions from the laboratory either (1) immediately cover the needle and send the entire syringe to the laboratory or (2) open the stoppers and immediately inject the aspirate into the anaerobic culture tube and quickly replace the double stoppers. If using an anaerobic culture tube, you must not open the stopper until you are ready to inject the specimen into the tube.
4. Properly discard gloves, swab, and any other objects that have touched the area.
5. Label the tube with the patient's name, time of collection, type of wound (e.g., puncture wound, decubitus ulcer, or surgical incision), probable source of infection, and whether the patient has received antibiotics. Transport immediately to the laboratory.
6. Dress the wound.

PATIENT TEACHING

Explain the purpose of the procedure, that it will take 1 to 2 minutes, and that there may be some discomfort.

GENITOURETHRAL AND RECTAL SPECIMENS

VAGINAL AND CERVICAL EXUDATES

Specimens for vaginal or cervical smears and cultures are obtained during the pelvic examination with the speculum in place. It is essential that only warm water is used for lubricant; any other lubricant will affect laboratory studies. If a Papanicolaou smear is ordered, it should be performed first, followed by vaginal and then cervical specimen collection.

COLLECTION PROCEDURES

1. Assemble this equipment (Figure 3-13): speculum, gloves, sterile cotton swabs, calcium alginate swab (for *Chlamydia*), glass slides with covers, saline and potassium hydroxide preparations, *Chlamydia* transport media, Thayer-Martin medium, and labels for identification.
2. With gloves on, insert speculum or separate labia.
3. Obtain specimen of vaginal secretions. Roll plain wooden end of sterile swab around in vaginal secretions for about 10 sec if testing for *Haemophilus*, *Candida*, or *Trichomonas*.

4. Obtain cervical specimen. Insert sterile cotton swab or calcium alginate swab into the opening of the cervical os (Figure 3-14). Move the swab from side to side for 10 to 30 seconds to allow good absorption of the specimen into the swab. If the patient is a child or a woman who has had a hysterectomy, obtain the specimen from the posterior vaginal vault or if the hymen is intact, the vaginal orifice.

5. Withdraw the swab and prepare the specimen (see Table 3-1 for microscopic examination; for gonorrhea see box on page 45; prepare with transport medium according to laboratory instructions for *Chlamydia*).

URETHRAL SPECIMENS

Urethral secretions are necessary for diagnosing a variety of infections, particularly gonorrhea and nongonococcal urethritis in the male patient. There are two methods for collecting these specimens.

COLLECTION PROCEDURES

For men:

1. Assemble this equipment: sterile cotton swab, culture medium for gonococcus, slide and appropriate liquid preparation, as indicated, gloves, and labels for identification.
2. Ask the patient to milk the urethra. This will bring the milky looking prostatic fluid to the urethral orifice.
3. While wearing gloves, collect the fluid with the cotton tip and prepare the specimen as described in the box on page 45.

For children, women, or men:

1. Assemble this equipment: either a special, thin urogenital alginate swab or a wire bacteriologic

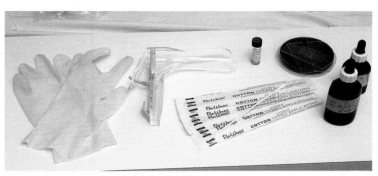

FIGURE 3-13
Equipment for collection of genitourethral and rectal specimens.

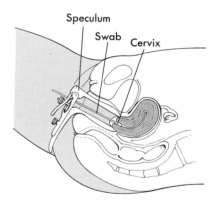

FIGURE 3-14
Obtaining cervical specimen.

loop, culture medium for gonococcus, slide and appropriate liquid preparation, as indicated, gloves, sterile gauze, cleansing agent, and labels for identification.

Table 3-1

PREPARATION OF SMEARS FOR MICROSCOPIC EXAMINATION

Type	Suspected organism	Preparation
Dry mount	*Haemophilus vaginalis*	Smear the specimen over a dry glass slide and cover immediately with the coverslip.
Wet mount	*Trichomonas vaginalis*	Smear the specimen over a dry glass slide and add 1 drop of saline. Mix together with wooden end of specimen swab. Cover with coverslip.
KOH (potassium hydroxide)	*Candida albicans*	Smear the specimen over a dry glass slide and add 1 drop of KOH. Mix together with wooden end of specimen swab. Cover with coverslip.

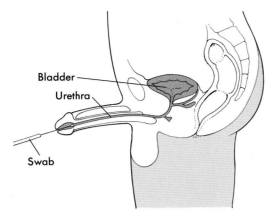

FIGURE 3-15
Obtaining urethral specimen.

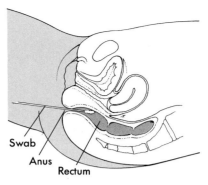

FIGURE 3-16
Obtaining specimen of exudate from rectum.

2. Place the patient in a supine position and drape.
3. While wearing gloves, clean the urethral meatus with sterile gauze.
4. Insert the swab or loop about 1 or 2 cm (⅜ or ¾ inch) into the meatus (Figure 3-15). Hold in place for 10 seconds, remove, and inoculate medium.

RECTAL SPECIMENS

The anal canal may be the primary site of gonorrhea infection, or the infection may spread from the genital tract. It is important to note that specimens for gonococcal cultures must not contain fecal material but only secretions from the anal crypts.

COLLECTION PROCEDURES

1. Assemble this equipment: sterile cotton tipped swab, culture medium (either Modified Thayer-Martin medium on a culture plate or Transgrow bottle), gloves, and labels for identification.
2. Position the patient in the left lateral recumbent position and drape.
3. Spread the buttocks and ask the patient to bear down to relax the external anal sphincter.
4. Insert the cotton tip approximately 2.5 cm (1 inch) into the anal canal (Figure 3-16). Move the swab from side to side, allowing 10 to 30 seconds for the swab to absorb organisms.
5. Remove the swab and inoculate culture medium.
6. Dispose of the swab and gloves properly.

GENITAL LESIONS

Cutaneous lesions may appear anywhere on the external genitalia in both women and men and even extend to the buttocks or thighs. Internal lesions may involve the vaginal walls, the cervix, or the anal canal. The appropriate method for collection and culturing depends on the suspected diagnosis.

Regardless of the type of lesion, the specimen must be collected from the exudate—not the surface of the lesion, which will usually yield only flora from the skin surface rather than the pathogen. Although there are minor variations among the procedures, collecting a specimen of a syphilis lesion is presented below.

Treponema pallidum, which causes syphilis, is identified by examination under a darkfield microscope. Because these organisms die quickly when removed from the body, microscopic examination must be done within 15 minutes, while they are still motile.

COLLECTION PROCEDURES

1. Assemble this equipment: sterile cotton swabs, saline, ether, pipette, slide with coverslip, gloves, and labels for identification.
2. While wearing gloves, clean the lesion with a saline-moistened swab to remove extraneous bacteria and debris.
3. Apply an ether-soaked swab to the lesion to release serum exudate.
4. Remove a sample of the exudate with a pipette.
5. Place the specimen on a dry slide and cover with the coverslip.
6. Discard gloves, swabs, and pipette appropriately.
7. Label the slide with the patient's name, time of collection, and location of the lesion.
8. Transport the slide immediately to the laboratory for examination.

PREPARATION OF GONOCOCCAL CULTURE SPECIMENS

Two methods are used for culturing *Neisseria gonorrhea:* modified Thayer-Martin medium and Transgrow bottles. The procedures for inoculation follow.

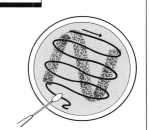

Modified Thayer-Martin medium

- After collecting the specimen with a sterile cotton swab, remove the plate cover.
- Spread the specimen over the medium in a large **Z** pattern while rotating the swab.
- Cover the plate and label it with the patient's name, age, site from which the specimen was obtained (e.g., cervix, vaginal wall, urethra, or anal canal), and the date and time of collection.
- Transport to the laboratory.

Transgrow bottle

- After collecting the specimen with a sterile cotton swab, remove the bottle cap. Be sure to keep the bottle upright throughout the procedure to prevent the loss of carbon dioxide.
- Insert the cotton swab into the bottle and allow it to absorb excess moisture.
- Roll the swab against the side of the bottle, starting at the bottom of the bottle and working toward the top.
- Replace the cap immediately and label the container with the patient's name, age, site from which the specimen was obtained (e.g., cervix, vaginal wall, urethra, or anal canal), and the time and date of collection.
- Transport to the laboratory.

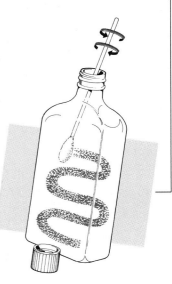

SKIN TESTS

Skin tests are based on the principle that an intradermal injection of either certain antigens or toxins produces a local (cell-mediated) reaction if the person has recently been infected with a particular pathogen. Injection of antigens will produce an inflammatory response if antibodies are present, and injection of toxins will produce a toxin neutralization response if the person has formed antitoxins.

A test volume, usually 0.1 ml, of the antigen is injected intradermally (Figure 3-17), and the size of induration at the injection site is measured at a specified time. A positive reaction suggests recent infection with a specific pathogen. Several skin tests are available to test for antibodies against tuberculosis. The Schick test for diphtheria and the Dick test for scarlet fever are examples of toxin tests.

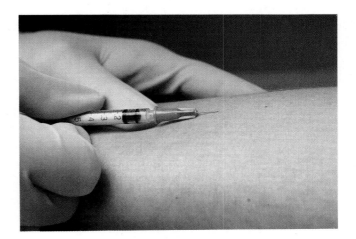

FIGURE 3-17
Administering intradermal injection for skin test. Note that the needle bevel is facing upward.

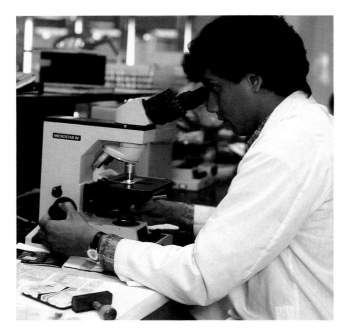

FIGURE 3-18
Microscope technician.

Microscopic Examination

Microscopic examination of a specimen is the only method of identifying parasites and ova, and it distinguishes tissue cells from microorganisms. Because most microorganisms and other cells appear colorless under a microscope, stains are added to highlight their structural characteristics. Microorganisms are classified partly according to their shape, size, and staining characteristics. Thus the type of organism can be identified (e.g., rods vs cocci, gram-positive vs gram-negative bacteria, and viruses vs bacteria) by microscopic examination. The results of microscopy are usually available within hours or even minutes, often permitting a presumptive diagnosis so that treatment can be initiated rapidly.

In addition to the basic brightfield microscope, several other microscopic techniques have been developed to identify specific organisms. They include electron, fluorescent, darkfield, and phase-contrast microscopy.

As soon as a specimen is obtained, it must be prepared immediately to preserve the pathogens and other cells for microscopic examination. Two basic methods are used for microscopy.

- **Wet mounts.** The specimen is smeared on a glass slide, and a liquid is added immediately. (The liquid used depends on the suspected diagnosis.) The specimen is protected with a coverslip for transport. Stains may be added in the laboratory to highlight the characteristics of the organisms. Wet mounts are used when diagnosis requires a

live organism (as in *T. palladium*) and for identifying yeasts, such as *Trichomonas vaginalis*.
- **Smears.** The specimen is smeared on a glass slide, allowed to air dry for a short period, and protected by a coverslip for transport. Stains are added to the smears to highlight cell structures. Smears are used to identify bacteria, viruses, normal tissue cells, and inflammatory cells.

GRAM'S STAIN

Gram's stains are one of the most useful procedures in microbiologic testing. This staining method consists of dropping first methyl violet and then iodine to the dried smear on a slide. Acetone is then added to wash excess stain away. Organisms that absorb the dye into their cell walls are gram positive and appear violet or blue when examined under the microscope. Gram-negative organisms easily give up the dye and can be counterstained with a red dye, such as fuchsin. Organisms that do not grow in culture, including some anaerobes, can often be identified by Gram's stain. In addition, this technique stains tissue cells, which allows a general evaluation of the patient's inflammatory response.

Finally, the quality of a specimen can be rapidly determined by Gram's staining before culturing. For example, if a "sputum" specimen is found to contain primarily normal flora of the nasopharyngeal tract and large numbers of epithelial cells, the laboratory can notify you that collection should be attempted again. Since cultures require from 24 hours to several weeks for development, microscopic assessment before culturing can save valuable time by excluding poor quality specimens that might grow little but normal flora.

OTHER STAINS

A multitude of other stains are available. Acid-fast stains can isolate *Mycobacteria*, a genus difficult to culture because of its slow growth, allowing a rapid diagnosis of tuberculosis. Periodic acid–Schiff (PAS) stain is used to identify fungi, and *Pneumocystis carinii*. Other commonly used stains include Giemsa stain and Wright's stain, silver stains, and trichrome stain.

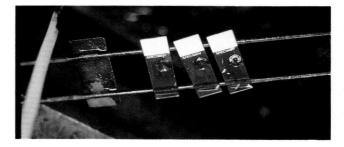

FIGURE 3-19
Gram's stain.

CULTURES

Bacteria, fungi, and some viruses are positively identified by culturing. Because many microorganisms have very specific requirements for growth, specimens are sent to the laboratory with instructions to culture the suspected pathogen(s). Several types of both liquid and solid culture media are available for supporting different types of organisms. In general, liquid medium is preferred for certain kinds of specimens, such as blood, because fewer microorganisms can be grown, whereas solid medium will grow mixed cultures.

In addition, some organisms have specific temperature, atmosphere, or pH requirements. For example, *N. gonorrheae* is sensitive to sudden temperature changes and will not grow when inoculated onto medium just removed from the refrigerator. Mycobacteria grow best when incubated with carbon dioxide. Anaerobic bacteria will not grow in the presence of oxygen.

Accurate results are obtained only when specimens are inoculated into culture media quickly. The bacterial population in room-temperature urine, for example, can quadruple within 60 minutes of voiding. As a result, culture growth will not reflect the actual bacterial level in the urinary tract.

In a few cases, notably when testing for gonorrhea, cultures must be inoculated immediately upon collection. Otherwise, most specimens are placed in a transport medium and sent to the laboratory. Transport media protect the microorganisms from drying, which results in death, and inhibit contaminants. As with culture media, the correct transport medium depends on the suspected pathogen. One method is to obtain the specimen with a polyester culture swab that comes in a plastic tube with an ampule containing the medium. This technique is obviously suitable only for collecting small quantities of exudates (e.g., from mucous membranes, the genitourinary tract, and wounds and lesions).

How quickly the pathogen can be recovered from cultures often depends on the type of microorganism, the type of specimen, and the stage of illness. Culture results are available in 24 to 48 hours on many of the

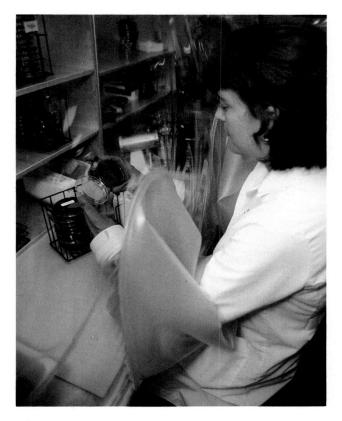

FIGURE 3-20
Culture under hood.

common pathogens, such as streptococci, staphylococci, and enterobacteria. Pneumococcal organisms grow cultures in 3 to 4 days. In contrast, mycobacteria require anywhere from 1 week to 2 months.

Some organisms are detectable in specimens from different sites at varying times. *Salmonella typhosa* is usually detected in blood cultures only during the first 10 days of fever, whereas the organisms appear in stool after 10 days and in urine at 2 or 3 weeks.

Serial cultures are mandatory for positively identifying some organisms. Because *M. tuberculosis* is shed intermittently, negative cultures are common in patients with active tuberculosis. Therefore culture specimens must be collected daily over a 4- to 6-day period.

IMMUNOLOGIC TESTS

Infectious agents cannot always be identified by the direct methods of microscopic examination or culturing. Pathogens that are antigenic stimulate antibodies, which can be detected in patients' serums by adding the specific antigen and observing the antigen-antibody reactions. Similarly, pathogens that release toxins are detected by adding antitoxins to serum. Several immunologic tests are available that measure antibody titers, the most common of which are described below.

It is important to note that the detection of antibodies is not diagnostic of current infection, since previous infection or immunization may account for the presence of antibodies in serum. Therefore antigen-antibody reactions must be evaluated over a period of time before a definite diagnosis can be made. IgM antibody production peaks during active infection and then decreases during the convalescent period. IgG antibodies peak during convalescence and last longer. A blood sample taken during acute infection is compared with a second sample obtained 2 to 3 weeks later. A fourfold rise in antibody titer (the measure of antigen-antibody reactions) during convalescence indicates concurrent infection.

AGGLUTINATION TESTS

Agglutination tests demonstrate the ability of antibodies and antigens to bind together, a "clumping" reaction that is observed in a test tube, slide, or other specially prepared surface. Several dilutions of the patient's serum are tested against constant amounts of antigen. The highest dilution that still demonstrates agglutination is the agglutination titer. A rise in titer between acute and convalescent serum is more diagnostic than a single high titer.

Two types of agglutination tests are used: direct and indirect. In direct agglutination tests, antibodies attach directly to antigens. In indirect tests, antigens must first be coated with chemicals that attract antibodies. Agglutination tests are used in blood typing and in identifying antibodies against many bacterial, fungal, and parasitic infections and a few viral infections. Table 3-2 lists the most common agglutination tests and their diagnostic applications.

COMPLEMENT FIXATION

Complement is a group of serum proteins that enter into antigen-antibody reactions, one of which is lysis of antigen cells. One or more of the complement components can be used (or fixed) in an antigen-antibody reaction, rendering complement unavailable for subse-

Table 3-2

AGGLUTINATION TESTS

Test	Diagnostic application
Antistreptodornase-B (Anti-DNase-B)	Detects antibodies against one streptococcal enzyme from group A-beta hemolytic streptococci
Antistreptolysin-O (ASO)	Detects antibodies against one enzyme released early in group A beta-hemolytic streptococcal infection
Bentonite flocculation	*Trichinella*, rheumatoid factor
Cold agglutinins	Mycoplasma pneumonia
Coombs' test	RBC agglutination, blood incompatibility
Febrile agglutinins	Agglutinins produced by fever from typhoid fever, paratyphoid, brucellosis, tularemia
Latex fixation	Rheumatoid factor
Hemagglutination	RBC incompatibility, amebae
Hemagglutination inhibition	Hepatitis B, rubella
Heterophil antibody titer (HAT) (Mono-Diff, Monospot, Monotest)	Epstein-Barr virus (mononucleosis)
Microhemagglutination-*Treponema pallidum* (MHA-TP)	*T. pallidum* (syphilis)
Rapid plasma reagin (RPR)	Syphilis
Streptozyme	Antibodies against five streptococcal enzymes
Venereal Disease Research Laboratory (VDRL)	Syphilis
Weil-Felix reaction	Agglutination of *Proteus DX-19* bacteria by serum from patients with typhus
Widal's reaction	Salmonellosis

quent reactions. Complement fixation (CF) is a multistage test that is based on this principle.

A known amount of complement is added to a patient's serum. Sheep red blood cells (SRBC), which are antigenic in human serum, are then added to the serum. Any unfixed complement will lyse the SRBC. Thus lysis occurs when complement is unfixed, indicating the serum lacks antigen or antibody. No lysis occurs if all complement are bound. CF test results are given in titers. The CF titer is the dilution of serum that completely fixes complement, with the higher dilutions indicating higher antibody titers.

The CF test detects antigens or antibodies associated with many bacterial, fungal, viral, and parasitic infections. The now obsolete Wassermann test for syphilis was based on complement fixation.

IMMUNODIFFUSION AND COUNTERELECTROPHORESIS

Immunodiffusion, electroimmunodiffusion, electrophoresis, counterimmunoelectrophoresis (CIE), and immunoelectrophoresis are assays that measure precipitation, which is the reaction that occurs when antigen-antibody complexes form and migrate across the test medium. The basic test is immunodiffusion, which uses agar or agarose gel and takes 48 to 96 hours to complete. Precipitin lines form when the concentrations of antigen and antibody are equal, indicating they have formed complexes.

The other four tests are electrophoretic variations on this basic test, in which an electric field is applied to the medium. These tests are much faster, requiring only 1½ to 4 hours to complete.

Precipitation assays detect a variety of viral, bacterial, fungal, and parasitic antigens and antibodies. The Western blot test is an immunoelectrophoresis assay for HIV.

ENZYME-LINKED IMMUNOABSORBENT ASSAY

Enzyme-linked immunoabsorbent assay (ELISA) is a complex and highly sensitive test that measures either antigens or antibodies. Commercial kits, containing specific antigens (or antibodies) that are labeled with an enzyme, provide a testing standard for comparison. The enzyme-labeled antigen (or antibody) is added to serum, where it competes with its unlabeled counterpart to bind to antibody (or antigen) present in the serum. A colorless substrate for the enzyme is added. The bound enzyme acts on the substrate to produce a color change, which can be read visually or with a spectrophotometer. Color increases as the amount of antibody fixed to antigen increases.

ELISA is more sensitive than CIE in detecting anti-

bodies or antigens in certain bacterial, fungal, parasitic, and viral infections. It is particularly useful in diagnosing HIV infection, hepatitis A and B, and rubella.

RADIOIMMUNOASSAY

In performing radioimmunoassay (RIA), a known amount of a specific antigen (or antibody) that is labeled with radioactive isotopes is added to the specimen, causing antigen-antibody complexes to precipitate. The radioactive count is measured in the precipitate and the result is converted to a titer measurement. RIA is highly sensitive and can detect small amounts of either antibody or antigen. This assay is useful in diagnosing hepatitis B.

IMMUNOFLUORESCENT ANTIBODY ASSAY

While performing an immunofluorescent antibody (IFA) assay, antigen-antibody binding can be observed under a fluorescent microscope when either antigens or antibodies are tagged with a fluorescent dye. Direct and indirect methods are used. Direct fluorescent antibody uses a specific, labeled antibody to identify viruses from a specimen. Indirect immunofluorescence tests unlabeled patient serum against labeled cell cultures. The highest dilution of patient serum that still shows fluorescence is the IFA titer.

Some commonly used IFA assays are the FTA-ABS (flourescent treponemal antibody-absorbed test) for syphilis, the IFA for toxoplasmosis, and the Micro-IF (micro-immunoflourescence) for *Chlamydia trachomatis*.

OTHER IMMUNOLOGIC TESTS

The limulus lysate assay detects endotoxins in CSF that are produced by gram-negative bacteria, including *E. coli*, *Neisseria meningitidis*, and *Haemophilus influenzae*. Although the limulus assay is not as specific as CIE and latex agglutination procedures, it is useful for the rapid diagnosis of gram-negative bacterial meningitis.

Three antigen-antibody reactions can be observed microscopically: immobilization, opsonization and phagocytosis, and capsular swelling (quellung reaction). The TPI (*T. pallidum* immobilization) test detects capsular swelling and is used in diagnosing syphilis.

Neutralization tests are sometimes used. A known antigen or toxin is incubated in test serum, which is then inoculated into tissue culture. Neutralizing antibodies or antitoxin, if present, will prevent tissue destruction. Because neutralizing antibodies persist for years, acute and convalescent serums must be compared to identify current infection.

Table 3-3

WHITE BLOOD CELL (WBC) COUNT AND DIFFERENTIAL IN A NORMAL ADULT AND IN ACUTE BACTERIAL INFECTION

Leukocyte	Normal adult	Adult with acute infection
Total WBC	$9,000/mm^3$	$15,000/mm^3$
WBC differential		
Bands*	3%	10%
Neutrophils	60%	72%
Eosinophils	5%	3%
Basophils	1%	1%
Lymphocytes	25%	10%
Monocytes	6%	4%

*Immature neutrophils.

HEMATOLOGIC TESTS

Routine hematology tests are an integral part of evaluating patients with infectious disease. Although these tests are nonspecific, they provide important information on the inflammatory response, general clues about the type of pathogen, and response to therapy.

The WBC count and differential are important in detecting the presence of infection. In noninfectious states, between 4,500 and $11,000/mm^3$ WBCs circulate in the blood. The total number of circulating leukocytes and the differential count (given as a percent of the total WBC count) may change during infection. For example, acute bacterial infection is typically accompanied by increased neutrophils and decreased lymphocytes, usually with an overall increase in total WBCs (Table 3-3). In contrast, some viral infections cause very little change in the WBC profile. The differential count may shift even when the total number of leukocytes remains within normal limits. The differential count also distinguishes the percent of immature vs mature forms (i.e., bands vs segments) of neutrophils, reflecting phagocytic activity.

The erythrocyte sedimentation rate (ESR) is elevated in acute inflammatory conditions that alter plasma proteins, especially fibrinogen. Fibrinogen increases 12 to 24 hours after the onset of acute inflammation, thus facilitating the clotting of red blood cells (RBCs). Anticoagulant is added to whole blood, and the ESR measures the clear plasma that remains after sedimentation of RBCs for a specified period in a calibrated tube. An elevated ESR occurs in tuberculosis, acute hepatitis, and many bacterial infections. The two methods for determining ESR are the Wintrobe method and the Westergren method.

C-reactive protein (CRP) appears in the circulation during acute inflammation or tissue destruction. Blood levels begin to rise 4 to 6 hours after onset of inflammation and decrease rapidly as the inflammation begins to resolve. CRP disappears altogether with steroid or antibiotic therapy.

Some intracellular enzymes can be detected in the serum following inflammation and tissue injury. Aspartate transferase (AST), alanine aminotransferase (ALT), and lactate dehydrogenase (LDH) levels are elevated with some acute infections.

Lactic acid levels increase in the presence of bacteria but not viruses. Therefore lactic acid determinations on CSF help differentiate bacterial from viral meningitis.

The ratio of immunoglobulin classes (IgG or IgM) aids in differentiating current infection from past infection or immunization. Serum IgM antibody levels generally peak 1 to 2 weeks after an antigen is introduced and then begin to decrease. IgG antibodies peak later and persist longer. Thus a high IgM level generally suggests recent infection, whereas a high IgG level indicates previous infection, placental transfer of maternal antibodies, or previous active or passive immunization.

ANTIBIOTIC SENSITIVITY TESTING

The growing number of pathogens that have developed resistance to antibiotics is a matter of great concern. The widespread, often inappropriate use of antibiotics since World War II has resulted in a varying degree of susceptibility among many species of bacteria. Resistance develops primarily in three ways: genetic mutation of the organism, transmissible genetic particles coding for drug resistance, and the production of beta-lactamase enzymes, which inactivate the drug.

Antibiotic sensitivity testing saves valuable time (and often lives) that might otherwise be wasted waiting for a clinical response. Antimicrobial drugs are added to a culture to determine whether the microorganism is inhibited from growing or is dead. Two methods are used for testing antibiotic sensitivity.

TUBE DILUTION

The tube dilution method uses either broth or agar as the medium, and different concentrations of an antibiotic are added to a known number of organisms to determine the amount of drug that will inhibit visible growth. This dose is termed the **minimum inhibitory concentration (MIC).**

The MIC is reported as the antibiotic concentration per milliliter of solution and compared with the achievable blood level of the antibiotic. An organism is considered sensitive to a drug if the antibiotic blood levels can be attained at two to four times the MIC. Laboratories may also report the **minimum bactericidal concentration (MBC),** the smallest concentration necessary to kill 99.9% of the organisms. This may or may not be higher than the MIC.

AGAR DIFFUSION

The agar diffusion method is more widely used. This involves exposing a pure culture of the microorganism to a paper disk impregnated with a known amount of antibiotic, which diffuses from the disk into the culture. MIC is measured by the size of the zone around the disk in which growth is inhibited. One advantage of the agar diffusion method is that several antibiotics can be tested on a single culture, allowing a rapid method of identifying the appropriate drug for organisms that are resistant to some antibiotic agents. This multidrug test is the Kirby-Bauer method of agar diffusion.

The results of agar diffusion tests are reported as "resistant" if growth is not altered, "sensitive" if growth is retarded, and "intermediate" if test results are uncertain. Some authorities believe that intermediate sensitivity should be classified as resistant.

CHAPTER 4

Central Nervous System Infectious Diseases

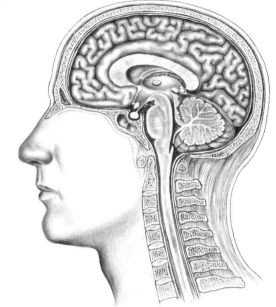

Meningitis

Meningitis is an inflammation of the meninges covering the brain and spinal cord. The inflammation may result from an acute infection of the meninges caused by the invasion of bacteria, viruses, fungi, or parasitic worms into the tissues or from the iatrogenic introduction of a substance that is irritating to the meninges. The forms of meningitis discussed in this section are those caused by bacterial and viral invasion (Table 4-1).

Meningococcal meningitis is an acute communicable inflammation of the meninges caused by *Neisseria meningitidis*. It frequently occurs in epidemic form.

Haemophilus meningitis is an acute communicable inflammation of the meninges caused by *Haemophilus influenzae*. It is the most common form of bacterial meningitis.

Pneumococcal meningitis is an acute inflammation of the meninges caused by *Streptococcus pneumoniae*. The meningitis frequently results from an extension of a primary infection in the upper respiratory tract. Patients infected with *S. pneumoniae* have a high risk of fatality.

Viral (aseptic or serous) meningitis is an acute meningeal inflammation that occurs as a sequela to many viral diseases. The condition is usually self-limited and benign.

Many bacteria are capable of producing a suppurative meningitis, but the most common forms are *Haemophilus*, meningococcal, and pneumococcal meningitides. They are discussed together, since their pathologic manifestations and symptoms are similar. Viral meningitis is discussed as a separate disease regardless of the viral disease that preceded the meningitis.

PATHOPHYSIOLOGY

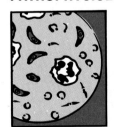

Bacteria causing the type of meningitis being considered here are inhaled in mucous droplets from infected persons or carriers, which invade the respiratory passages and are disseminated by way of the blood to meninges of the brain and spinal cord. The respiratory phase is generally subclinical in meningococcal meningitis, although organisms present in respiratory secretions can be transmitted to another host. The respiratory phase is usually symptomatic in pneumococcal and *Haemophilus* meningitides. The bacteremia produced during dissemination causes toxic manifestations. In the case of meningococcus the organism penetrates and damages vascular endothelium. This results in petechial and purpuric lesions of the skin.

Table 4-1

OVERVIEW OF MENINGITIS

	Meningococcal meningitis	Pneumococcal meningitis	Haemophilus meningitis	Viral meningitis (aseptic)
Occurrence	Endemic and epidemic; worldwide; greatest during winter and spring; greatest in males, in children less than 5 yr, and in persons in crowded living conditions	Endemic; greatest in infants, elderly persons, and alcoholics; follows pneumococcal pneumonia	Worldwide; most common bacterial meningitis in children 2 months to 3 yr	Worldwide; epidemics and sporadic cases associated with other infections
Etiologic agent	*Neisseria meningitidis,* with many subgroups	*Streptococcus pneumoniae,* many serotypes	*Haemophilus influenzae,* six serotypes; type B responsible for 90% of *Haemophilus* meningitis	Most viruses (e.g., mumps, herpes, and polio) produce the syndrome
Reservoir	Humans	Humans; many carriers	Humans	Humans
Transmission	Direct contact with droplets from respiratory passages of infected persons and carriers	Direct and indirect contact with discharges from respiratory passages	Direct contact with droplets from respiratory passages	Not transmitted at this stage
Incubation period	2-10 days; usually 3-4 days	1-3 days for pneumonia	2-4 days	Depends on virus and associated viral disease
Period of communicability	Until organism is not present in discharges: within 24 h of treatment with sulfonamides	Until organism is not present in respiratory discharges: 24-48 h after antibiotic treatment	Prolonged; until organism is not present in nasal discharge	
Susceptibility and resistance	Susceptibility to clinical disease is low; many carriers; group-specific immunity of unknown duration follows infection	Infants and elderly most susceptible; immunity for specific type persists for years	Children most susceptible; otitis media may be a precursor; immunity of unknown duration follows infection	Children, elderly and immunocompromised patients, and those unimmunized against vaccine-preventable viral diseases.
Report to local health authority	Mandatory case report	Only epidemics; no individual case reports	Yes, in certain endemic areas	Yes, in endemic areas

Data from Benenson.[3]

The invasion may produce a primary or secondary infection. Some bacteria produce a primary focal infection in the meninges. Such is the case with *N. meningitidis* and *H. influenzae,* which cause meningococcal and *Haemophilus* meningitides, respectively. Other bacterial and viral pathogens are capable of producing a secondary infection in the meninges following hematogenous dissemination from a primary focal infection elsewhere in the body. *H. influenzae, S. pneumoniae* (pneumococcal meningitis), many viruses, and other bacteria have this pathogenic potential.

Bacteria in the meninges elicit an inflammatory response and the production of an exudate consisting of leukocytes, fibrin, and bacteria in the subarachnoid space. Cerebrospinal fluid may be thin or thick and have plaquelike accumulations, and high leukocytosis with the majority of the leukocytes being neutrophils. In untreated disease the cerebrospinal fluid may achieve a thickness that interferes with its circulation and reabsorption. An internal or external hydrocephalus may result. Extension of the bacteria into brain tissue may produce a bacterial encephalitis.

Meningococcal infections may be so severe in the systemic stage that they produce an acute meningococcemia that leads to death or the initiation of therapy before meningeal involvement. Meningococcemia may become chronic, with toxic symptoms persisting intermittently for weeks or months. Recurrent meningitis is usually of the pneumococcal form and is frequently associated with an undetected skull fracture.

Complications of bacterial meningitis include internal hydrocephalus, deficits of cranial nerve function that lead to blindness and deafness, arthritis, myocarditis, pericarditis, and neuromotor and intellectual deficits. Symptomatic and asymptomatic infection with bacterial meningitis results in a protective immune response of unknown duration.

Aseptic (viral, serous, or nonsuppurative) meningitis is a syndrome generally associated with an existing systemic viral disease, the most common one being mumps. Inflammation and lymphocytic infiltration of the meninges occur with a wide gradient in clinical severity, depending on the infectious agent. Toxic and meningeal symptoms are usually less severe than in suppurative meningitis; cerebrospinal fluid leukocytes are less and primarily consist of lymphocytes. This form may also progress to clinical encephalitis. The disease is usually self-limited with complete recovery, although patients may experience muscle weakness and malaise during a prolonged convalescence.

NURSING CARE

See pages 58 to 65 for nursing care for meningitis.

COMPLICATIONS

Bacterial meningitis:
Internal hydrocephalus
Cranial nerve function deficits that lead to blindness and deafness, arthritis, myocarditis, pericarditis, and neuromotor and intellectual deficits
Aseptic meningitis:
Clinical encephalitis
Muscle weakness and malaise during prolonged convalescence

DIAGNOSTIC STUDIES AND FINDINGS

Diagnostic Test	Findings
Cerebrospinal fluid (CSF) examination	
Gross appearance	Bacterial: turbid
	Viral (aseptic): clear
Leukocytes	Bacterial: 500 to 20,000/mm^3
	Viral: 10 to 500/mm^3
Cell types	Bacterial: neutrophils
	Viral (aseptic): lymphocytes
Protein	Increased for both
Glucose	Bacterial: low to normal
	Viral (aseptic): normal
Cerebrospinal fluid culture or Gram's stain or serologic techniques	Positive for bacteria
	Absence of bacteria with CSF cell changes suggest viral (aseptic) meningitis
Gram's stain of scrapings from petechial skin lesions	Positive for meningococci
Culture of respiratory secretions	Positive for *H. influenzae*, *N. meningitidis*, or *S. pneumoniae*
Blood culture	Positive for *H. influenzae* or *N. meningitidis* (meningococci)
Serology	Increase in antibody titer with specific viral infections

---

MEDICAL MANAGEMENT FOR MENINGITIS

DRUG THERAPY

Antiinfective agents for bacterial menigitides: Initial therapy until organism is identified: Ampicillin, 200 mg/k/24 h IV plus cholramphenicol if *H. influenzae* is suspected for patients >2 mos.

Antiinfective agents for meningococci or pneumococci: Ampicillin (Amcill), 200 mg/kg/24 h IV, or chloramphenicol (Chloromycetin), 100 mg/kg/24 h IV to a maximum of 4 g.

Antiinfective agents for *H. influenzae*: Ampicillin or chloramphenicol, 100 mg/kg/24 h IV to a maximum of 4 g. All of the above are administered by rapid IV infusion; initial dose should be ⅓ of daily dose, the remainder divided into six equal doses; therapy should continue for 5 days after temperature is normal and clinical signs have cleared; barbiturates may be given for seizures.
Analgesics prescribed for headache and muscle pain (nonnarcotic).
Immunologic agents prescribed for prevention of bacterial meningitides (see also Chapter 13).
Meningococcal polysaccharide vaccine used against group A and C serotypes for patients >2 yrs at risk for epidemic disease; group A serotype given to children 3 mos to 2 yr. Routine immunization of civilians is not recommended.
Pneumococcal polysaccharide vaccine given to patients at high risk for pneumococcal pneumonia and subsequent systemic complications.
H. influenzae type B conjugate vaccine now recommended for all children > 15 months.

Antiinfective agents for meningococcal contacts: Rifampin (Rifamycin, others), 600 mg bid (adults) for 2 days Sulfadiazine, 1 g bid for 3 days for mass prophylaxis during meningococcal epidemics or for close patient contacts if strain is proved susceptible

Antiinfective agents for *H. influenzae* household contacts (excluding pregnant women): Rifampin, 20 mg/kg/day (maximum daily dose of 600 mg) for 4 days as soon as possible after contact.
Osmotic agents (e.g., Dexamethasone) for cerebral edema.

GENERAL MANAGEMENT

Intratracheal intubation
Ventilatory assistance
IV therapy and dopamine if shock is present
Fluid restriction to ⅔ of daily needs if excess secretion of antidiuretic hormone (ADH)
Control of intracranial pressure
Close monitoring for early diagnosis of patient contacts

References: 3, 17, 27, 32, 44, 152.

Encephalitis

Encephalitis is an inflammation of the tissues of the brain and spinal cord, resulting in altered function of various portions of these tissues. Encephalitis is frequently accompanied by signs of systemic infection. Clinical disease manifestations range from mild to severe to death, and disease may be followed by temporary or permanent neurologic sequelae or complete recovery.

Similar to meningitis, encephalitis may result from at least four causes: a toxemia accompanying an infectious disease, an allergic response to microbial antigens, direct invasion of central nervous system tissue by pathogens as a primary focal infection, or direct invasion of central nervous system tissue secondary to hematogenous dissemination from a primary focal infection elsewhere in the body. Direct invasion, either primary or secondary, is usually caused by a virus, a great many of which are capable of producing encephalitis.

The majority of viruses producing encephalitis as a primary focal infection are transmitted by mosquitoes and are discussed together. Encephalitides occurring secondary to other viral diseases are discussed as infectious encephalitis. A rarer form of meningoencephalitis caused by direct invasion of an ameba is also discussed (Table 4-2).

Table 4-2

OVERVIEW OF ENCEPHALITIS

	Viral encephalitis	Mosquito-borne viral encephalitides (equine and St. Louis encephalitis)	Amebic meningoencephalitis
Occurrence	Worldwide; epidemic and sporadic; associated with other viral diseases	Warm, moist climates; summer and early fall when mosquitoes are greatest	Worldwide, but rare; greatest in young persons, in warm climates, and during summer
Etiologic agent	A variety of viruses, commonly the *Herpesvirus*	A variety of diseases, each caused by a different virus	*Naegleria fowleri; Acanthamoeba culbertsoni*
Reservoir	Humans	Birds, rodents, bats, reptiles, and amphibians; differing for each virus	Amebae that are free living in water and soil
Transmission	Direct contact with droplets from respiratory passages or other excretions harboring the virus	Bite of infective mosquitoes	Water infected with *N. fowleri* forced into nasal passages while swimming; *Acanthamoeba* enters a skin lesion
Incubation period	Depends on viral disease	5-15 days	3-7 days or longer
Period of communicability	Depends on viral disease	Not communicable person to person; mosquitoes are infective for life	Not communicable person to person
Susceptibility and resistance	Depends on viral disease	Highest susceptibility to clinical disease is infancy and old age; in endemic areas, adults are immune to local strains of virus because of subclinical infections	Unknown; immunosuppressed persons are susceptible to infection with *Acanthamoeba*
Report to local health authority	In select endemic areas	Mandatory case report	Only for means of surveillance

Data from Benenson.[3]

Infectious viral encephalitides are acute inflammations of the central nervous system that are associated with and sequelae to systemic viral infections; they are commonly caused by the genus *Herpesvirus.*

Mosquito-borne viral encephalitides are a group of acute inflammatory diseases of the brain, spinal cord, and meninges caused by a variety of viruses transmitted to humans through bites from infected mosquitoes.

Amebic meningoencephalitis is an acute and severe inflammation of the brain and meninges caused by invasion of the tissues by a free-living ameba usually found in water, soil, and decaying vegetation. The disease is frequently fatal.

PATHOPHYSIOLOGY
Infectious encephalitis

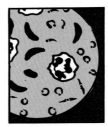

A variety of directly transmittable viruses is capable of producing encephalitides either as a concomitant to or as a sequela of clinical viral diseases (e.g., measles, mumps, rubella, and chickenpox) or as a result of a subclinical viral infection such as herpes. In both cases the pathologic manifestations of the encephalitis may result from a postinfection autoimmune response to the virus or from direct invasion of the central nervous system by the virus. Timing of the onset of central nervous system manifestations in relationship to the associated disease symptoms and the ability to isolate the virus from cerebrospinal fluid allow differentiation as to postinfection or direct invasion encephalitis.

Disease onset may be acute or insidious, and disease severity may be mild to severe depending on the virus and the distribution, location, and concentration of the neuronal lesions. Mumps virus usually produces a more benign disease, whereas herpes encephalitis is frequently fatal. Permanent neurologic sequelae are also more common in herpes infections.

Mosquito-borne viral encephalitis

A variety of viruses capable of infecting animals and birds can be carried to humans by vector mosquitoes that feed on infected animals. The virus, injected into humans from a mosquito bite, rapidly localizes in the central nervous system and produces congestion, edema, and small hemorrhages in the brain. Neuronal lesions with nerve cell necrosis and destruction and foci of cellular infiltration are widespread throughout the brain and spinal cord. Disease severity depends on the virus and on host resistance factors. Generally, older persons are more severely affected and have the highest fatality. Disease onset may be acute or insidious, depending on the virus involved. Infants generally have a more acute-onset encephalitis than do other age groups. Infants and children are also more likely to develop motor and mental disabilities (e.g., seizures, hydrocephalus, and mental retardation) as a sequela to mosquito-borne encephalitis.

An antibody response can be seen within 7 days. Duration of the disease is variable, depending on the virus. Blood leukocyte levels are generally normal or slightly elevated with some viruses. The virus cannot be recovered from blood, secretions, or discharges and is therefore not communicable from person to person.

Amebic meningoencephalitis

Two types of amebae, *Naegleria* and *Acanthamoeba*, are capable of producing meningoencephalitis in humans. *Naegleria* infection is caused when water containing the pathogen is forced into the nasal passages, usually by diving or swimming in water containing large amounts of organic matter. The organism colonizes and invades the mucosa, travels along olfactory nerves to the meninges and brain, and produces a severe and rapidly fatal fulminating pyogenic meningoencephalitis. *Acanthamoeba* colonizes a skin lesion and travels to the central nervous system along peripheral nerves to produce a meningoencephalitis with a more insidious onset and prolonged course. Immunologic investigations have shown many people to have a natural antibody against these organisms, suggesting that more subclinical than clinical infections may occur.

COMPLICATIONS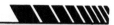

Infectious encephalitis:
Permanent neurologic sequelae are more common in herpes infections
Mosquito-borne viral encephalitis:
Motor and mental disabilities (e.g., seizures, hydrocephalus, and mental retardation), more likely in infants and children
Amebic meningoencephalitis:
Severe and rapidly fatal fulminating pyogenic meningoencephalitis

DIAGNOSTIC STUDIES AND FINDINGS

Diagnostic Test	Findings
Cerebrospinal fluid (CSF) examination	Viral: 50-500/mm^3 leukocytes (predominately lymphocytes); many RBCs, normal glucose; elevated protein: 50-150 mg/dl
	Mosquito-borne: 50-500/mm^3 leukocytes (up to 1000/mm^3 in infants) (usually lymphocytes); rare to have RBCs; normal to high glucose; elevated protein
	Amebic: polymorphonuclear leukocytes; RBCs; low to normal glucose; elevated protein
Culture and/or microscopic examination of CSF	All: negative for bacteria
	Viral: virus can sometimes be isolated
	Mosquito-borne: virus can sometimes be isolated
	Amebic: mobile amebae can be visualized on a wet mount
Serology	Viral and mosquito-borne: fourfold increase in antibody titer between early disease and convalescence
Immunofluorescent staining of biopsied brain tissue	Viral: positive for specific viruses
Hematology: (WBC)	Mosquito-borne: range from 10,000-66,000/mm^3, depending on virus

---

MEDICAL MANAGEMENT FOR ENCEPHALITIS

DRUG THERAPY

Antiinfective agents: Amebic meningoencephalitis: combination of the following drugs (individual dose calculation)
>   Amphotericin B (Fungizone), IV
>   Sulfadiazine, IV
>   Miconazole (Monistat), IV
>   Rifampin (Rifamycin; others), PO
>Mosquito-borne: no specific treatment
>Infectious viral encephalitides: no specific treatment except for herpes infections; adenine arabinoside (Vidarabine, ara-A), IV 15 mg/kg/24 h for 10 days; Acyclovir

GENERAL MANAGEMENT

Tracheostomy
Assisted ventilation
Suction
Sedatives for hyperexcitability and seizures
IV fluids and electrolytes
Nasogastric tube feedings

References: 56, 88, 100.

---

1   ASSESS

ASSESSMENT	OBSERVATIONS	
	MENINGITIS	ENCEPHALITIS
History	Recent upper respiratory or ear infection; contact with person with rhinitis or meningitis Pneumonia and otitis media frequently precede *Pneumococcal* and *Haemophilus* meningitis	Viral: systemic viral infection Mosquito-borne: exposure to mosquitos Amebic: swimming and diving in fresh water
Subjective symptoms	Severe throbbing headache, muscle pains, stiff neck, backache, chills, expressions of fear Malaise and irritability in chronic meningococcemia	Severe frontal headache, nausea and vomiting, dizziness, fever and chills
Body temperature	38°-41° C (100°-106° F), starting in systemic phase; flushed, hot, dry skin; perspiration Intermittent low-grade fever in chronic meningococcemia	39°-41° C (102°-106° F); may be acute-onset fever accompanying CNS symptoms or a 1- to 4-day prodromal period with fever and chills before CNS symptoms

ASSESSMENT	OBSERVATIONS	
	MENINGITIS	ENCEPHALITIS
Vital signs	Pulse may be slow as intracranial pressure increases; BP increases with intracranial pressure	Tachypnea, tachycardia
Level of consciousness	Alert early in disease but may show delirium progressing to deep coma later	Alterations in consciousness—mild listlessness progressing to confusion, stupor, and eventual coma May be extremely irritable; bizarre behavior with temporal lobe involvement of herpes encephalitis; seizures, particularly in infants with postinfectious encephalitis
Neurologic	Reflex changes: absence of abdominal reflexes, absence of cremasteric reflexes in male, alteration of tendon reflexes Resistance to neck flexion Brudzinski's sign positive (attempted flexion of neck will elicit flexion of knees and hips) Kernig's sign positive (limitation in angle at which a straight leg may be raised with patient supine) Bulging fontanel in infants	Focal neurologic signs, aphasia, olfactory hallucinations Nuchal rigidity (if meningeal irritation) Weakness, accentuated deep tendon reflexes, extensory plantar response Ataxia, spasticity, tremors Herpes encephalitis: may be a flaccid paralysis and depression of tendon reflexes with spinal cord involvement and bowel and bladder paralysis Postinfectious encephalitis: motor signs may not manifest
Fluids and electrolytes	Poor skin turgor; decreased urine output	Excess or deficient ADH secretion
Musculoskeletal	Chronic meningococcemia: Swelling and pain in large joints (especially knees and ankles)	
Skin	Meningococcemia: Petechia and purpura lesions preceded by a rash resembling measles on trunk and extremities (recurring with chronic meningococcemia); large ecchymotic lesions on face and extremities in severe disease	

→ > >

2 DIAGNOSE

NURSING DIAGNOSIS	SUPPORTIVE ASSESSMENT FINDINGS
Potential for infection related to presence of pathogen in CSF and respiratory secretions	Laboratory findings positive for infectious agent; upper respiratory exudates; history of repiratory infection or recent exposure to person with rhinitis or meningitis; history of systemic viral infection; history of immunosuppression
Hyperthermia related to infection	Body temperature 38° to 41° C (100° to 106° F); flushed, hot, dry skin; excess perspiration; tachycardia and tachypnea; seizures; chills, feels hot or cold
Pain related to inflammation of meninges and brain	Swelling and pain in large joints, particularly knees and ankles; nuchal rigidity; restlessness; severe throbbing headache; muscle pains; stiff neck; backache
Altered cerebral tissue perfusion related to inflammation and edema of brain and meninges	Malaise; irritability; altered consciousness; confusion, delirium, or coma; seizures; bizarre behavior; nausea, vomiting, or dizziness; reflex changes; focal neurologic signs in encephalitis; signs of intracranial pressure increases (bradycardia and increased BP); severe throbbing headache
Altered peripheral tissue perfusion related to infection with meningococcus	Petechial and purpuric skin lesions preceded by rash on trunk and extremities; large ecchymotic lesions on face and extremities
Ineffective breathing pattern related to altered level of consciousness	Depressed respiratory effort; recent diagnosis of pneumonia
Ineffective airway clearance related to altered level of consciousness	Stasis of respiratory secretions; unable to cough or clear secretions
Potential fluid volume deficit related to fever and vomiting	Fever, perspiration, nausea and vomiting, decreased fluid intake; feels thirsty
Fluid volume deficit related to fever and vomiting	Decreased skin turgor, decreased and concentrated urinary output; hot, dry skin
Potential fluid volume excess related to excess ADH secretion	Sodium retention related to increased ADH secretion; increased confusion or lethargy
Fear related to severity of condition	Muscle rigidity or tension; restlessness; inability to sleep; fear of pain, death, or long-term disability
Self-care deficit related to CNS alteration	Unable to feed, toilet, bathe, or dress self without help; unable to move in bed or get out of bed (related to loss of consciousness, pain, or fatigue); fatigue and pain on movement
Potential for injury related to altered level of consciousness	Alteration in consciousness; uncontrolled seizure activity

3 PLAN

Patient goals

1. Patient will be free of infection. Complications of bacterial meningitis will be prevented by early and effective therapy.
2. Infection will not be transmitted to patient contacts.
3. Body temperature will be maintained within normal range. Comfort and safety will be maintained for patient experiencing fever.
4. Patient will obtain relief from pain.
5. Patient will demonstrate improved tissue perfusion and cellular oxygenation.
6. Patient will demonstrate normal respiratory pattern and blood gases. Aspiration of secretions is avoided.
7. Fluid and electrolyte balance will be maintained.
8. Patient will demonstrate reduction in fear of disease condition and residual disability.
9. Patient will have daily living needs met while acutely ill and will return to preillness level of function.
10. Patient will not experience injury.
11. Patient will have information to prevent future mosquito-borne or amebic encephalitis.
12. Patient and family will be aware of rehabilitation needs and will use resources.

4 IMPLEMENT

NURSING DIAGNOSIS	NURSING INTERVENTIONS	RATIONALE
Potential for infection related to pathogen in CSF and respiratory secretions	Assist in collection of CSF. Record amount and character of CSF. Administer antiinfective agents as soon as ordered.	To provide for laboratory diagnosis of infectious agent and to prevent transmission.
	Employ respiratory isolation for 24 h after initiation of antibiotic therapy for bacterial meningitis.	Early antibiotic therapy is essential to prevent complications of bacterial meningitis. Every hour is important. Encephalitis is frequently fatal. Early treatment for amebic encephalitis is particularly important.
	Employ secretion precautions for duration of hospitalization for viral meningitis and viral encephalitis.	To prevent transmission of pathogen during this highly contagious time.
	Encourage patient contacts to be examined and immunized or treated.	To prevent transmission of pathogen and decrease risk for infection of patient contacts.
Hyperthermia related to infection	See inside back cover (Interventions 1-15).	
Pain related to inflammation of meninges and brain	Administer analgesics as prescribed. (Do not give narcotics or sedatives that will depress vital functions in patients with increased intracranial pressure). Provide moist heat (in absence of high fever). Place blanket roll under knees (in absence of elevated intracranial pressure).	To relieve muscle aches and pains. To relieve pain in back and joints.
	Darken room and provide ice pack for head.	To relieve headache.

→ → →

NURSING DIAGNOSIS	NURSING INTERVENTIONS	RATIONALE
Altered cerebral tissue perfusion related to inflammation and edema of brain and meninges	Monitor patient carefully, particularly after lumbar puncture. Have patient lie flat for 4-6 h or as ordered after lumbar puncture.	To prevent headache associated with alterations in CSF pressure.
	Monitor for signs of intracranial pressure throughout course of disease (e.g., slowing of pulse, increased BP, decreased level of consciousness (LOC), arrhythmic breathing, altered pupillary response, and facial weakness.	To detect signs of shock, which must be reported to physician for early intervention.
	Monitor vital signs and neurologic findings every 5-30 min for patient with intracranial pressure. Report changes to physician immediately.	These changes indicate alterations in intracranial pressure and necessitate early intervention.
	Avoid bent leg positions or movement of patient; provide bed rest.	To prevent increased intracranial pressure.
	Elevate patient's head slightly. Prevent any sudden or unnecessary movements of head and neck and avoid neck flexion; use log roll to turn.	To decrease intracranial pressure.
	Assist patient with all activities and movements. Administer stool softeners as prescribed (avoid enemas). Instruct patient to exhale while turning or moving in bed. Position to avoid knee or hip flexion.	To prevent muscle straining, which leads to increased intracranial pressure.
	Time nursing procedures to coincide with periods of relaxation or sedation; avoid unnecessary environmental stimuli.	To prevent excitation, which stimulates the already irritated brain and leads to seizures.
	Administer hypertonic agents or steroids, as prescribed.	To lower intracranial pressure.
	Give clear, concise explanations to confused patient; interpret environment to patient and reorient confused patient.	To lessen disorientation and to clarify impaired sensory perceptions.
	Evaluate during convalescence for motor, sensory, and intellectual impairment.	To refer for rehabilitation.
Altered peripheral tissue perfusion related to infection with meningococcus	Monitor peripheral circulation, pulses, purpura.	To detect increased vascular permeability.
	Administer range of motion exercises to patients with no sign of elevated intracranial pressure; frequently change position.	To prevent contractures and pressure on skin; to stimulate peripheral circulation.

NURSING DIAGNOSIS	NURSING INTERVENTIONS	RATIONALE
Ineffective breathing patterns related to altered LOC	Monitor depth and rate of respiration, breath sounds, and blood gases.	To detect altered oxygenation.
	Oxygenate before suctioning, and limit suctioning to 10-15 sec for apneic patients; employ mechanical ventilation if necessary.	Transportation of oxygen to the brain is decreased because of diminished blood flow.
Ineffective airway clearance related to altered LOC	Continually monitor delirious or convulsive patient; maintain fully patent airway for patient with increased intracranial pressure; suction secretions; perform endotracheal care.	To prevent aspiration.
Potential fluid volume deficit related to fever and vomiting	Monitor intake and output, urine specific gravity, and weight loss.	Accurate measurement is essential in proper administration of fluids.
	Administer frequent oral or continuous IV fluids. (Administer IV fluids **carefully** to prevent overload if fluid retention is likely.)	To prevent dehydration related to fever or decreased input or loss related to vomiting.
	Monitor vital signs.	Decreasing BP may indicate bleeding.
Potential fluid volume excess related to excess secretion of ADH	Monitor intake and output, serum electrolytes and weight; restrict IV fluids to ⅔ of needs if signs of fluid retention occur.	To detect signs of fluid retention and prevent increasing intracranial pressure.
	Test urine specific gravity.	Concentrated urine may indicate excess secretion of ADH.
	Administer osmotic agents as prescribed.	To decrease fluid overload.
Fear related to severity of of condition	Allow patient and significant others to verbalize fears.	To foster confidence in care.
	Instruct patient and family regarding disease course, diagnostic procedures, and treatments. Inform patient that symptoms are temporary and recovery is usually complete.	To relieve fear of unknown and provide a sense of comfort to patient and family.
Potential for injury related to altered LOC	Continually supervise patient who has convulsions or is delirious; pad bed and provide restraints for delirious patient; keep side rails up; prevent aspiration or injury during convulsions.	To protect from injury.
	Maintain quiet environment.	Excessive stimuli may induce seizures.
Self-care deficit related to CNS alterations	Provide all feeding and hygiene measures.	To conserve energy.
	Maintain indwelling catheter if necessary.	To empty bladder of unconscious patient.

→ › ›

5   EVALUATE

PATIENT OUTCOME	DATA INDICATING THAT OUTCOME IS REACHED
Patient is free of infection and complications of meningitis and encephalitis.	CSF findings: <30 cells/mm³; glucose, protein, and pressures are normal; cultures are negative for bacteria; color is clear. Neurologic signs are normal. Pupils are equal and reactive to light. Neck flexion unimpaired. Straight legs may be raised from the bed from a prone position. Abdominal, cremasteric, and tendon reflexes are normal. Patient able to walk and perform all functions without residual weakness or impairment. No skin petechiae or purpura. Blood cultures negative for bacteria. Patient is alert, responds appropriately to questions and environmental stimuli, is oriented to person and place, and has memory of recent and past events.
Infection was not transmitted to patient contacts.	Hospital personnel and patient contacts are free of infection.
Body temperature is maintained within normal range; comfort and safety maintained during fever.	Absence of flushing, chills, seizures; body temperature maintained 35.8° to 37.3° C. Vital signs within normal limits for patient.
Relief from pain obtained.	Verbalizes relief; alternates periods of activity and rest; sleeps 3-4 h at a time.
Improved tissue perfusion and oxygenation demonstrated.	Vital signs are within normal limits; shock has been avoided. No petechiae or purpura. Patient is alert and oriented to person, place, and time and exhibits recall of recent and past events. Affect is appropriate to environmental stimuli. Adults demonstrate cognitive ability, ability to problem solve, concentration, and attentiveness.
Normal respiratory pattern and blood gases demonstrated. Secretions have not been aspirated.	Breathing patterns are normal. Blood levels (O_2 saturation, CO_2, and P_{O_2}) are normal. Skin is warm and a normal color. No signs of pneumonia.
Fluid and electrolyte balance is maintained.	No excessive thirst or weight loss; serum electrolytes within normal limits. I & O balanced; urine specific gravity within normal limits (1.01-1.025); skin turgor good. No restlessness or confusion.
Fear of disease and disability is reduced.	Patient and significant others trust care providers, are participating in treatment, and have realistic expectations of recovery. Patient sleeps.
Activities of daily living have been performed for patient while ill and will be managed after hospital discharge	Patient has not lost weight; skin is intact; urinary and bowel elimination are normal. If patient cannot manage ADL at home, care has been arranged.

PATIENT OUTCOME	DATA INDICATING THAT OUTCOME IS REACHED
No injury experienced.	Seizures have been prevented or no trauma has resulted from seizures.
Patient or family is aware of needs and able to use resources.	Patient or family with a residual limitation in physical or mental function has been referred for appropriate therapy during convalescence. Family of disabled person has been given an opportunity to express concerns and has been referred for counseling and to support groups if necessary.

PATIENT TEACHING

1. Inform patient of the diagnostic procedures that may be performed:
   - Neurologic assessment and eye examination
   - Cultures of blood, CSF, and respiratory secretions to identify the causative organism
   - Serologic tests of blood to identify viral antibodies
   - Lumbar puncture to abtain spinal fluid for analysis
2. Instruct patient to lie flat for 24 hours following lumbar puncture (see Chapter 3) and to report change in symptoms.
3. Explain purposes of antibiotic therapy to patients receiving antibiotic therapy. Discuss dosage, time, rationale, route of administration, and side effects for each prescribed drug. Antiinfective therapy for bacterial meningitis must be continued as prescribed for 5 days after temperature returns to normal. Exacerbation of symptoms should be reported to the physician immediately.
4. Instruct patients who have positive sputum cultures about respiratory isolation procedures (Chapter 13).
5. Explain to patient and family that convalescence is of variable duration, depending on the severity of the disease. Patients should allow adequate time for recovery before resuming full activities. Exacerbation of symptoms should be reported to the physician immediately.
6. Recovery is usually complete in meningitis, however, neurologic sequelae do occur. The patient should be evaluated during convalescence for functional and neurologic deficits and should participate in rehabilitation if prescribed.
7. Sequelae of encephalitis include mental deterioration, paralysis, and possible convulsive disorders, particularly in children. Families should be informed of the need for periodic evaluation and long-term physical therapy and of potential resources to help them cope with a handicapped family member.
8. Prophylactic measures should be initiated for close patient contacts, as described in the Medical Management on page 55. Patient contacts should be evaluated medically for early detection and treatment of bacterial meningitis.
9. Amebic meningoencephalitis can be prevented by swimming in chlorinated pools only. Mosquito-borne encephalitis can be prevented by environmental control of mosquitoes, particularly through elimination of stagnant pools of water (where mosquitoes breed), and by wearing protective clothing, screening living quarters, and using repellents.

Gastrointestinal Infectious Diseases

A wide range of gastrointestinal (GI) infectious diseases are caused by pathogens that are ingested in contaminated food or water. These are presented in five sections in this chapter as follows:

1. Food poisoning caused by pathogens that have already multiplied in the food at the time of ingestion:
   Staphylococcal food poisoning
   Botulism
   Food poisoning: enteric infections
     Bacillus cereus
     Clostridium perfringens
     Vibrio parahaemolyticus
2. Acute gastroenteritis produced by bacteria and viruses that multiply in the gastrointestinal tract after ingestion:
     Campylobacter
     Escherichia coli
     Shigella
     Norwalk virus
     Rotavirus
3. Parasitic enteritis caused by parasites that multiply in the colon after ingestion:
     Amebiasis
     Giardiasis
4. *Salmonella* infections caused by ingested food- or water-borne *Salmonella:*
     Salmonellosis
     Typhoid fever
     Paratyphoid fever
5. Parasitic worm infections:
     Ancylostomiasis (hookworm)

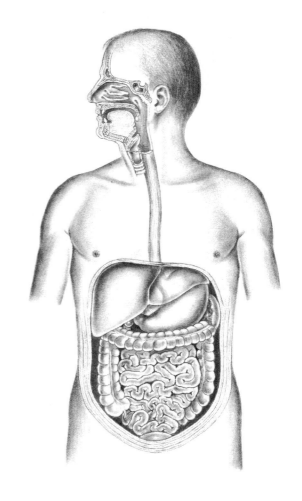

     Ascariasis (roundworm)
     Enterobiasis (pinworm)
     Strongyloidiasis (threadworm)
     Taeniasis (tapeworm)
     Toxocariasis
     Trichinosis
     Trichuriasis (whipworm)

Food Poisoning

Food poisoning is the generic term applied to illnesses acquired through consumption of food or water contaminated with chemicals, bacteria and bacterial toxins, or organic poisons naturally present in some edible substances.

The food poisonings caused by bacteria and bacterial toxins are discussed here. In all cases disease is produced in the host shortly after ingestion of food containing bacteria that have already multiplied in the food. These diseases are not directly communicable. If the bacteria have produced a toxin in the food, the resulting disease in the host is intoxication, as in staphylococcal food poisoning and botulism. If the bacterial cells are antigenic, they produce an infection in the host, such as those caused by *Clostridium perfringens* and *Vibrio parahaemolyticus* (Table 5-1).

Table 5-1

OVERVIEW OF FOOD POISONING: INTOXICATIONS AND ENTERIC INFECTIONS

	Intoxications		Enteric infections		
	Staphylococcal food poisoning	**Botulism**	***Clostridium perfringens***	***Vibrio parahaemolyticus***	***Bacillus cereus***
Occurrence	Widespread and frequent; one of the principal acute food poisonings in the United States	Sporadic; family-grouped cases occur	Widespread and frequent in countries with cooking practices that favor growth of organism	Sporadic cases and outbreaks occur in warm months of the year	Outbreaks in Europe and United States
Etiologic agent	Several enterotoxins of staphylococci; stable at boiling temperature	Toxins produced by *Clostridium botulinum* in anaerobic conditions; destroyed by boiling	Type A strains of *C. perfringens* (*C. welchii*)	*V. parahaemolyticus* (many types)	*B. cereus*, an aerobic spore former that produces two enterotoxins—one heat stable, causing vomiting, and one heat labile, causing diarrhea
Reservoir	Humans; cows with infected udders; dogs and fowl	Soil, water, and intestinal tract of animals and fish	Soil and gastrointestinal tract of humans and animals	Marine silt, coastal waters, fish, and shellfish	Soil; commonly found in raw, dried, and processed foods
Transmission	Ingestion of food containing staphylococcal toxin, which formed while food was held at room temperature	Ingestion of food in which toxin has formed; generally home-canned vegetables, fruits, and meats; also onions and potatoes cooked and held at room temperature	Ingestion of food, especially meat, contaminated by soil or feces; spores survive normal cooking temperatures, germinate, and multiply during cooking and reheating	Ingestion of raw or undercooked contaminated seafood; food contaminated with seawater	Ingestion of food that has been kept at ambient temperatures after cooking, permitting multiplication of the organism
Incubation period	30 min-7 h, usually 2-4 h	12-36 h	6-24 h; usually 10-12 h	4-96 h; usually 12-24 h	1-6 h for disease causing vomiting; 6-20 h for disease causing diarrhea
Period of communicability	Noncommunicable	Noncommunicable	Noncommunicable	Noncommunicable	Noncommunicable
Susceptibility and resistance	General; no immune response	General; no immune response	General; no resistance develops from exposure	General	Unknown
Report to local health authority	Prompt report of outbreaks	Report of cases and outbreaks	Prompt report of outbreaks	Report outbreaks	Report cases and outbreaks

Data from Benenson.[3]

STAPHYLOCOCCAL FOOD POISONING

Staphylococcal food poisoning is an enteric intoxication of acute onset. Symptoms are severe nausea, intestinal cramps, vomiting, diarrhea, prostration, and occasionally subnormal temperature and hypotension. The intensity of the disease depends on the quantity of the ingested toxin and host susceptibility. The duration of the illness is 1 to 2 days, and recovery is generally complete.

PATHOPHYSIOLOGY

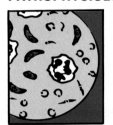 The ingested enterotoxin acts on the abdominal viscera, creating a sensory stimulus that reaches the vomiting center of the brain by way of the vagus and sympathetic nerves. The action of the enterotoxin on the gastric mucosa produces a patchy hyperemia, erosions, petechiae, and a purulent gastric exudate. Diarrhea results from inhibition of water absorption from the intestinal lumen and from increased transport of fluid into the lumen.

COMPLICATIONS

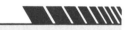

Dehydration ⎤ particularly in infants
Prostration ⎦ and older adults

BOTULISM

Botulism is a severe neurointoxication with a wide range of neurologic symptoms and severity of symptoms. In the United States 10% of cases under treatment result in death, primarily from respiratory failure. Three types of botulism have been recognized: foodborne, wound, and infant botulism.

PATHOPHYSIOLOGY

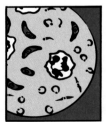 *Clostridium botulinum,* a spore-forming anaerobe capable of withstanding boiling, produces a potent toxin in anaerobic conditions. A common source of botulinal toxin is improperly processed canned foods. Less commonly, *C. botulinum* enters the body through a wound and produces toxin in traumatized, necrotic tissue. Inges-

tion of *C. botulinum* spores does not result in toxin production in adults and children but does cause toxin production in the bowel lumen of some infants, producing infant botulism.

The botulinal toxin is hematogenously disseminated to peripheral cholinergic synapses, where it becomes irreversibly bound. This action blocks the release of acetylcholine, producing impaired autonomic and voluntary neuromuscular transmission and muscular paralysis. Gradual recovery occurs over a period of weeks from the regeneration of terminal motor neurons to reinnervate noncontracting muscle fibers.

Intestinal stasis predisposes to the colonization of any ingested viable spores of *C. botulinum.* Additional toxin is produced in vivo, prolonging the course of the disease.

COMPLICATIONS

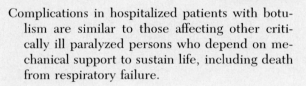

Complications in hospitalized patients with botulism are similar to those affecting other critically ill paralyzed persons who depend on mechanical support to sustain life, including death from respiratory failure.

FOOD POISONING: ENTERIC INFECTIONS

The three enteric infections discussed here are all caused by ingestion of food contaminated with specific bacteria that have already multiplied in the food. Disease occurs in the host shortly after ingestion of the food and manifests as symptoms of gastroenteritis.

C. perfringens generally causes a mild intestinal infection characterized by sudden onset of abdominal colic, nausea, and diarrhea. Fever and vomiting are rare.

V. parahaemolyticus is a moderately severe intestinal infection characterized by sudden-onset abdominal cramps and watery diarrhea lasting 1 to 7 days. Nausea, vomiting, fever, and headache may be present.

B. cereus food poisoning is a gastrointestinal infection characterized by sudden-onset nausea and vomiting or colic and diarrhea, lasting no longer than 24 hours.

PATHOPHYSIOLOGY

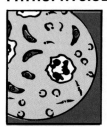

C. perfringens, a spore former widely distributed in feces, soil, and water, multiplies rapidly in foods that have been cooled and reheated. The organism produces an enterotoxin in the intestinal tract within 6 to 24 hours after ingestion. The enterotoxin acts on the epithelial layer of the ileum, increasing the secretion of sodium, chloride, and fluid, and inhibiting the absorption of glucose.

V. parahaemolyticus multiplies in uncooked, contaminated seafood. When ingested, the pathogen directly invades intestinal tissue to produce necrosis, ulceration, possible hemorrhage, and granulocytic infiltration of the mucosa. Disease intensity ranges from asymptomatic to severe; duration ranges from 2 hours to 10 days.

The spores of *B. cereus* survive cooking and multiply in food held at room temperature. One type of enterotoxin that is heat stable attacks the gastric mucosa. Another type, which is heat labile, affects the intestinal mucosa. Thorough reheating of food destroys the heat-labile enterotoxin but not the enterotoxin that causes vomiting.

COMPLICATIONS

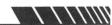

Dehydration
Prostration
} particularly in infants and older adults

DIAGNOSTIC STUDIES AND FINDINGS

Diagnostic Test	Findings
Culture of stomach contents, feces, or suspected food	10^5 enterotoxin-producing staphylococci per g of specimen, positive for *C. botulinum;* $>10^5$ spores of *C. perfringens* or *B. cereus* per g of specimen; or positive for *V. parahaemolyticus*
Serum	Positive for botulinal toxins; circulating toxins found in about ⅓ hospitalized patients with botulism

MEDICAL MANAGEMENT

DRUG THERAPY FOR BOTULISM Trivalent (ABE) botulinal antitoxin (not used for infants) administered IV or IM as soon as possible after onset of symptoms.

Antiinfective agents: Penicillin for wound botulism; agent-specific antiinfective agents for secondary bacterial infection.

GENERAL MANAGEMENT

For botulism: Gastric lavage initially
Mechanical ventilation in the event of respiratory paralysis
Suction of secretions
Intubation or tracheostomy
Nasogastric feedings
IV fluid and electrolytes
Must be reported to local health authority immediately
All patient contacts known to have eaten the same food should have gastric lavage, high enemas, and cathartics, and should be kept under close medical supervision.

For staphylococcal poisoning and enteric infection: Oral fluids if tolerated; IV fluids and electrolytes if needed

References: 3.

1 ASSESS

ASSESSMENT	OBSERVATIONS		
	STAPHYLOCOCCAL FOOD POISONING	BOTULISM	ENTERIC INFECTIONS
History	May have eaten within past 7 h at a picnic or large gathering where food has been sitting unrefrigerated	Consumption of home-canned food within past 36 h	Ingestion within past 24 h of high-risk food (e.g., raw seafood or cooked meat dishes held at room temperature)
Subjective symptoms	Weakness; prostration	Vertigo and neurologic symptoms	Nausea and abdominal pain
Gastrointestinal	Acute-onset nausea, vomiting, intestinal cramps, and diarrhea	Vomiting, diarrhea, and constipation	Acute-onset nausea, abdominal cramping, and diarrhea in *C. perfringens* infections. Diarrhea may be watery and bloody and persist up to 7 days in *V. parahaemolyticus* infections. Acute-onset nausea and vomiting or colic and diarrhea in *B. cereus* infections
Vital signs	Subnormal temperature; hypotension	Normal	Usually normal
Head and neck		Abrupt onset, bilateral and symmetric: ptosis, blurred vision, diplopia, dry mouth, dysphagia, dysphonia, dysarthria, and nasal regurgitation	
Respiratory		Paralysis of muscles of respiration	
Large muscles		Symmetric flaccid paralysis; motor disturbances but no sensory disturbances	

2 DIAGNOSE

NURSING DIAGNOSIS	SUPPORTIVE ASSESSMENT FINDINGS
Fluid volume deficit related to vomiting and diarrhea	Vomiting; diarrhea; weakness and prostration; nausea
Diarrhea related to pathogens and their toxins in the intestinal tract	Persistent watery stools

NURSING DIAGNOSIS	SUPPORTIVE ASSESSMENT FINDINGS
Diagnoses specific to botulism:	
Ineffective airway clearance related to neurologic effects of botulinal toxin	Dry mouth
Impaired swallowing related to neurologic effects of toxin	Dysphagia; nasal regurgitation
Ineffective breathing pattern related to neurologic effects of toxin	Paralysis of muscles of respiration; cyanosis
Impaired physical mobility related to neurologic effects of toxin	Symmetric flaccid paralysis
Sensory/perceptual alteration (visual) related to neurologic effects of toxin	Abrupt onset, bilateral and symmetric: ptosis, blurred vision, diplopia
Impaired verbal communication related to neurologic effects of toxin	Dysarthria, dysphonia

3 PLAN

Patient goals

1. Patient's fluid and electrolyte balance will be maintained.
2. Patient will return to normal pattern of bowel elimination.
3. Patient will have information to prevent further episodes of food poisoning.

Patient goals specific for botulism in addition to the above:

4. Patient's airway will be patent, and aspiration of secretions will be avoided.
5. Patient will maintain adequate fluid and nutrition intake while swallowing is impaired; oral intake will improve during convalescence.
6. Patient will demonstrate normal respiratory pattern, oxygen intake, and blood gasses.
7. Patient will maintain function, comfort, and skin integrity while immobile and will demonstrate increasing strength and movement during convalescence.
8. Patient will not be confused or frightened by environmental stimuli during time of alteration in vision; visual function will return to normal.
9. Patient will communicate needs; speech will return to normal.

4 IMPLEMENT

NURSING DIAGNOSIS	NURSING INTERVENTIONS	RATIONALE
Fluid volume deficit related to vomiting and diarrhea	Monitor fluid and electrolyte balance, intake and output, urine specific gravity, moisture of skin and mucous membranes, skin turgor, frequency of vomiting and diarrhea, vital signs, and weight loss.	Fluids, sodium, and potassium lost through diarrhea and vomiting must be replaced.
	Encourage small amounts of oral fluids as tolerated. Administer IV fluids and electrolytes as prescribed.	To maintain adequate intake and replace those lost in vomitus and diarrhea.

→ → →

NURSING DIAGNOSIS	NURSING INTERVENTIONS	RATIONALE
Diarrhea related to pathogens and toxins in the intestinal tract	Collect fecal specimen (as described in Chapter 3).	Incorrect collection and handling of specimens may destroy the pathogen or contaminate the specimen with environmental organisms, interfering with accurate diagnosis and treatment. Improper handling can also contaminate the health care worker.
	Monitor frequency and characteristics of stool.	To detect complications.
	Provide air circulation and room deodorization.	To eliminate odors.
	Wash hands and lubricate anal opening frequently.	To prevent irritation of skin around anal opening.
For botulism: **Ineffective airway clearance** related to neurologic effects of botulinal toxins	Monitor cough and gag reflexes.	To detect and report loss of patency of airway.
	Suction secretions.	To prevent aspiration.
	Have tracheostomy tray available for emergency use. Provide tracheostomy care.	To maintain patent airway.
Impaired swallowing related to neurologic effects of toxins	Assess ability to swallow.	To prevent aspiration of oral fluids or food.
	Administer nasogastric tube feeding or alimentation as prescribed; offer frequent, small oral feedings as patient tolerates.	To maintain adequate intake.
Ineffective breathing pattern related to neurologic effects of toxins	Monitor for signs of respiratory paralysis and oxygen insufficiency; initiate mechanical ventilation and oxygen as prescribed.	To assist breathing; to ensure adequate oxygen intake.
	Monitor patient on respirator for signs of hyperventilation or hypoventilation.	To prevent or detect early signs of respiratory acidosis or alkalosis.
Impaired physical mobility related to neurologic effects of toxins	Position in proper body alignment.	To prevent contractures and foot drop.
	Assist with range of motion exercises.	To prevent joint stiffness.
	Turn q 2 h.	To prevent skin pressure sores and pooling of secretions.
	Provide total hygienic care as needed.	To prevent skin breakdown.
Sensory/perceptual alterations (visual) related to neurologic effects of toxins	Interpret environment and stimuli for patient whose vision is altered.	To minimize injury.
	Explain that condition is not permanent.	To relieve fear associated with vision changes.
	Minimize stimuli.	To prevent confusion.

NURSING DIAGNOSIS	NURSING INTERVENTIONS	RATIONALE
Impaired verbal communication related to neurologic effects of toxins	Anticipate patient's needs and provide necessary care. Explain that loss of speech is not permanent.	To relieve anxiety of patient who cannot communicate.
Knowledge deficit	See Patient Teaching and Patient Teaching Guide on Food Safety, page 299.	

5 EVALUATE

PATIENT OUTCOME	DATA INDICATING THAT OUTCOME IS REACHED
Fluid and electrolyte balance is maintained.	Skin turgor is good. Urine output equals intake. Urine specific gravity is normal. Measurements of sodium, potassium, chloride, magnesium, and calcium in blood are normal.
Patient returns to normal pattern of bowel elimination.	Stools are soft, formed, and normal colored. Abdomen is soft; bowel sounds normal. Patient tolerates regular diet. Weight returns to normal. Stool specimens are negative for any pathogen.
Patient has information to prevent further episodes of food poisoning.	Patient discusses proper food-handling practices to prevent contamination of food.
Airway is patent and aspiration of secretions is avoided.	Airway is open. Secretions are thin and easily coughed up by patient. Patient swallows without difficulty. Breathing is quiet.
Adequate fluid and nutrition intake is maintained	Skin turgor is good; secretions are thin. Urine output equals intake. Weight loss is avoided. Energy improves and patient eats regular diet during convalescence.
Patient demonstrates normal respiratory pattern, oxygen intake, and blood gas levels.	Respiratory rate is normal. Respirations are of normal depth. There is no dyspnea. Skin and mucous membranes are warm and moist with normal color. O_2 saturation, CO_2, P_{O_2} and P_{CO_2} are normal.
Patient maintains function, comfort, and skin integrity and demonstrates increasing strength and movement.	Patient moves extremities and changes position in bed. During convalescence, patient sits, stands, and walks without signs of contractures, foot drop, or pain.
Patient is not confused or frightened by environmental stimuli; visual function returns to normal.	There are no startle responses to environmental stimuli. During convalescence, the patient correctly identifies letters on a Snellen eye chart from a distance of 20 ft. Pupils are normal and reactive.
Patient communicates needs; speech returns to normal.	Health care workers and visitors respond to patient's nonverbal cues. Patient speaks audibly during convalescence.

PATIENT TEACHING

Provide patient with the following instructions:

1. These conditions are transmitted by contaminated food and can be prevented by proper food handling.
2. Cooked foods should not be held at room temperature; they should be kept hot (140° F) or should be refrigerated. Reheating should be done rapidly and completely.
3. All seafood should be cooked at a temperature above 60° C (140° F) for 15 minutes.
4. Keep all seafood, raw or cooked, adequately refrigerated before eating.
5. Handle cooked seafood to avoid its contamination with raw seafood or with contaminated seawater.
6. All persons should wash hands thoroughly following defecation and before handling food.
7. Destroy all canned food and containers from same batch that contained the *C. botulinum* by burying deep in soil or boiling 3 minutes before discarding. Commercial canned foods should be submitted for laboratory examination. Contaminated cooking utensils should be sterilized by boiling for 3 minutes before reuse.

8. No questionable canned food should ever be tasted. Foods containing *C. botulinum* do not necessarily have "off" odors or a spoiled taste.
9. Recommended processing times and temperatures for home canning must be followed to ensure killing of all *C. botulinum* spores. This information is available through state agricultural extension services.
10. Home-canned vegetables and meats should be boiled for 3 minutes to destroy botulinal toxin.
11. Honey must not be given to infants under 1 year of age.
12. Fluids should be encouraged and food may be eaten when tolerated.
13. Report the following symptoms of complication to a physician: vomiting and diarrhea persisting beyond 1 to 2 days; alteration in consciousness; loss of skin turgor, particularly in infants and children; fever; absence of urination; and severe prostration.
14. Explain that food poisonings are self-limiting.

Acute Bacterial and Viral Gastroenteritis

Many forms of **acute gastroenteritis** are caused by ingestion of food and water contaminated with pathogenic agents or by fecal-oral transmission directly or indirectly from an infected person. These infections differ from the food poisonings previously discussed in the following ways:

- The pathogenic agents causing these diseases invade, colonize, and multiply in the human intestinal tract.
- The incubation periods are slightly longer, ranging from 1 day to several weeks.
- Direct and indirect fecal-oral transmission is possible.
- Acquired immunity of varying duration results from many of these infections.

In addition, the predominant manifestation of these diseases is acute-onset diarrhea of varying intensity and duration. The bacterial- and viral-caused gastroenteri-

tises are usually self-limited diseases (Table 5-2).

Campylobacter **enteritis** is an acute bacterial enteric infection lasting from 1 to 10 days and is considered to be an important cause of "traveler's diarrhea."

Escherichia coli diarrhea is another cause of "traveler's diarrhea." Three types of pathogenic *E. coli* are capable of producing a self-limited enteritis of varying intensity.

Shigellosis (bacillary dysentery) is an acute bacterial infection of the large intestine, with severity ranging from asymptomatic infection to fulminating diarrheal disease and death.

Epidemic viral gastroenteritis is usually a self-limited, mild gastric and intestinal infection lasting 24 to 48 hours. Disease often occurs in outbreaks.

Rotavirus gastroenteritis is a sporadically occurring gastric and intestinal infection of infants and young children ranging in severity from asymptomatic to severe disease and occasionally to death.

Table 5-2

OVERVIEW OF ACUTE BACTERIAL AND VIRAL GASTROENTERITIS

	Campylobacter enteritis (traveler's diarrhea)	*E. coli* diarrhea (traveler's diarrhea)	Shigellosis (Bacillary dysentery)	Epidemic viral gastroenteritis	Rotavirus gastroenteritis
Occurrence	Worldwide; common-source outbreaks occur; highest in warmer months	Worldwide; common-source outbreaks occur; high in areas of poor sanitation and during warm months	Worldwide; highest in children under 10 yrs old; outbreaks common in crowded living conditions, day care	Worldwide and common; epidemics and outbreaks occur; affects infants and adults	Worldwide; sporadic and in outbreaks; highest in infants and young children
Etiologic agent	*Campylobacter jejuni* and *C. coli*	Enterotoxigenic, invasive, or enteropathogenic strains of *E. coli*	Four different groups of *Shigella* bacteria, with many strains	Many viruses; Norwalk virus most common	Many types of rotaviruses
Reservoir	Domestic and wild animals and birds	Humans, who are often asymptomatic; cattle	Humans	Humans	Humans; pathogenicity of animal viruses undetermined
Transmission	Ingestion of water, food, or raw milk contaminated with organism from feces; contact with infected animals or infants; fecal-oral	Fecal contamination of food, water, baby formula, or fomites; transmitted to infant during delivery; fecal-oral, by hand	Direct or indirect fecal-oral transmission from infected person or carrier, usually by hand	Fecal-oral route; food-borne and water-borne transmission	Fecal-oral; possibly fecal-respiratory
Incubation period	3-5 days; range: 1-10 days	10-72 h	12-96 h	Usually 24-48 h; range: 10-50 h	24-72 h
Period of communicability	Several days to weeks throughout course of infection; usually 2-7 wks; carriers are rare	Duration of fecal excretion of organism, possibly weeks	During acute infection to 4 wks after illness; carrier state may persist for months	During acute stage and up to 48 h after diarrhea stops	During acute stage and as long as virus is shed (up to 30 days)
Susceptibility and resistance	General	Infants very susceptible; travelers to developing countries; duration of acquired immunity unknown	General; more severe in children and elderly and debilitated individuals; strain-specific antibodies develop	General; short-term (14 wks) immunity may follow infection with specific serotypes	By age 3 yrs most individuals have acquired antibodies against most serotypes
Report to local health authority	Report cases	Report epidemic only	Report cases	Report epidemic only	Report epidemic only

Data from Benenson.[3]

PATHOPHYSIOLOGY

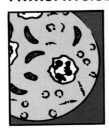

Bacterial and viral agents that produce gastroenteritis produce pathologic conditions in one of three ways:

- Toxigenic agents, such as some *Shigella* stains and enterotoxigenic *E. coli*, release an enterotoxin that acts on the small intestine to produce a local inflammation and a secretory diarrhea with rapid loss of electrolytes.
- Invasive pathogens, such as *Shigella*, *Campylobacter*, and invasive strains of *E. coli*, penetrate the small or large intestine, producing cellular destruction, necrosis, and potential ulceration. The diarrheal stools in these conditions frequently contain leukocytes and erythrocytes.
- Some pathogens, such as the rotaviruses, attach to the mucosal epithelium without invasion. They destroy cells of the intestinal villi, resulting in malabsorption of electrolytes and the potential for electrolyte imbalance.

Fluid and electrolyte loss in other forms of gastroenteritis may develop more gradually or may not occur at all. Infants, small children, and debilitated individuals are at greater risk for severe dehydration.

The attachment of the pathogens to the mucosa may be altered by nonspecific resistance factors in the host:

- The normal bacterial flora of the intestinal tract prevents attachment by competing for attachment sites or by production of volatile organic acids. If the normal flora is diminished as a result of antibiotic therapy or malnutrition, this host defense is ineffective.
- The pH of the gastrointestinal tract impedes the growth of some microbes. Altering the pH through the ingestion of antacids reduces the effectiveness of this defense.
- Normal gastrointestinal motility purges the intestinal tract of many pathogens, and interference with this function increases the risk for invasion of pathogens.
- Specific immune responses of varying duration occur in the host following infection with *Shigella*, parovirus-like agents, rotavirus, and *E. coli*.

COMPLICATIONS

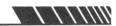

Dehydration
Electrolyte imbalance
Circulatory failure and death

MEDICAL MANAGEMENT

DRUG THERAPY

Agents that suppress intestinal motility are not given for bacterial gastroenteritis.

Antiinfective agents for shigellosis: Trimethoprim-sulfamethoxazole (Septra, Bactrim), 1 tablet (80 mg trimethoprim and 400 mg sulfamethoxazole) q 12 h for 5 days.

Antiinfective agents for prevention of *E. coli* diarrhea: Trimethoprim-sulfamethoxazole, 160 mg of TMP to 800 mg of SMX/day, or doxycycline (100 mg/day) PO for 2 wks before travel to a high-risk area.

GENERAL MANAGEMENT

IV fluids and electrolyte replacement:
For shock: rapid infusion of 20 to 30 ml/kg of Ringer's lactate, isotonic saline, or similar isotonic solution given within 1 hr.
For complete rehydration after circulation is restored: glucose electrolyte solution (oral or IV hypotonic electrolyte solutions in amounts equal to estimated fluid loss).

References: 3, 102.

DIAGNOSTIC STUDIES AND FINDINGS

Diagnostic Test	Findings

The diagnosis of these conditions relies on identification of the pathogen in a specimen of feces and by a fourfold or greater rise in serum antibody titer between acute disease and convalescence.

Campylobacter

Direct examination of stool with phase-contrast microscopy	Positive for leukocytes and erythrocytes and *C. jejuni*
Serology immunoflourescence or agglutination tests	Fourfold increase in antibody titer

***E. coli* diarrhea**

Stool culture	Positive for enterotoxigenic or invasive strains of *E. coli*
Serology	Fourfold increase in antitoxic antibodies

Shigellosis

Examination of stool specimen	Pus cells in specimen
Fecal culture	Positive for *Shigella*

Epidemic viral gastroenteritis

Immune electron microscopy or radioimmunoassay of feces specimen	Positive for virus
Serologic tests using immune electron microscopy, immune adherence hemagglutination assay, or radioimmunoassay	Fourfold or greater increase in antibody titer

Rotavirus gastroenteritis

Electron microscopy or immunologic examination of feces or rectal swabs	Positive for rotavirus (10^6/g of feces)
Serology: complement fixation, ELISA, or immunoflourescent techniques	Fourfold increase in antibody titer; 80%-90% of children have detectable antibodies by 3 yrs

1 ASSESS

ASSESSMENT	OBSERVATIONS				
History	Travel to another country; ingestion of questionable food or water during past wk; eating food contaminated by person with diarrheal disease during past wk				
Subjective	Myalgia, headache, malaise, prostration				
Fluids and electrolytes	Anytime during disease: poor skin turgor, dry mucous membranes, faint pulse, hypotension	Anytime during disease: poor skin turgor, dry mucous membranes, faint pulse, hypotension	Days 2-5: loss of turgor, oliguria, hypotension, weak pulse, shock	Usually no alteration in fluid balance	Days 2-8: severe dehydration possible
Body temperature	38°-41° C (100°-105° F); febrile convulsions	Low-grade fever on day 1 or 2	Days 1-5: 38°-41° C (101° to 105° F)	Low-grade fever	Day 1: usually low-grade fever (up to 39° C [102° F])

→ > >

ASSESSMENT	OBSERVATIONS				
	Campylobacter	*E. coli* diarrhea	Shigellosis	Epidemic viral gastroenteritis	Rotavirus gastroenteritis
Gastrointestinal	Days 1 and 2: nausea, vomiting, abdominal pain Days 2-4 (maybe 10): foul-smelling or liquid diarrhea; sometimes 20-30 stools/day; blood in stools after day 4 Day 7: ulcerative colitis may occur	Day 1: vomiting Day 2 (lasting 7-10 days); mucous and bloody diarrhea or profuse watery diarrhea without blood or mucus	Day 1: nausea, abdominal pain, colic, vomiting, painful diarrhea Days 2-5: stools contain blood, pus, and mucus; rectal irritation and tenesmus	Day 1 (lasts 24-48 h): nausea, vomiting, diarrhea, abdominal pain	Day 1: vomiting for 48 hrs Days 2-8: watery diarrhea; rectal bleeding may occur
Respiratory					Anytime during disease: pharyngeal exudate, cough, and rhinitis may be present

2 | DIAGNOSE

NURSING DIAGNOSIS	SUPPORTIVE ASSESSMENT FINDINGS
Potential fluid volume deficit related to vomiting and diarrhea	Nausea; vomiting on day 1 for all these infections Diarrhea lasting 2-8 days Anytime during disease: poor skin turgor, dry mucous membranes, faint pulse, hypotension Days 2-5: loss of turgor, oliguria, hypertension, weak pulse, shock
Diarrhea related to pathogenic activity in GI tract	Frequent liquid stools lasting 1-10 days (see Assessment); colic
Hyperthermia related to infection	Fever; headache, malaise
Potential for infection (patient contacts) related to presence of pathogen in stool	Stool culture positive for pathogen Serologic evidence of recent antibody response History of exposure to contaminated food and water or infected persons

3 | PLAN

Patient goals

1. Fluid and electrolyte balance will be maintained.
2. Patient will return to normal pattern of bowel elimination.
3. Patient's body temperature will be maintained within the normal range; comfort and safety will be maintained for patients experiencing fever.
4. Patient's infection will not be transmitted to contacts.
5. Patient will have information to prevent further episodes of gastroenteritis caused by *Campylobacter, E. coli, Shigella,* and viruses.

4   IMPLEMENT

NURSING DIAGNOSIS	NURSING INTERVENTIONS	RATIONALE
Potential fluid volume deficit related to vomiting and diarrhea	Monitor for symptoms of dehydration and electrolyte imbalance (e.g., oliguria and loss of skin turgor).	To detect early signs of dehydration for early intervention.
	Measure all fluid output (emesis, urine, and diarrhea); measure all intake.	To determine if intake compensates for output.
	Monitor blood pressure, temperature, pulse, and respirations.	To detect symptoms of circulatory collapse early.
	Administer liquids frequently as tolerated.	To maintain adequate intake.
	Administer electrolytes as prescribed.	To replace those lost during diarrhea.
	Provide oral glucose electrolyte solution as soon as patient can take oral fluids.	Oral fluids can usually be tolerated once electrolyte balance is corrected.
	Gradually add clear fluids and soft foods (milk and cream products should be avoided at first; apple juice and white soda [7-Up] are usually well-tolerated).	Clear carbohydrates (fluids and foods) are easier to tolerate with nausea.
Diarrhea related to pathogenic activity in GI tract	Obtain stool specimens for culture.	To identify pathogen.
	Measure watery diarrhea output.	To estimate rapidity of fluid loss.
	Cleanse perianal area and lubricate after each diarrheal stool.	To prevent irritation of skin.
	Provide adequate air circulation, room de-	To control odors and prevent embarrass-
Hyperthermia related to infection	(See inside back cover, interventions 1-15).	
Potential for infection (patient contacts) related to presence of pathogen in stool	Collect fecal specimen (as described in Chapter 3).	Incorrect collection and handling of specimens may destroy the pathogen or contaminate the specimen with environmental organisms, interfering with accurate diagnosis and treatment. Improper handling of specimens can also contaminate the health care worker.
	Use enteric precautions until 3 fecal cultures are negative for infecting *Shigella* organism; use enteric precautions for duration of illness for others.	To prevent transmission to health care workers, other patients, and patient contacts.
	Report **Shigellosis** to local health authority.	Required by law for public health monitoring and control of outbreaks.
Knowledge deficit	See Patient Teaching and Patient Teaching Guide, page 299.	

➜ ❯ ❯

5　EVALUATE

PATIENT OUTCOME	DATA INDICATING THAT OUTCOME IS REACHED
Fluid and electrolyte balance is maintained	Blood pressure and pulse are normal. Skin turgor is good. Mucous membranes are moist. Urine output is equal to intake. Blood levels of sodium, potassium, chloride, magnesium, and calcium are normal. Urine specific gravity is normal. Secretions are thin.
Patient returns to normal pattern of bowel elimination	Stools are soft, formed, and brown colored. Abdomen is not distended. There is no cramping.
Body temperature is within normal range; comfort and safety are maintained	See inside back cover.
Infection is not transmitted to patient's contacts	Patient care staff members wash hands after providing care to each patient and follow universal blood and body secretion procedures with all patients. Appropriate isolation procedures are implemented soon after infection is confirmed.
Patient has information to prevent further episodes of food-borne gastroenteritis	Patient or family describes transmission of the pathogen. Patient or family demonstrates proper procedures for handling infective materials and proper handwashing and other behaviors necessary to prevent transmission.

PATIENT TEACHING ▪

Provide patient with the following instructions:

1. These conditions are transmitted by food or water contaminated with organisms from feces of infected person.
2. They are communicable while the organisms are in the feces (usually from onset of diarrhea until up to 7 weeks).
3. Disease onset is between 1 to 7 days from exposure to the infection (see Overview, page 74 for specifics for each disease).
4. Transmission of the infection to others can be prevented by thorough handwashing before eating and after bowel movements, changing diapers, or handling feces.
5. For patients cared for at home, teach the family:

   ▪ Signs of dehydration and the importance of prompt medical attention should dehydration occur.

   ▪ Measurement of intake and measurement or estimation of output.
   ▪ Maintenance of oral fluid intake equal to output.
   ▪ Types of clear, high-glucose oral fluids that may be tolerated (apple juice; mildly carbonated beverages, such as 7-Up).
   ▪ Scrupulous handwashing; avoidance of food contamination.

6. Persons with *Shigella* infections should not be permitted to handle food or provide child care until two successive fecal samples or rectal swabs are free of *Shigella* organisms.
7. Child day-care programs should provide for:

   ▪ Frequent handwashing of workers.
   ▪ Separate areas for food preparation and diaper changing.
   ▪ Separate rooms for children of different age groups.

- Routine exclusion of children with diarrhea.

8. Most acute gastroenteritis can be prevented by:

  - Thorough handwashing after toileting, handling feces, or contact with animals.
  - Thorough cooking of all food derived from animals, and avoidance of recontamination within the kitchen after cooking.
  - Using pasteurized milk and chlorinated water.
  - Maintaining food at hot or cold temperatures.

9. Report the following symptoms of complications to physician:

  - Dry mucous membranes, loss of skin turgor, listlessness or change in level of consciousness, or absence of urination.
  - Continuation of diarrhea or blood in urine.
  - Increase in colic or pain.
  - Increase in fever or convulsions.

Acute and Chronic Parasitic Enteritis

Parasitic enteritis is similar to the bacterial and viral forms of gastroenteritis; however, these infections may become chronic (Table 5-3).

Amebiasis (amebic dysentery) is an infection with an ameba. This parasite may form a commensal relationship with the host or invade the intestinal mucosa, producing an enteritis ranging from asymptomatic to fulminating diarrheal and systemic disease. The parasite may persist in the host for years.

Giardiasis is a protozoan infection of the upper intestinal tract ranging in severity from asymptomatic infection to chronic damage to the duodenal and jejunal mucosa resulting in a malabsorption syndrome.

PATHOPHYSIOLOGY
Amebiasis

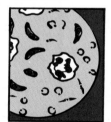

Ingested cysts of *Entamoeba* develop into trophozoites that penetrate the mucosa and submucosa of the large intestine by mechanical and proteolytic activity. Edema, fibrin formation, and necrosis occur, creating necrotic lesions that may extend laterally in the submucosa, giving a flasklike appearance. These discrete lesions appear primarily in the cecal area, sigmoid colon, and rec-

Table 5-3

OVERVIEW OF ACUTE AND CHRONIC PARASITIC ENTERITIS

	Amebiasis	Giardiasis
Occurrence	Widespread; higher in areas with poor sanitation, in homosexual communities, and in institutions	Worldwide; more common in children, institutions, and where sanitation is poor
Etiologic agent	*Entamoeba histolytica* (a parasitic ameba)	*Giardia lamblia* (a protozoan)
Reservoir	Humans, usually an asymptomatic carrier	Humans; possibly beaver and other animals
Transmission	Water contaminated with human feces of infected persons; fecal-oral by hand or contaminated food; oral-rectal sexual contact	Ingestion of contaminated water; fecal-oral by hand contamination or by oral-rectal sexual contact; cysts in water are not killed with chlorine
Incubation period	Variable: 3 days to months; usually 2-4 wks	5-25 days; median 7-10 days
Period of communicability	As long as cysts are in feces, probably years	Entire period of infection; could persist for months
Susceptibility and resistance	General, although most people harboring the organism do not develop disease	General; asymptomatic carrier rate is high
Report to local health authority	In some endemic areas	Case report in endemic areas

Data from Benenson.[3]

tum. Hematogenous dissemination may occur to the liver, peritoneum, pleura, lung, pericardium, vagina, cervix, skin, and brain, with microabscesses produced in those tissues. Symptomatic onset may be acute or ill defined, or the infection may be asymptomatic. Untreated persons develop symptoms similar to a chronic persistent colitis.

Giardiasis

Ingested cysts of the *Giardia lamblia* protozoan develop into trophozoites that attach by a powerful ventral sucker to the mucosa of the jejunum and ileum without producing an inflammatory response. Diarrhea and malabsorption are thought to occur as a result of mechanical obstruction in the intestinal mucosa. Trophozoites and cysts are both excreted in the stool of ill individuals. Cysts may continue to be excreted for months in untreated persons. The disease is characterized by acute-onset diarrhea that may progress to a chronic intermittent diarrhea with malabsorption of fats and the fat-soluble vitamins. There is no invasion beyond the bowel lumen.

COMPLICATIONS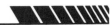

Amebiasis
Perforated bowel
Hemorrhage
Systemic deterioration
Anemia
Extraintestinal disease resulting from abscesses in other organs and tissue
Giardiasis
Chronic diarrhea
Malabsorption

MEDICAL MANAGEMENT

DRUG THERAPY

Amebiasis: treatment regimens depend on the severity of the illness and the location and dissemination of the parasite; some combination of the following amebicides and antibiotics is used; the number of drugs and potency of the drug used increase with the severity of the symptoms.

Antiinfective agents: Emetine hydrochloride, 1 mg/kg IM (not to exceed 65 mg/24 h) for 7-10 days; not to be repeated for 8 wks; dehydroemetine, 1.5 mg/kg (not to exceed 80 mg/24 h); chloroquine (Aralen) (to be used concurrently with one of the above), 0.25 g qid for first day; 0.5 g/24 hrs for next 14 days (adults); metronidazole (Flagyl), 750 mg PO tid for 10 days (adults); diiodohydroxyquin (Diodoquin), 650 mg PO tid for 20 days (adults); diloxanide furoate (Furamide), 0.5 g PO tid for 10 days (adults); tetracycline, 250 mg PO q 6-8 h for 10 days (adults).
Giardiasis

Antiinfective agents:
Quinacrine hydrochloride (Atabrine), 100 mg PO tid for 7 days (adults); furazolidone suspension for children; metronidazole (Flagyl), 250 mg tid for 7 days (is not currently licensed for giardiasis use).

GENERAL MANAGEMENT

Household and sexual contacts should be examined and treated; pregnant women should be treated only if they show significant symptoms and then should not be given metronidazole or dehydroemetine during the first trimester.

SURGERY

Aspiration of abscesses.

References: 3, 88, 155.

DIAGNOSTIC STUDIES AND FINDINGS

Diagnostic Test	Findings
Amebiasis	
Microscopic examination of feces, rectal secretions, aspirates of abscesses, or tissue sections	Positive for trophozoites or cysts of protozoan
Serology: agglutination tests	Increased titer may persist for some time after infection
Liver scan	Detection of abscesses
Giardiasis	
Examination of feces or duodenal contents	Positive for cysts or trophozoites of the *G. lamblia* protozoan

1 ASSESS

ASSESSMENT	OBSERVATIONS
History	Travel within past 4 wks to area where sanitation is poor; drinking untreated water; oral-rectal sexual contact; fecal-oral indirect contact
Gastrointestinal	**Amebiasis** Nondysenteric colitis: recurring episodes of loose stools; vague abdominal pain; tenesmus; hemorrhoids with occasional rectal bleeding; constipation alternating with diarrhea Dysenteric colitis: intense, intermittent, bloody, mucous diarrhea Rigid abdomen symptomatic of appendicitis Enlarged, tender liver (with hepatic abscess) May have ulceration of perianal area
	Giardiasis Acute: explosive, foul-smelling diarrheal stool (frothy appearance with steatorrhea); abdominal cramping and flatulence; nausea (no vomiting) Chronic: intermittent loose stools; increased flatulence and distention; vague abdominal discomfort
Systemic manifestations	Signs of dehydration, anemia, or hemorrhage; may have fever and chills
Respiratory	Expectoration of reddish-brown, odorless pus, suggesting rupture of hepatic abscess to lung

2 DIAGNOSE

NURSING DIAGNOSIS	SUPPORTIVE ASSESSMENT FINDINGS
Potential for infection (patient contacts) related to presence of pathogens in stool	Microscopic examination of feces, rectal secretions, aspirates of abscesses, or tissue secretions; positive for trophozoites or cysts of protozoan

➔ ➢ ➢

NURSING DIAGNOSIS	SUPPORTIVE ASSESSMENT FINDINGS
	Examination of feces or duodenal contents; positive for cysts or tropho-zoites of the *G. lamblia* protozoan Exposure to contaminated food or water; fecal-oral contact (indirect); oral-sexual contact (direct)
Diarrhea related to pathogenic activity in colon	Amebiasis—recurring episodes of loose stools Giardiasis—acute: explosive, foul-smelling diarrheal stool; chronic: inter-mittent loose stools
Potential fluid volume deficit related to diarrhea	Diarrhea; signs of dehydration
Potential for poisoning related to chemotherapeutic agent	Patient is perscribed an amebicide, which is extremely toxic

3 PLAN

Patient goals

1. Patient will be free of infection and complications of amebiasis or giardiasis. Infection is not transmitted to patient's contacts.
2. Patient will return to normal pattern of bowel elimina-tion.
3. Fluid and electrolyte balance will be maintained.
4. Patient will take antiinfective agents as prescribed.
5. Patient will have information to prevent further epi-sodes of infection.

4 IMPLEMENT

NURSING DIAGNOSIS	NURSING INTERVENTIONS	RATIONALE
Potential for infec-tion related to pres-ence of pathogens in stool	Obtain stool specimen for examination. (Specimen obtained within 3 days of a barium enema or of a soapsuds, oil, hy-pertonic, or water enema cannot be ex-amined.)	Specific pathogen must be identified for effective treatment. (Specimen must be collected properly to identify the patho-gen.)
	Employ enteric precautions for duration of the infection.	To prevent transmission of the pathogen.
	Assess patient or family's understanding of the transmission of the infection. Provide information necessary so that contacts can be adequately examined and treated.	Patient contacts must be treated or they will reinfect the patient.
	Instruct patient or family how to handle in-fective secretions, excretions or exudates, proper handwashing, and safe sexual practices.	To prevent contamination of the environ-ment or transmission to others.
Diarrhea related to pathogenic activity in colon	Monitor frequency and characteristics of stool. Observe stool for signs of bleeding.	To detect symptoms of perforation, ob-struction, or liver disease.
	Cleanse perianal area and lubricate after each diarrheal stool.	To prevent irritation of the skin.

NURSING DIAGNOSIS	NURSING INTERVENTIONS	RATIONALE
	Provide adequate air circulation and room deodorization.	To remove odors.
Potential fluid volume deficit related to diarrhea	Monitor for signs of dehydration.	To replace fluids.
	Encourage oral fluids as tolerated. Administer IV line as prescribed.	To prevent dehydration. To replace fluids.
	Provide patient with oral glucose electrolyte solution as soon as patient can take oral fluids.	Oral fluids can usually be tolerated once electrolyte imbalance is corrected.
	Gradually add clear fluids and soft foods (milk and cream products should be avoided at first; apple juice and 7-Up are usually well-tolerated).	Clear carbohydrates (fluids and food) are easier to digest.
Potential for poisoning related to chemotherapeutic agent	Administer amebicide therapy as prescribed.	Amebicides are extremely toxic.
	Monitor for symptoms of toxicity to GI, cardiovascular, muscular, and neurologic systems.	To provide supportive management and to be prepared to intervene if complications occur.
	Enforce restricted activities during amebicide therapy.	To decrease additional metabolic demands.
Knowledge deficit	See Patient Teaching and Patient Teaching Guide: Food Safety, page 299.	

5 EVALUATE

PATIENT OUTCOME	DATA INDICATING THAT OUTCOME IS REACHED
Patient is free of infection and complications of amebiasis or giardiasis.	Stool culture is negative for protozoan cysts. There are no signs of hepatic abscesses. There are no skin, vaginal, or lung abscesses or drainage. Body temperature is normal. Weight and energy level are now normal. WBC is normal.
Infection is not transmitted to patient's contacts.	Enteric isolation procedures are implemented soon after infection is confirmed. Reportable infections are reported to the local health department. Patient contacts have been examined and treated for infection. Patient or family demonstrates proper handwashing and other behaviors necessary to prevent transmission.
Patient returns to normal pattern of bowel elimination.	Stools are soft, formed, and normal colored. Abdomen is soft and nontender. Liver is normal sized. Bowel sounds are normal.
Fluid and electrolyte balance is maintained.	Skin turgor is good. Mucous membranes are moist. Urine output is normal. Secretions are thin. Blood levels of sodium, potassium, chloride, magnesium, and calcium are normal. Urine specific gravity is normal (1.01-1.025).

→ > >

PATIENT OUTCOME	DATA INDICATING THAT OUTCOME IS REACHED
Patient self-administers antiinfective agents as prescribed.	Patient completes full course of antiinfective therapy. No preventable drug interactions or allergic reactions are experienced. If untoward reactions are experienced, the patient discontinues the drug and contacts the physician immediately.
Knowledge deficit resolved.	Patient discusses measures to avoid reinfection.

PATIENT TEACHING

1. Instruct patients taking amebicides on the medication name; purpose; correct dose, time, and route of administration; length of time the medication is to be taken; behaviors to avoid while taking the medication; medication side effects; and untoward reactions and responses to report to physician. Write all responses for patient. Assess patient or family's understanding of the information and ability to administer medication as prescribed.
2. Patients taking amebicides should restrict their activity during treatment.
3. Patients taking metronidazole (Flagyl) should abstain from alcohol during treatment.
4. Relapses after treatment for amebiasis and giardiasis are common. Patient should be monitored by a physician at 6 weeks and 6 months.
5. Cyst passers must wash their hands thoroughly after defecating to prevent recontamination or transmission to others.
6. Travelers to areas where the water supply is not chemically treated or protected from sewage contamination should boil all water used in cooking, drinking, or making ice.
7. Backpackers should be prepared to boil water obtained from streams. Adding chlorine to drinking water may not be protective.
8. Instruct patient and sexual contacts on safe sex.
9. Household and sexual contacts should seek medical examination and treatment.
10. Protect food supplies from fly contamination.

Water-borne and Food-borne *Salmonella* Infections

Salmonella bacteria multiply in food and water contaminated with feces from an infected person, carrier, or, in the case of salmonellosis, an animal. Person-to-person transmission is least common. Once ingested, the organisms invade and multiply in the gastrointestinal mucosa, producing systemic and enteric pathologic findings and symptoms.

Three disease processes are identified based on the type of *Salmonella* ingested (Table 5-4). Any one of four overlapping clinical entities are possible, depending on the type of *Salmonella* ingested and on host defenses. They are acute gastroenteritis, enteric fever, septicemia with or without localized infection, and asymptomatic carrier state.

Salmonellosis is manifested by an acute gastroenteritis and sometimes a septicemia. It is frequently classified as a food poisoning because of the short incubation period following ingestion of food contaminated with *Salmonella*. The greater the number of organisms present in the food, the shorter the incubation period.

Paratyphoid fever is an acute systemic infection manifested by an enteric fever generally of less severity than typhoid fever. Mild and asymptomatic infections occur.

Typhoid fever is an acute enteric fever manifested by a sustained bacteremia, reticuloendothelial involvement, and microabscess formation and ulceration of the distal ileum. Gastrointestinal symptoms generally follow the systemic manifestations. Mild and asymptomatic infections occur. Acute typhoid is less common than other *Salmonella* infection.

Table 5-4

OVERVIEW OF WATER-BORNE AND FOOD-BORNE *SALMONELLA* INFECTIONS

	Salmonellosis	**Paratyphoid fever**	**Typhoid fever**
Occurrence	Worldwide; frequently classi-fied as a food poisoning; small outbreaks in institu-tions; 2 million cases per year in the United States; increasing	Worldwide; sporadic cases and small outbreaks	Worldwide; rare; sporadic cases occur in the United States; usually associated with unsanitary conditions
Etiologic agent	2,000 serotypes of *Salmonella,* a bacterium	*Salmonella paratyphi* with many serotypes	96 types of *Salmonella typhi* (the typhoid bacillus)
Reservoir	Humans and domestic and wild animals	Humans	Humans; carriers are common
Transmission	Ingestion of food contami-nated with feces from an in-fected person or animal; ingestion of meat and animal products (commonly chickens and chicken eggs); handling infected animals; fecal-oral contact	Ingestion of food, particularly milk, and water contami-nated with feces or urine from an infected person or carrier; direct or indirect contact with urine or feces	Ingestion of food or water contaminated with feces or urine from infected person or carrier; sewage-contaminated shellfish; food contaminated with feces carried by flies
Incubation period	6-72 h; usually 12-36 h	1-10 days	1-3 wks
Period of communicability	Throughout infection; days to weeks; temporary carrier state may continue up to 1 yr	As long as bacilli are in ex-creta; weeks to months; com-monly 1-2 wks after recovery	As long as bacilli are in ex-creta; first week to 3 months; 2%-5% of cases become per-manent carriers
Susceptibility and resistance	General; increased risk for those with achlorhydria, ant-acid therapy, gastrointestinal surgery, and immunosup-pression	General; some immunity fol-lows infection	General; increased risk with gastric achlorhydria; suscepti-bility usually declines with age; lifelong immunity some-times follows infection as long as antibiotic therapy was not used
Report to local health author-ity	Mandatory case report	Mandatory case report	Mandatory case report

Data from Benenson.[3]

PATHOPHYSIOLOGY

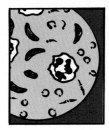

Salmonella organisms ingested in contaminated food or water invade and multiply in deep mucosal layers of the stomach and small intestine, lodging in the lamina propria. An in-flammatory response in the tissue with many polymorphonuclear leu-kocytes produces a gastroenteritis if the *Salmonella* is not S. *typhi* or S. *paratyphi*. The me-senteric lymph nodes become edematous, and the Pey-er's patches show edema and superficial ulceration. The disease may be contained here, or the organism may in-vade beyond the lymph system and be disseminated into the vascular circulation, producing a septicemia or lesions in other organs.

S. *typhi* and S. *paratyphi* stimulate a mononuclear leukocyte reaction in the lamina propria, facilitating early hematogenous dissemination of the organisms. Disease is manifest as an enteric fever. Invasion of other organs results in lesion formation, with disease manifestations dependent on the organ involved. En-docarditis, meningitis, pneumonia, pyelonephritis, os-teomyelitis, cholecystitis, and hepatitis may result from the invasion of any type of *Salmonella.*

Complications of gastroenteritis may include intesti-nal perforation and hemorrhage. Secondary infections, such as otitis media, pneumonia, skin infections, and septicemia, sometimes occur with all types of *Salmo-nella.*

Several nonspecific host defenses affect the type and severity of clinical disease produced by *Salmonella.*

Gastric acidity impedes *Salmonella* growth, and persons with hypochlorhydria or achlorhydria or who have had gastric surgery are more susceptible to infection. Normal intestinal peristalsis, intact mucous membranes, and the normal intestinal flora all act to prevent invasion. Anything interfering with these defenses increases the risk for more severe infection.

Cellular and humoral immunity appears also to interfere with invasion of *Salmonella*, and persons with an impaired immune system are more susceptible to systemic disease with *Salmonella*. In addition, systemic focal lesions most commonly appear in those tissues that are damaged or devitalized or in those persons with altered immune systems.

About 2% of acute cases of typhoid fever result in the chronic carrier state (excreting *S. typhi* for 12 months or longer following infection). Subclinical infections or other *Salmonella* disease may also result in the chronic carrier state. Relapse is common in treated and untreated typhoid and paratyphoid fevers.

COMPLICATIONS

Endocarditis
Meningitis
Pneumonia
Pyelonephritis
Osteomyelitis
Cholecystitis
Hepatitis
Intestinal perforation and hemorrhage
Septicemia

DIAGNOSTIC STUDIES AND FINDINGS

Diagnostic Test	Findings
Culture of feces	Positive for *Salmonella* during first week
Culture of feces and/or urine	Positive for *S. typhi* or *S. paratyphi* during second week
Culture of blood	Positive for *S. typhi* or *S. paratyphi* during first week
Serology: Widal's agglutination test	Not specific for *Salmonella* organisms and not used for salmonellosis
	Increase in antibody titer to the O antigen after 10 days-2 wks
	Titer greater than or equal to 1:160 or fourfold increase to 1:640 by 4 wks is presumptive
	Initial high antibodies to H antigen suggests past infection
	Gradual increase during acute disease suggests concurrent infection
WBC count	Salmonellosis: 10,000 to 15,000 WBC/mm³
	Typhoid and paratyphoid: leukopenia
	Typhoid: anemia; 50,000 platelets/mm³

MEDICAL MANAGEMENT[3,51,100,117,131]

DRUG THERAPY

Antiinfective agents:* Chloramphenicol (Chloromycetin), 100 mg/kg/day in four divided doses IV or PO until defervescence; then 50 mg/kg/day until a total 14-day course has been completed; ampicillin, 1-2 g IV qid for 2 wks (adults), ampicillin, 8 g/day PO in divided doses for 6 wks for carrier state; trimethoprim-sulfamethoxazole (for organisms resistant to above drugs); corticosteroids—prednisone, 40-50 mg/day for 3 days (adults). Large prolonged doses of ampicillin and surgical removal of gallbladder, if it is the site for focal infection, for treatment of carriers.

Typhoid vaccine given in a primary series of two subcutaneous 0.5 ml injections, 4 wks apart, with boosters in 3 yrs; or 4 capsules taken orally on alternate days; recommended only for those living in or traveling to areas of high endemicity; confers only partial immunity

GENERAL MANAGEMENT

IV fluids and electrolytes
Bed rest
Hyperalimentation
Treatment of complications, such as perforation and hemorrhage
Avoidance of antispasmodics, laxatives, and salicylates
Prevention of carriers from handling food for general consumption

*For typhoid fever and paratyphoid fever (anti-infective agents are not used with salmonellosis unless there is systemic disease).

1 ASSESS

ASSESSMENT	OBSERVATIONS		
	SALMONELLOSIS	TYPHOID FEVER	PARATYPHOID FEVER
History	Ingestion of undercooked meat or eggs	Ingestion of undercooked meat, eggs, or contaminated water	Ingestion of undercooked meat, eggs, or contaminated water
Onset	Acute abdominal symptoms	Gradual onset of symptoms; early: headache, malaise, and anorexia	Some symptoms of salmonellosis and some of typhoid fever
Gastrointestinal	Acute onset: abdominal pain, diarrhea, nausea, and vomiting, persisting for several days Stool is greenish-brown, slimy, watery, and foul; may contain mucus, pus, or blood Bloody diarrhea more common in children	Constipation more common than diarrhea; acute cholecystitis is a complication; enlarged spleen; abdominal pain; distention	Similar to salmonellosis; early: nausea and vomiting in children; abdominal pain and diarrhea in adults; abdominal distention; enlarged spleen
Body temperature	Low-grade fever to 41° C (105° F); chills; lasting 2-7 days	Stair-step rise in temperature during first week to 40° C (104° F) (slightly lower in morning); sustained at 40° C (104° F) for 3-4 wks	Acute-onset fever 39°-40° C (102°-104° F), spiking to 41° C (105.8° F)
Pulse		Slower than expected with fever	
Fluids and electrolytes	Dehydration may be severe in infants: loss of skin turgor, dry mucous membranes, prostration, circulatory collapse, and death are possible		
Skin	May have rose spots on trunk	Discrete rose spots that blanch on pressure, found on trunk after first week; secondary skin infections frequently occur	
Neurologic	Vertigo	Central nervous system: delirium to stupor; personality change; catatonia; aphasia	Meningeal symptoms similar to typhoid
Respiratory	Possible cough	Nonproductive cough	Possible cough
Sensory	May have slight deafness or otitis media	May have slight deafness or otitis media	May have slight deafness or otitis media
Musculoskeletal		Pain in joints	

→ ❯ ❯

ASSESSMENT	OBSERVATIONS		
	SALMONELLOSIS	TYPHOID FEVER	PARATYPHOID FEVER
Urinary tract		Urinary retention	Urinary retention
Cardiovascular	Tachycardia, hypotention, and shock if hemorrhage, secondary infection, or septicemia develops		

Septicemia with localized infection: Symptoms depend on site of systemic lesions caused by any of the *Salmonella* organisms (appendicitis, cholecystitis, peritonitis, otitis media, meningitis, pneumonia, osteomyelitis, pyelonephritis, cystitis, and endocarditis)

Septicemia without localized infection: Symptoms—Intermittent fever, chills, anorexia, and weight loss

2 DIAGNOSE

NURSING DIAGNOSIS	SUPPORTIVE ASSESSMENT FINDINGS
Potential for infection (patient contacts) related to presence of *Salmonella* in stool and urine	Culture of feces, urine, and/or blood positive for *Salmonella*
Hyperthermia related to infection	Chills, fever, lasting 2-7 days (salmonellosis) to 3-4 wks (typhoid)
Diarrhea related to infection in intestinal tract	Diarrhea and vomiting persisting for several days
Potential fluid volume deficit related to vomiting and diarrhea	Signs of dehydration, particularly in infants: loss of skin turgor, dry mucous membranes, prostration, circulatory collapse
Constipation related to invasion of *Salmonella* in intestinal mucosa	Abdominal pain, abdominal distension; absence of bowel elimination
Urinary retention related to *Salmonella* in urinary tract	Urinary output absent or less than intake; bladder distension

Other related diagnoses
Further diagnoses depend on whether bacteremia, septicemia, or systemic focal abscesses are present and where they are located. These may include altered cerebral tissue perfusion, decreased cardiac output, and potential impaired skin integrity.

3 PLAN

Patient goals
1. Patient will be free of infection and complications of *Salmonella* infections.
2. Infection will not be transmitted to patient's contacts.
3. Body temperature will be maintained within the normal range; comfort and safety will be maintained for patients experiencing fever.
4. Patient will return to normal pattern of bowel elimination.
5. Fluid and electrolyte balance will be maintained.
6. Constipation will be relieved.
7. Urine will be eliminated, and patient will resume normal voiding patterns.

4   IMPLEMENT

NURSING DIAGNOSIS	NURSING INTERVENTIONS	RATIONALE
Potential for infection (patient contacts) related to presence of *Salmonella* in stool and urine	Collect blood, stool, or urine specimen (as described in Chapter 3).	Incorrect collection and handling of specimens may destroy the pathogen or contaminate the specimen with environmental organisms, interfering with accurate diagnosis and treatment. Improper handling can also contaminate the health care worker.
	Administer antiinfective therapy as ordered. Initiate universal blood and body secretion precautions and other isolation procedures as indicated.	Antiinfective therapy and isolation procedures should be initiated as soon as possible to prevent transmission to health care workers, other patients, and patient contacts.
	Employ enteric precautions for duration of diarrhea with salmonellosis.	To prevent transmission.
	Employ enteric precautions until 3 consecutive fecal cultures, after cessation of antibiotic therapy, are negative for *S. typhi* and *S. paratyphi.*	To prevent transmission of pathogen (see Chapter 13).
	Utilize protective isolation procedures as indicated. Prevent patient exposure to infected visitors/staff. Limit visitors, if necessary.	To limit the exposure of patients to additional pathogens.
	Participate in follow-up of patient contacts.	To ensure that they are examined and treated.
	Report all *Salmonella* infections to the local health authority.	Reporting is required by law to facilitate public health monitoring and control of outbreaks.
	Teach safe food handling practices, proper hygiene, nutritional and fluid requirements, and handwashing after defecating or handling raw foods or feces.	To prevent recurrence of infection.
Hyperthermia related to infection	See back cover, interventions 1-15.	
	Do not administer aspirin.	Potential exists for GI hemorrhage with these conditions.
Diarrhea related to infection in intestinal tract	Measure output.	To replace fluids equal to output.
	Apply heating pad to abdomen.	To help cramping (antispasmodic agents should be avoided).
	Use room deodorizers and adequate ventilation.	To remove odors.

➜ ❯ ❯

NURSING DIAGNOSIS	NURSING INTERVENTIONS	RATIONALE
	Obtain stool specimen for culture.	To detect pathogen present.
	Wash and lubricate skin around anal opening frequently.	To prevent irritation and skin breakdown.
Potential fluid volume deficit related to vomiting and diarrhea	Assess for symptoms of dehydration (e.g., oliguria and loss of skin turgor).	To intervene early.
	Give oral fluids as tolerated.	To maintain adequate intake.
	Administer IV fluids and electrolytes as prescribed. (Once circulation is stabilized, the initial rate of IV infusion and type of IV electrolytes may be altered.)	To provide for rehydration.
	Measure all fluid output (emesis, urine, diarrhea). Measure all intake.	To ensure that fluid intake compensates for output.
Constipation related to invasion of *Salmonella* in intestinal mucosa	Observe stool.	To detect blood.
	Monitor for signs of perforation and hemorrhage.	For immediate medical intervention.
	Check for and prevent abdominal distension.	Unresolved distension adds to the risk of perforation of the intestines.
	Administer small low enema or glycerin suppositories as ordered (do not give laxatives).	To relieve distension.
Urinary retention related to *Salmonella* in urinary tract	Monitor for bladder distension. Measure output.	To detect urinary retention.
	Catheterize if necessary.	To empty bladder.
Knowledge deficit	See Patient Teaching and Patient Teaching Guide, page 299.	

5   EVALUATE

PATIENT OUTCOME	DATA INDICATING THAT OUTCOME IS REACHED
Patient is free of infection and complications of *Salmonella*.	Vital signs are within normal limits. Blood, stool, or urine cultures are negative for Salmonella. Blood count is within normal limits. Hemorrhage has been avoided.
Infection is not transmitted to patient's contacts.	Patient care staff members wash hands after providing care to each patient and follow universal blood and body secretion procedures with all patients. Enteric isolation procedures are implemented soon after infection is confirmed. Patient or family describes transmission of the pathogen and demonstrates proper procedures for handling infective materials and proper handwashing and other behaviors necessary to prevent transmission. Infection has been reported to local health department. Patient contacts have been examined and treated. Patient completes full course of antiinfective therapy.

PATIENT OUTCOME	DATA INDICATING THAT OUTCOME IS REACHED
Body temperature is maintained within the normal range.	See inside back cover.
Patient returns to normal pattern of bowel elimination.	Patient eats without nausea, vomiting, or abdominal distension. Stools are soft, formed, and brown. Abdomen is soft and nondistended. No cramping or pain occurs.
Fluid and electrolyte balance are maintained.	Skin turgor is good. Mucous membranes are moist. Urine output is normal. Secretions are thin. Blood levels of sodium, potassium, chloride, magnesium, and calcium are normal. Urine specific gravity is normal.
Patient experiences relief from constipation.	Patient has bowel movement at least every 3 days. Stools are soft and pass easily.
Urine is eliminated and patient resumes normal voiding pattern.	There is no distension. Urine output equals fluid intake.

PATIENT TEACHING

Provide patient with the following information:

1. These conditions are transmitted by contaminated food or water or direct fecal-oral route.
2. These conditions are communicable as long as the infective organism is in the feces or urine, which may persist for up to 1 year.
3. Transmission of the infection to others can be prevented by handwashing after defecating and urinating and through proper disposal of excretions so as to not contaminate food or water supply.
4. Follow enteric isolation procedures (Chapter 13).
5. This disease can be prevented by drinking chlorinated water, eating thoroughly cooked food and shellfish, screening food from flies, and other methods listed below.
6. Manage fever with antipyretics, tepid sponge baths, minimal clothing, and by maintaining a cool environment. Avoid chilling and aspirin. Encourage intake of fluids and food as tolerated. Popsicles and soda may appeal to young children.
7. Manage other symptoms with bedrest; avoid laxatives or antispasmodics.
8. Report the following to a physician: signs of dehydration, any bleeding, or recurrence of symptoms.
9. Refer to Patient Teaching Guides for fever, page 302 and Food Safety, page 299.

Important:

1. Scrupulous handwashing after defecation and before preparing food is necessary.
2. Carriers must not handle food for consumption by others until six consecutive fecal and urine cultures taken 1 month apart are negative for *S. typhi* and *S. paratyphi*.
3. Family and close contacts should be examined and treated if specimens from them are positive for any *Salmonella* bacilli.
4. All foods of animal origin, including eggs, must be thoroughly cooked; cross contamination of cooked and uncooked foods must be avoided; and foods must be refrigerated below 8° C (46° F) to avoid infection with *Salmonella*.
5. Protect food and water supply from contamination with sewage containing *S. typhi*. Screen food against flies or other mechanical vectors.
6. Frozen meat, particularly poultry, should be defrosted in the refrigerator.
7. All milk should be pasteurized, and water should be chlorinated.
8. Children should be protected from handling pet turtles and should be taught to wash hands after touching any animal.
9. Relapse is common following typhoid and paratyphoid fevers. Recurrence of symptoms should be reported to physician immediately.

Intestinal Parasitic Worm Infections

Ancylostomiasis (hookworm) is a chronic debilitating disease manifest as an iron deficiency anemia and hypoproteinemia that result from intestinal blood loss to the hookworm.

Ascariasis (roundworm), the most common roundworm infection of the small intestine, is a chronic infection, producing vague gastrointestinal symptoms and sometimes acute and severe manifestations of infection in other organs, commonly the lung. Bowel obstruction is a potential complication.

Enterobiasis (pinworm) is a mild infection of the cecum and colon, producing mild symptoms of anal pruritus.

Strongyloidiasis (threadworm) is a chronic, frequently asymptomatic infection of the duodenum and upper jejunum manifest as (1) a dermatitis in which lar-

Table 5-5

OVERVIEW OF INTESTINAL PARASITIC WORM INFECTIONS

	Ancylostomiasis (hookworm)	Ascariasis (roundworm)	Enterobiasis (pinworm)	Strongyloidiasis (threadworm)
Occurrence	Endemic in tropic and subtropic areas where disposal of human feces is inadequate	Worldwide and common; in the United States, most common in the South; greatest in moist, tropic areas; greatest in children	Worldwide and very high in some areas; most common helminth infection in United States; highest in school- and preschool-aged children and in mothers of infected children	Common in warm wet climates; endemic or epidemic where hygiene is poor, particularly in institutions
Etiologic agent	*Necator americanus, Ancylostoma duodenale, A. ceylanicum*	*Ascaris lumbricoides,* and *A. suum*	*Enterobius vermicularis*	*Strongyloides stercoralis*
Reservoir	Humans, cats, and dogs	Humans	Humans; pinworms of animals not transmitted to humans	Humans, dogs, cats, and primates
Transmission	Infective larvae in soil penetrate skin, usually the foot, and migrate through the blood to the intestines; may be ingested directly	Ingestion of infective eggs from soil contaminated with feces	Direct transmission of infective eggs from anus to mouth; indirect transmission through contaminated food, clothing, or dust	Infective larvae in soil penetrate skin (usually the foot) migrate through the blood to the lungs, migrate up to the pharynx, and are swallowed to the intestines
Incubation period	Weeks to months, depending on health status of host	Worms reach maturity 2 mo after ingestion	Life cycle of worms requires 2-6 wks	2-3 wks
Period of communicability	Infected persons can excrete larvae for years; larvae remain infective in soil for weeks	As long as mature, fertilized female lives in intestine (12-24 months); eggs viable in soil for years	As long as gravid females are depositing eggs on perianal skin; continuous reinfection occurs	As long as living worms remain in the intestines; up to 35 yrs
Susceptibility and resistance	General; immunity unknown	General	General	General; no acquired immunity has been demonstrated
Report to local health authority	No	No	No	No

Data from Benenson.[3]

vae penetrate the skin, (2) respiratory symptoms caused by migration through the lungs, and (3) GI symptoms.

Taeniasis (tapeworm) is a mild infection of the small intestine, occurring with the adult stage of the large tapeworm. It is manifest as variable GI symptoms and loss of weight.

Toxocariasis is a chronic and usually mild infection of young children with systemic and local symptom manifestation, depending on the organs and tissues to which the nematode has migrated.

Trichinosis is a chronic disease, ranging from asymptomatic to acute, caused by migration of the *Trichinella* larvae to striated muscles (where they become

encapsulated). Severity of symptoms depends on the number of larvae and the organ system involved.

Trichuriasis (whipworm) is an infection of the cecum and colon resulting in enteritis and potential rectal prolapse.

Helminths (worms) differ from other agents pathogenic to humans in the following ways: they are large enough to be seen directly; they migrate within the host; their life cycles are more complex; they replicate by means of eggs, which are shed through the feces; and they are capable of producing an eosinophilia. Portal of entry into the host is by ingestion, skin penetration, or injection into the blood by an insect (Table 5-5).

Taeniasis (tapeworm)	Toxocariasis	Trichinosis	Trichuriasis (whipworm)
Particularly high where beef and pork are eaten raw or under-cooked; pork tapeworm rare in the United States	Worldwide; highest in children 14-40 mos; some infection in adults	Worldwide in areas where pork is eaten	Common in warm, moist regions
Taenia saginata (beef tapeworm); *T. solium* (pork tapeworm)	*Toxocara canis* and *T. cati*, predominantly the former	Larvae of *Trichinella spiralis*	*Trichuris trichiura* (human whipworm)
Humans, swine, and cattle	Dogs and cats; almost 100% of newborn puppies are infected	Swine, rats, dogs, cats, and many wild animals	Humans
Ingestion of inadequately cooked, infected meat; anal-oral transfer from person to person; contaminated food or water with eggs from feces	Direct or indirect transmission of eggs in soil (from animal feces) to mouth	Ingestion of inadequately cooked flesh of infected animals	Ingestion of eggs from soil contaminated with human feces
8-14 wks	Weeks or months	5-45 days; usually 8-15 days	Indefinite; eggs appear in feces 90 days after ingestion; symptoms may be earlier
As long as worm is in intestine; up to 30 yrs; not directly communicable	Not directly communicable	Not directly communicable; animal hosts are infective for months	As long as eggs reach the soil, probably years; not directly communicable
General; no resistance follows infection	Adults have lower exposure or decreased susceptibility	General; infection probably results in immunity	General
Report cases in some areas	No	Report cases	No

PATHOPHYSIOLOGY

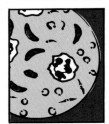

The helminths discussed here produce pathologic conditions in the human by one or more of the following ways: feeding on the host's blood, resulting in anemia; feeding on nutrients in the intestinal tract, which deprives the host of those nutrients; growing in numbers or size, which causes blockage in the intestinal tract or ducts in other organs where they have migrated; causing inflammation and necrosis in tissue; or causing an allergic response in tissue, with a resulting eosinophilia. The site of their damage depends on their life cycle migratory patterns within the host, which is specific for each type of helminth. The extent of pathologic findings is greatly affected by the number of helminths present in the host. Unless treated, helminths remain for long periods. Reinfection or autoinfection greatly adds to the worm burden in the host, particularly in a host whose defenses are compromised by the presence of the worms, malnutrition, and debilitation.

In both **ancylostomiasis** and **strongyloidiasis,** the larvae of the respective hookworm and threadworm, present in the soil, penetrate the host's skin. An erythema and papular vesicular rash appear at the site of the penetration, possibly resulting in a generalized uticaria. The larvae migrate through the blood to the lungs, producing an eosinophilia and transitory respiratory inflammation. From the lungs the larvae migrate to the pharynx and are swallowed to the small intestine. There the hookworms attach and the threadworms burrow in the intestinal mucosa. Localized irritation is manifest as symptoms of burning or colicky abdominal pain and diarrhea. The adult hookworm may remain attached to the intestinal mucosa for as long as 5 years. It ingests 15 ml of the host's blood per worm per day, resulting in weight loss, anemia, and hypoalbuminemia. Eggs from the hookworm pass through the feces as long as the hookworm is attached. The threadworm produces the same pathologic findings as the hookworm, with the additional ability to lay eggs that hatch within the mucosa of the duodenum and upper jejunum. The larvae may be excreted in the feces or may invade the bloodstream directly from the mucosa, reinitiating the life cycle to produce an autoinfection. Septicemia and death may be complications of threadworm infections in immunosuppressed individuals.

In **ascariasis** the eggs of the roundworm are ingested, hatch in the small intestine, penetrate the mucosa, and migrate by way of the blood to the lungs. There they produce inflammation, transitory respira-

tory symptoms, and an eosinophilia similar to that produced by the hookworm and threadworm. The larvae then penetrate the alveoli and migrate to the pharynx, where they are swallowed to the small intestine. They attach to the mucosa, where they impair digestion and protein absorption. They may also travel to the biliary duct and attach there. The irritating presence of the worms may produce vomiting, abdominal distention, and cramps. Blockage of the biliary duct results in colicky epigastric pain, nausea, and vomiting. Because of the size of these roundworms, a large mass may obstruct the bowel lumen.

The roundworms causing **enterabiasis** (pinworm) and **trichuriasis** (whipworm) have simpler life cycles in the human host. Ingested eggs hatch in the small intestine, and larvae migrate directly to the cecum. The tiny gravid female pinworm migrates at night to the perianal area to deposit eggs, which embryonate within 6 hours. Perianal and perineal irritation and pruritus are the only symptoms. Occasionally appendicitis, salpingitis, or ulcerative lesions result from migrating pinworms. Embryonated eggs remain infective on the skin, clothing, and bedclothes for 29 days and may be reingested by the host.

Once in the cecum, the whipworm larvae embed their heads in the mucosa and consume 0.005 ml of blood per worm per day, producing a mild anemia. In 1 to 3 months the adult female worms discharge eggs, which are eliminated in the feces.

The roundworms causing **toxocariasis** and **trichinosis** produce more severe systemic pathologic findings because of the ability of the larvae to invade and encyst in organs beyond the intestinal tract. In toxocariasis eggs from animal feces (particularly puppies) are ingested and hatch in the intestinal tract. The larvae penetrate the intestinal mucosa and migrate through the blood to the eye, skin, liver, lung, kidney, brain, or muscles. The larvae invade those tissues, producing a localized inflammatory reaction and granulomatous nodules. The larvae remain viable in the nodules for years. Systemic manifestations include an eosinophilia $(3,000/\text{mm}^3)$; a leukocytosis $(100,000/\text{mm}^3)$; an increase in IgG, IgM, and IgE antibodies; and an increase in isoagglutinin titers to A and B blood group antibodies. Specific pathologic findings depend on the organ sites of invasion but may include hepatomegaly, an elevated SGOT, respiratory symptoms, blindness, and central nervous system manifestations.

In **trichinosis** the ingested larvae from improperly cooked infected meat attach to the intestinal mucosa within 2 to 3 weeks after infection. The body responds by producing an inflammatory exudate, containing polymorphs, eosinophils, lymphocytes, and macrophages. Intestinal symptoms may be present. Each female *Trichinella* releases about 500 larvae over a 2-week period. The adult females are then discharged in the feces. The larvae penetrate into the bloodstream, migrate, and invade striated muscle. There they increase in length tenfold during a 3-week period. Muscle fibers become edematous, lose their cross-striations, and undergo basophilic degeneration and nuclear proliferation. An acute toxemia results from inflammatory destruction of larvae in the blood. The toxemia subsides when the larvae become encysted in the muscles during the fourth to sixth weeks. Although most infections are subclinical, disease manifestations may be severe, depending on the numbers and sites of invading larvae. Muscles and organs most frequently affected are the intercostal, diaphragm, eye, masseter, neck, pectoral, and limb flexors. Laboratory findings show an eosinophilia and an increase in serum creatinine phosphokinase and lactic dehydrogenase, indicating muscle destruction. Death may result from respiratory failure or pneumonia, myocarditis, or encephalitis caused by the toxemia.

Taeniasis (tapeworm) infections may be local or systemic. If eggs of the pork tapeworm are ingested, they hatch in the intestine, and the larvae penetrate the intestinal mucosa and migrate and form cysts in subcutaneous tissue, striated muscles, or other vital organs. Disease may be severe if larvae localize in the eye, central nervous system, or heart. When larvae from the beef or pork tapeworm are ingested directly, the larvae attach to the intestinal mucosa where they feed and grow. The adult may remain attached for more than 30 years, discharging segments (proglottids) containing eggs into the feces. This form of the disease is less severe than the systemic form.

MEDICAL MANAGEMENT[3,104,148,151].

DRUG THERAPY

Antiinfective agents: Antihelminthic agents are toxic substances and should not be used for small worm burdens.
Ancylostomiasis (hookworm): Mebendazole (Vermox),* 100 mg bid for 3 days or pyrantel pamoate (Antiminth), single oral dose of 11 mg/kg up to total of 1 g/day.
Ascariasis (roundworm): Mebendazole (Vermox),* 100 mg bid for 3 days or piperazine citrate (Antepar), 150 mg/kg initially followed by six doses of 65 mg/kg for 12 h through nasogastric tube for intestinal or biliary obstruction.
Enterobiasis (pinworm): Mebendazole (Vermox),* 100 mg PO one time, or pyrantel pamoate (Antiminth), or pyrvinium pamoate (Povan), or piperazine citrate (Antepar); treatment should be repeated after 2 wks.
Strongyloidiasis (threadworm): Thiabendazole (Mintezol), 25 mg/kg bid for 2 days, or mebendazole (Vermox),* 100 mg bid for 3 days; repeated treatment may be required.
Taeniasis (tapeworm): Niclosamide (Yomesan), 2 g in one dose (adults), or paromycin (Humatin), 1 g q 4 h for 4 doses (adults), or quinacrine (Atabrine), 800 mg in one dose or 400 mg in two doses; 30 min apart for adults.
Toxocariasis: Diethylcarbamazine (Banocide), 5 mg/kg/day for 2-3 wks.
Thiabendazole (Mintezol), 50 mg/kg/day for 7-10 days (questionable effectiveness; infections recur after treatment).
Trichinosis: Thiabendazole (Mintezol) (within 24 h of eating infected meat), 25 mg/kg/day for 1 wk. No treatment available once larvae are in bloodstream and muscle.
Trichuriasis: Mebendazole (Vermox),* 100 mg bid for 3 days PO.

GENERAL MANAGEMENT

Iron therapy to correct anemias
Nutritional supplements
Follow-up examination of stool
Examination and treatment of contacts

*Contraindicated during pregnancy.

DIAGNOSTIC STUDIES AND FINDINGS

Diagnostic Test	Findings

The diagnosis of the parasitic infections where the worm localizes in the intestinal tract is confirmed when eggs or larvae are detected in a fecal specimen or at the anal opening. Toxocariasis and trichinosis are confirmed by biopsy of affected tissue together with the demonstration of elevated serum antibodies.

Ancylostomiasis

Microscopic examination of cultured specimen	Positive for larva; 1,200 hookworm eggs/ml

Ascariasis

Fecal specimen	Eggs of *A. lumbricoides*

Enterobiasis

Fecal specimen	Adult pinworms
Transparent adhesive tape to perianal region	Eggs can be visualized; five examinations will detect 99% of infections

Strongyloidiasis

Fecal specimen	Motile threadworm larvae; after 24 h adults may be visualized
Differential WBC	Increase in eosinophils

Taeniasis

Fecal specimen	Visualizes worm segments (proglottids)

Toxocariasis

Liver biopsy	*Toxocara* larvae in about 20% of cases
Serology: ELISA	Increase in IgG, IgM, and IgE antibodies

Trichinosis

Skeletal muscle biopsy	*Trichinella* larvae 10 days after exposure
Serology: complement fixation, precipitin, and fluorescent antibody	Fourfold increase in antibody titer 2 wks after infection
Bentonite flocculation	Antibody titer greater than 1:5
Differential WBC count	Increase in eosinophils

Trichuriasis

Fecal specimen	Lemon-shaped eggs of whipworm
Sigmoidoscopy	Visualizes adult worms attached to colon wall

1 ASSESS

ASSESSMENT	OBSERVATIONS						
	ANCYLOSTO-MIASIS (HOOK-WORM)	STRONGYLOI-DIASIS (THREAD-WORM)	ASCARIASIS (ROUND-WORM)	TRICHUR-IASIS (WHIP-WORM)	TAENIASIS (TAPEWORM)	TRICHINOSIS	ENTERO-BIASIS (PINWORM)	TOXOCAR-IASIS
History	Walked barefoot in sewage-contaminated soil within past month		Ingested inadequately washed vegetables grown in soil with human or animal fertilizer		Ingested inadequately cooked meat within past 2 mo		Contact with person with pinworms	Contact with feces of newborn puppies or kittens
Skin	Erythematous papular or vesicular eruption at site of invasion (generally soles of feet); may become generalized	No signs	No signs	No signs		Petechial rash; periorbital edema	Pruritis and erythema of perianal area	Pallor; nodular skin eruptions
Respiratory	Transitory cough and irregular respirations (Löffler's syndrome) during migration of larvae	Wheezing, coughing	No signs	No signs		During third to sixth wk: shortness of breath; painful breathing; dysphagia; cough	No signs	Continual cough; rales; rhonchi
Gastrointestinal	Colicky abdominal pain; diarrhea	Vomiting; abdominal distension; cramps; acute abdominal symptoms	Bloody diarrhea; rectal prolapse	Mild abdominal discomfort		Abdominal discomfort and diarrhea (first week only)	No signs	Abdominal pain; hepatomegaly
Body temperature	Fever during migration of larvae through lungs	Fever during lung migration	No fever	No fever		Fever during second week (40° C [104° F]); profuse sweating	No fever	Fever throughout infection
Systemic manifestations	Anemia; weight loss; impaired growth	Anemia; weight loss; impaired growth			Anemia; weight loss; impaired growth	Weakness and headache persisting for vary-	No signs	Weakness and malaise

→ → →

ASSESSMENT	OBSERVATIONS							
	ANCYLOSTO-MIASIS (HOOK-WORM)	STRONGYLOI-DIASIS (THREAD-WORM)	ASCARIASIS (ROUND-WORM)	TRICHUR-IASIS (WHIP-WORM)	TAENIASIS (TAPEWORM)	TRICHINOSIS	ENTERO-BIASIS (PINWORM)	TOXOCAR-IASIS
						ing periods of time beyond migratory phase of larvae; prostration during acute phase		
Central nervous system	No signs	No signs	No signs	No signs	Seizures; psychiatric symptoms; systemic manifestations	During third to sixth week: symptoms of encephalitis	No signs	Seizures
Sensory	No signs	No signs	No signs	No signs	No signs	Periorbital edema; subconjunctival, subungual, and retinal hemorrhage; photophobia	No signs	Strabismus; loss of vision
Musculoskeletal	No signs	No signs	No signs	No signs	No signs	Edema and pain in affected muscles, including the eye, diaphragm, intercostal, pectoral, masseter, neck, and lumbar muscles and limb flexors	No signs	No signs

2 DIAGNOSE

NURSING DIAGNOSIS	SUPPORTIVE ASSESSMENT FINDINGS
Potential for infection (patient contacts) related to presence of eggs or larvae in feces	Fecal specimen contains eggs or larvae of hookworm, threadworm, roundworm, whipworm, tapeworm, or pinworm
Hyperthermia related to infection with ascariasis and trichinosis	Elevated body temperature
Ineffective breathing pattern related to:	
Ancylostomiasis, strongyloidiasis, and ascariasis	Transitory cough and irregular respirations (Löffler's syndrome) during migration of larvae
Trichinosis	Dysphagia; cough; painful breathing, SOB during third to sixth week
Toxocariasis	Continual cough; rales; rhonchi
Altered cerebral tissue perfusion related to toxocariasis	Seizures
Trichinosis	During third to sixth week: symptoms of encephalitis
Taeniasis (systemic)	Seizures and psychiatric symptoms
Altered nutrition, less than body requirements related to ancylostomiasis, strongyloidiasis, trichuriasis, ascariasis, and taeniasis	Anemia; abdominal discomfort and pain; weight loss; impaired growth
Pain related to trichinosis	Pain, edema in affected muscles, including eye, diaphragm, intercostal, pectoral, masseter, neck, and lumbar muscles and limb flexors
Sensory/perceptual alterations (visual) related to:	
Toxocariasis	Strabismus; loss of vision
Trichinosis	Periorbital edema; subconjunctival, subungual, and retinal hemorrhage; and photophobia

3 PLAN

Patient goals

1. Patient will be free of infection and complications of helminth infections. Infection will not be transmitted to patient's contacts.
2. Patient's body temperature will be maintained within normal range; comfort and safety will be maintained for patients experiencing fever.
3. Patient will demonstrate normal respiratory pattern, oxygen intake, and blood gasses.
4. Patient will demonstrate improved cerebral tissue perfusion and cellular oxygenation.
5. Patient's weight, RBC count, hemoglobin, and energy will return to normal.
6. Patient will obtain relief from pain.
7. Patient will not be confused or frightened by environmental stimuli during time of alteration in vision; visual function returns to normal.
8. Patient will describe measures to prevent reinfection with worms.

→ › ›

4 IMPLEMENT

NURSING DIAGNOSIS	NURSING INTERVENTIONS	RATIONALE
Potential for infection (patient contacts) related to presence of worm eggs or larvae in feces	Collect stool specimen (as described in Chapter 3).	Incorrect collection and handling of specimens may destroy the pathogen or contaminate the specimen with environmental organisms, interfering with accurate diagnosis and treatment. Improper handling can also contaminate the health care worker.
	Administer antiinfective therapy as ordered. Initiate universal blood and body secretion precautions; wash hands thoroughly after handling feces. No other isolation precautions are required.	Antiinfective therapy and isolation procedures should be initiated as soon as possible to prevent transmission to health care workers, other patients, and patient contacts.
	Participate in follow-up of patient contacts.	To ensure that they are examined and treated.
	Report trichinosis and taeniasis to local health authority.	Reporting is required by law to facilitate public health monitoring and control of outbreaks.
	Teach safe food handling practices, proper hygiene, and nutritional and fluid requirements.	Helminth infections are transmitted by the fecal-oral route and contaminated food and soil. Malnutrition and dehydration increase the severity of GI infections.
Potential for infection (patient) related to debilitated condition	For patients debilitated because of ancylostomiasis, trichuriasis, ascariasis, and taeniasis: utilize protective isolation procedures as indicated. Prevent patient exposure to infected visitors and staff. Limit visitors if necessary.	To limit the exposure of patients to additional pathogens.
Hyperthermia related to infection	See inside back cover, interventions 1-15.	
Ineffective breathing pattern related to ancylostomiasis, ascariasis, strongloidiasis, toxocariasis, and trichinosis	Monitor for signs of pneumonia.	For early intervention.
	Administer oxygen and respiratory assistance if required.	To maintain adequate oxygen intake.
	Aid patients to breathe deeply.	To prevent atelectasis.
Altered cerebral tissue perfusion related to toxocariasis, trichinosis, and taeniasis (systemic).	Monitor for signs of central nervous system involvement.	To report to physician.
	Closely supervise patient.	To protect from injury.
	Have available padded tongue blade, padded headboard, and side rails.	To protect from injury.

NURSING DIAGNOSIS	NURSING INTERVENTIONS	RATIONALE
Altered nutrition: less than body requirements related to ancylostomiasis, trichuriasis, ascariasis, and taeniasis	Administer iron and nutritional supplements as prescribed. Encourage frequent high-protein feedings. (Blood transfusions may be necessary in ancylostomiasis.)	To replace those absorbed by parasite.
	Assess abdomen for bowel sounds, distension, and pain. Report to physician symptoms of acute abdominal pain and distension that may suggest obstruction.	To start early intervention.
Pain related to trichinosis	Encourage rest.	To relieve muscle pain.
	Administer analgesics as prescribed.	To provide pain relief.
Sensory/perceptual alterations (visual) related to toxocariasis and trichinosis	Reassure patient that visual symptoms will disappear in 3 months.	To relieve anxiety about future.
	Assist patient as needed with mobility.	To protect from injury.
Knowledge deficit	See Patient Teaching and Patient Teaching Guide on Food Safety, page 299.	

5 EVALUATE

Patient is free of infection and complications of helminth infections. Infection is not transmitted to patient's contacts.	Vital signs are within normal limits. Stool specimen is negative for larvae of pinworms or threadworm; negative for eggs of hookworm, ascariasis, and whipworm; and negative for tapeworm segments. There is no perianal pruritis. WBC count is within normal limits. For toxocariasis and trichinosis, SGOT, CPK, and lactic dehydrogenase levels are normal. Patient or family describes transmission of the pathogen and demonstrates proper procedures for handling infective materials and proper handwashing and other behaviors necessary to prevent transmission. All patient contacts are examined and treated for infection. Patient self-administers antiinfective agents as prescribed.
Body temperature is maintained within the normal range; comfort and safety are maintained for patients experiencing fever.	See inside back cover.
Patient demonstrates normal respiratory pattern, oxygen intake, and blood gasses.	Respiratory patterns are normal without cough, rales, or rhonchi.
Patient demonstrates improved cerebral tissue perfusion and cellular oxygenation.	Patient is mentally alert and oriented, can concentrate, and does not experience seizures, personality changes, or alterations in affect. There are no signs of myocarditis, encephalitis, meningitis, or visual loss. Body temperature is normal.

→ > >

PATIENT OUTCOME	DATA INDICATING THAT OUTCOME IS REACHED
Nutritional intake is adequate for needs.	Energy is at preinfection level. The patient is mentally alert. Growth, development, and weight are normal for patient's age. Skin and mucous membranes are warm and moist, with natural color. Skin turgor is good. Abdomen is soft, and stools are soft, formed, and normal colored. Spleen and liver are not palpable. For ancylostomiasis, trichuriasis, ascariasis, and taeniasis, hemoglobin, hematocrit, and erythrocyte levels are normal.
Patient obtains relief from pain.	Patient expresses relief of muscle pain or headache and rests quietly.
Patient is not confused or frightened by environmental stimuli during time of alteration in vision; visual function returns to normal.	These are no startle responses to environmental stimuli. During convalescence, the patient correctly identifies letters on a Snellen eye chart at 20 ft. Pupils are normal and reactive.

PATIENT TEACHING

Provide patient with the following information:

1. Follow-up examination of stools 2 weeks after therapy is necessary in ascariasis, ancylostomiasis, strongyloidiasis, and taeniasis. Monthly examinations for 3 months are necessary for taeniasis.
2. Toxocariasis and strongyloidiasis tend to recur following treatment. Monitoring by a physician is recommended.
3. Anemias and protein deficiencies from ancylostomiasis, trichuriasis, ascariasis, and taeniasis may take time to correct. Nutrition counseling and taking iron and vitamin supplements until deficiencies are corrected is recommended.
4. Treatment for enterobiasis should be repeated in 2 weeks following first treatment. Daily machine washing of underwear and bedclothes with hot water is necessary during that time.
5. Family members and close contacts of patients with any of these intestinal parasitic infections should be examined and treated for parasites.
6. Thorough handwashing after defecation is vital.
7. Treatment of puppies for worms may prevent toxocariasis in humans.
8. Prevent children from eating dirt.
9. Proper cooking of pork to 65.6° C (150° F) is necessary.
10. Home freezing of meat for 3 weeks at −25° C (−13° F) destroys larvae.
11. Employ sewage disposal of contaminated feces. No human feces should be used as fertilizer.
12. Wear shoes in areas where human or animal feces may be on soil.
13. Bury animal feces deep in an area where children do not play.

CHAPTER 6

Hepatitis and Hematolymphatic Infectious Diseases

Viral Hepatitis

Viral hepatitis refers to several distinct infections of the liver, each caused by a different hepatitis virus. Depending on the etiologic agent, the diseases differ in their mode of transmission and in their immunologic, pathologic, and clinical characteristics. Treatment is similar for each disease, but prevention and control vary greatly.

To date, five types of primary hepatitis viruses have been identified. These are hepatitis A, B, C, D, and E. The hepatitis virus category "non-A, non-B" is used to refer to the hepatitis viruses that are yet to be identified. Hepatitis can also occur as a secondary infection during the course of diseases associated with cytomegalovirus, Epstein-Barr, herpes simplex, varicella-zoster, coxsackievirus B, and rubella viruses (Table 6-1).

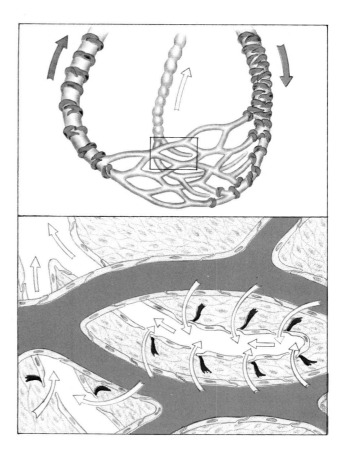

PATHOPHYSIOLOGY

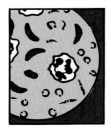

Although the etiologic agents, mode of transmission, and course of the disease vary with each type of hepatitis, the pathologic condition produced in the liver is the same with all types. The similarities in pathologic findings for each type are presented first, followed by the variations.

The hepatitis virus, regardless of its mode of transmission, invades, replicates, and produces damage only in the liver. Inflammation and mononuclear cell infiltration in the parenchyma and portal ducts, hepatic cell necrosis, proliferation of Kupffer cells, cellular collapse, and accumulation of necrotic debris in the lobules and portal ducts all act to produce architectural changes in the lobules and portal ducts. The result is disturbance in bilirubin excretion.

Table 6-1

OVERVIEW OF VIRAL HEPATITIS

	Hepatitis A	Hepatitis B	Hepatitis C	Hepatitis D	Hepatitis E
Occurrence	Worldwide; sporadic and epidemic, with a tendency toward cyclic recurrence; outbreaks in institutions	Worldwide; endemic; highest in young adults, homosexual men, heterosexuals with multiple sex partners, parenteral drug users, and health care and public safety workers	Worldwide; accounts for 90% of posttransfusion hepatitis in the United States	Worldwide; occurs epidemically and endemically in populations at risk for HBV infection	Epidemic and sporadic cases, particularily in developing countries; highest in young adults; rare in children or elderly
Etiologic agent	Hepatitis A virus (HAV)	Hepatitis B virus (HBV) Delta agent may coinfect with HBV	Hepatitis C virus (HCV)	A viruslike particle (HDV, or the delta agent); coinfects with HBV	Viruslike particle (HEV)
Reservoir	Humans and captive primates	Humans and possibly captive primates	Humans, chimpanzees	Humans, chimpanzees	Humans, chimpanzees
Transmission	Person to person by fecal-oral route; contaminated food, water, shellfish	Direct and indirect contact with blood, saliva, and semen; sexual contact; perinatal	Percutaneous exposure to blood; person-to-person and sexual transmission have not been defined	Similar to HBV, including sexual contact	Contaminated water; person to person by fecal-oral route
Incubation period	15-50 days; average: 28-30 days	45-180 days; average: 60-90 days	2 wks to 6 months; commonly 6-9 wks	2-10 wks	15-64 days; average: 26-42 days
Period of communicability	Latter half of incubation period to 1 wk after onset of jaundice	During incubation period and throughout clinical course of disease; carrier state may persist for years	From 1 or more wks before symptom onset, indefinitely during chronic and carrier states	Throughout acute and chronic disease	Not known; probably similar to HA
Susceptibility and resistance	Usually affects children and young adults; immunity after infection probably lasts for life; 45% of population has hepatitis A antibodies	All age groups; disease is mild in children; lifetime immunity follows infection if antibody to HBsAg develops and HBsAg is negative	All age groups; degree of immunity following infection is unknown	All persons susceptible to HB, HBV carriers; disease is severe in children	Unknown; no explanation for epidemics among young adults; pregnant women have highest fatality
Report to local health authority	Mandatory case report	Mandatory case report	Mandatory case report	Mandatory case report	Mandatory case report

Data from Benenson.[3]

Cellular regeneration and mitosis are usually concurrent with hepatocyte necrosis; complete regeneration usually occurs within 2 to 3 months. Failure of the liver cells to regenerate while the necrotic process progresses results in a severe, fulminant, frequently fatal hepatitis. This occurs more often in hepatitis B.

For photograph of hepatitis virus, see color plate 1, page x.

Continuation of the inflammatory response and necrosis, also more common in types B, E, and non-A, non-B, results in active chronic or persistent chronic hepatitis. In active chronic hepatitis the necrotic process, fibrosis, and architectural destruction continue throughout the hepatic lobes and portal ducts. In persistent chronic hepatitis the inflammatory process is limited to the portal tracts with little or no evidence of hepatocellular necrosis. There is a great deal of variability in clinical manifestations of hepatitis. All types of hepatitis may be present with or without icterus and may have a clinical severity ranging from subclinical infection to acute fulminating disease. Only hepatitis A does not lead to chronic disease or the chronic carrier state. All types stimulate an antibody response specific to the type of virus causing the disease.

Hepatitis A virus (HAV) is acquired by ingestion of the HAV in food, water, or uncooked shellfish contaminated with feces containing the virus or by direct fecal-oral transmission. The virus localizes in the liver, replicates, enters the bile, and is carried to the intestinal tract, where it is shed in the feces. Fecal shedding occurs late in the incubation period, usually before onset of clinical symptoms. Antibodies (anti-HAV) develop during acute disease and later during convalescence.

Hepatitis B virus (HBV) is viable in blood and in secretions containing serum (oozing cutaneous lesions) or derived from serum (e.g., saliva, semen, and vaginal secretions). Transmission may be by one of five routes: (1) direct percutaneous inoculation of infective serum or plasma by needle or transfusion of infective blood or blood products; (2) indirect percutaneous introduction of infective serum or plasma, such as through minute skin cuts or abrasions; (3) absorption of infective serum or plasma through mucosal surfaces, such as those of the mouth or eye; (4) absorption of other potentially infective secretions, such as saliva or semen through mucosal surfaces, as might occur during vaginal, anal, or oral sexual contact; and (5) transfer of infective serum or plasma via inanimate environmental surfaces or possibly vectors. Fecal transmission of HBV does not occur. HBV may be transmitted transplacentally, or the infant may become contaminated with the mother's infective blood at birth.

HBV is composed of three antigens: the core antigen (HBcAg), an outer surface antigen (HBsAg), and a soluble antigen (HBeAg). HBV antigens infect the blood within 30 to 60 days of exposure to HBV and are at their peak before disease onset. They persist for varying lengths of time, and their presence is useful for determining the course of the disease and the carrier state. Antibodies specific for the antigens develop at different times during convalescence. Detection of serum antibodies is useful for predicting the course of the disease and for determining immune status.

The identification of serologic markers for type-specific virus antigens and antibodies has been important in the diagnosis, prevention, and control of viral hepatitis. The standard nomenclature and abbreviation with characteristics and implications are presented here for easy reference (Table 6-2).

A viral-like particle called the **delta agent** has recently been identified. This agent is pathogenic only with HBV, causing coinfection with the HBV or superimposing infection on an inapparent HBV carrier state. Prolongation or an increase in severity of an HBV infection may be attributable to the delta agent.

Hepatitis C virus (HCV) is a parenterally transmitted non-A, non-B (PT-NANB) hepatitis virus that causes a disease similar to hepatitis B (i.e., prolonged incubation period, insidious onset, and potential chronicity). Diagnosis currently depends on exclusion of HAV, HBV, and the delta particle. HCV can stimulate an antibody response. A screening test for the antibody has recently been developed and is used for screening blood donors.

Hepatitis E virus (HEV) is an enterically transmitted non-A, non-B (ET-NANB) hepatitis virus that causes disease with a clinical course similar to hepatitis A (i.e., shorter incubation period, acute onset, and complete recovery). Disease may be more severe in pregnant women, particularly in the third trimester. A serologic test for HEV antibodies is being developed.

COMPLICATIONS

Fulminant, frequently fatal, hepatitis
Chronic hepatitis infection
Hepatic carcinoma

Table 6-2

STANDARD NOMENCLATURE, ABBREVIATIONS, AND CHARACTERISTICS OF HEPATITIS

Abbreviation	Term	Characteristics and implications
HAV	Hepatitis A virus	Etiologic agent with one serotype
Anti-HAV	Antibody to HAV	Detectable at onset of symptoms and persists for lifetime; probably confers lifetime immunity
IgM	Immunoglobulin M (antibody to HAV)	The anti-HAV is present early in the infection; it represents current infection and is used to establish the diagnosis; serum levels drop during convalescence and disappear in 4-6 months
IgG	Immunoglobulin G (antibody to HAV)	The anti-HAV that develops late in the infection and persists for years; its presence in serum indicates past infection and present immunity
HBV	Hepatitis B virus	Etiologic agent of hepatitis B; also called **Dane particle**
HBsAg	Hepatitis B surface antigen	Previously known as Australian antigen; large quantities detectable in serum 2-7 wks before and during acute clinical disease, during chronic disease, and in carriers; its presence indicates infectious blood
HBeAg	Hepatitis B e antigen	Soluble antigen that correlates with HBV replication; indicates a high titer of HBV in serum and consequent infectivity of serum; it rises 2-7 wks before clinical disease onset and usually drops before acute disease; its persistence is associated with progression to chronic hepatitis; found only in HBsAg-positive serum
HBcAg	Hepatitis B core antigen	Found in liver cells; cannot be detected in sera with present technology
Anti-HBs	Antibody to HBsAG	Rises in serum during convalescence; its presence indicates immunity to HBV from past infection, passive antibody from HBIG, or active immune response from HBV vaccine
Anti-HBe	Antibody to HBeAg	Its presence in serum of person with continuing levels of HBeAg suggests chronic presence of HBV and infectivity of blood
Anti-HBc	Antibody to HBcAg	Increases during clinical disease, peaks during convalescence, and persists for years; presence indicates past infection with HBV
IGM anti-HBc	IGM antibody to HBcAg	Indicates recent infection with HBV; positive for 4-6 months after infection
IG	Immunoglobulin	Formerly called **immune serum globulin (ISG)** or **gamma globulin;** given before and within 2 wks after exposure to HAV and NANB
HBIG	Hepatitis B immune globulin	Contains a higher titer of HB immune globulins than does IG; preferred for use after exposure to HBV
HB vaccine	Hepatitis B vaccine	Inactivated vaccine prepared from carriers of HBsAg; stimulates production of anti-HBs; series of three injections recommended for those at risk for hepatitis B
PT-NANB	Parenterally transmitted non-A, non-B hepatitis	Diagnosed by exclusion; At least 2 viruses, one of which is hepatitis C; shares features with Hepatitis B
ET-NANB	Enterically transmitted non-A, non-B	Diagnosed by exclusion; fecal, oral, or water-borne transmission
HDV	Hepatitis D virus	Etiologic agent of delta hepatitis; may only cause infection in presence of HBV
HDAg	Delta antigen	Detectable in early, acute delta infections
Anti-HDV	Antibody to delta antigen	Indicates past or present infection with delta antigen

Reference: 41.

DIAGNOSTIC STUDIES AND FINDINGS

Diagnostic Test	Findings
Serum enzymes	
Asparate aminotransferase (AST, SGOT) and alanine aminotransferase (ALT, SGPT)	At least eight times normal during clinical disease; indicators of liver damage; peak at onset of jaundice and fall during recovery; may be 20-50 times normal for hepatitis B and 10-20 times normal for non-A, non-B hepatitis, persisting at 2-5 times normal for months
Alkaline phosphatase	1 to 3 times normal
Lactic dehydrogenase (LDH)	1 to 3 times normal
Creatine phosphokinase (CPK)	Normal
Serum bilirubin	Elevated: measures extent of liver dysfunction; ratio of direct to indirect fraction—1:1
Prothrombin time	Normal; elevated only in severe fulminating hepatitis
VDRL	False positive
Hepatitis A	
Stool specimen: immune electron microscopy, radioimmunoassay, or enzyme immunoassay	Positive for HAV 2-4 wks after exposure, remains until onset of clinical disease, then is negative HAV may be absent from stool by time patient is hospitalized
Serology: radioimmunoassay (RIA) or ELISA test	Fourfold rise in anti-HAV antibodies between early disease and convalescence Identification of IgM antibodies during early disease indicates present infection; peaks at 3 months and then drops IgG peaks after clinical disease and persists for life; high levels indicate past infection and present immunity
Hepatitis B	
Serum antigen tests: radioimmunoassay, enzyme immunoassay	HBeAg and HBsAg in serum 1-2 wks after exposure and 2-7 wks before onset of clinical disease; peaks and begins to drop during clinical disease HBsAg remains in serum of chronic carriers for life; positive tests indicate present infection or carrier state Positive test in carrier with disease symptoms may misdiagnose infection with HAV or NANB
Serum antibody tests: radioimmunoassay	Anti-HBe increases during clinical disease and peaks during convalescence; anti-HBe begins rising during convalescence; both persist and gradually decrease over time; anti-HBs rises rapidly during late convalescence and persists Carriers are always HBeAg positive and/or HBsAg positive and anti-HBs negative For screening purposes: anti-HBs >10 RIA sample ratio units indicates immunity
Non-A, non-B hepatitis	
If above tests are negative in patient with clinical symptoms of viral hepatitis, non-A, non-B is suspected	
Hepatitis C	
One serologic test for parenterally transmitted hepatitis C is recently available	

RECOMMENDED DOSES AND SCHEDULES OF CURRENTLY LICENSED HB VACCINES

	Vaccine					
	Heptavax-B*†		Recombivax HB*		Engerix-B*‡	
Group	Dose (μg)	(ml)	Dose (μg)	(ml)	Dose (μg)	(ml)
Infants of HBV-carrier mothers	10	(0.5)	5	(0.5)	10	(0.5)
Other infants and children <11 years	10	(0.5)	2.5	(0.25)	10	(0.5)
Children and adolescents 11-19 years	20	(1.0)	5	(0.5)	20	(1.0)
Adults >19 years	20	(1.0)	10	(1.0)	20	(1.0)
Dialysis patients and other immunocompromised persons	40	(2.0)§	40	(1.0)‖	40	(2.0)§¶

Reference: 41.

*Usual schedule: three doses at 0, 1, 6 months.

†Available only for hemodialysis and other immunocompromised patients and for persons with known allergy to yeast.

‡Alternative schedule: four doses at 0, 1, 2, and 12 months.

§Two 1.0-ml doses given at different sites.

‖Special formulation for dialysis patients.

¶Four-dose schedule recommended at 0, 1, 2, and 6 months.

MEDICAL MANAGEMENT

DRUG THERAPY

There is no direct chemotherapeutic treatment for viral hepatitis (there is no evidence that corticosteroids are helpful); however supportive medications may be used for fulminating hepatitis.

Antiinfective agents: Neomycin (Mycifadrin), 1-1.5 g q 6 h orally until loose stools are achieved.
    Histamine-receptor antagonist: cimetidine (Tagamet), 300-500 mg IV q 6 h or vigorous antacid therapy for GI bleeding.

Hepatitis A: Prevention: preventive medications may be used for < 2 months for preexposure prophylaxis against hepatitis A (HAV) for those traveling to high-risk areas outside tourist routes.
Immunologic agent:
    Immune globulin (IG), 0.02 ml/kg in a single dose IM.
Immunologic agent for prolonged travel:
    Immune globulin (IG), 0.06 ml/kg IM in a single dose q 5 months.
Postexposure prophylaxis within 2 wks of close personal contact with hepatitis A-infected person in the home, day-care center, institution for custodial care, or hospital.
Immunologic agent:
    Immune globulin (IG), 0.02 ml/kg in a single dose IM.

Hepatitis B: Preexposure prophylaxis against hepatitis B (HBV) for high-risk groups (health care workers in contact with blood or blood products, clients, and staff of institutions for the mentally retarded, hemodialysis patients, heterosexuals with multiple sexual partners, homosexual males, illicit injectable drug users, patients with clotting disorders who receive factor VII or IX concentrates, household and sexual contacts of HBV carriers, classroom contacts of deinstitutionalized mentally retarded carriers, and inmates of long-term correctional facilities).
Prevaccination serologic screening to identify HBV carriers and those already immune; one anti-HBc test will identify both; anti-HBs test will identify those immune but will not identify carriers.

MEDICAL MANAGEMENT—cont'd

GENERAL MANAGEMENT

For nonfulminating hepatitis:

Hospitalization for those with bilirubin concentrations >10 mg/dl or >10 times normal and for those with a prolonged prothrombin time; bed rest until symptoms subside; diet as tolerated: small, frequent, low-fat, high-carbohydrate feedings may be better tolerated; symptomatic treatment for nausea (avoid chlorpromazine); symptomatic treatment for pain (acetaminophen preferred over aspirin); avoid all unnecessary medications, particularly sedatives.

For fulminating hepatitis:

Hospitalization and bed rest; low-protein diet: 20 to 30 mg protein/day; enemas; discontinue any sedatives; IV fluids and electrolytes; central venous pressure line; nasogastric tube feedings; urinary catheter; fresh frozen plasma to correct coagulation defects.

References: 37, 41, 96, 105, 123.

POSTEXPOSURE PROPHYLAXIS

RECOMMENDATIONS FOR HEPATITIS B PROPHYLAXIS FOLLOWING PERCUTANEOUS OR PERMUCOSAL EXPOSURE

Exposed person	Treatment when source is found to be:		
	HBsAg-positive	HBsAg-negative	Source not tested or unknown
Unvaccinated	HBIG × 1* and initiate HB vaccine†	Initiate HB vaccine†	Initiate HB vaccine†
Previously vaccinated known responder	Test exposed for anti-HBs 1. If adequate,‡ no treatment 2. If inadequate, HB vaccine booster dose	No treatment	No treatment
Known nonresponder	HBIG × 2 or HBIG × 1 + 1 dose HB vaccine	No treatment	If known high-risk source, **may treat as if source were HBsAg-positive**
Response unknown	Test exposed for anti-HBs 1. If inadequate,‡ HBIG × 1 + HB vaccine booster dose 2. If adequate, no treatment	No treatment	Test exposed for anti-HBs 1. If inadequate,‡ HB vaccine booster dose 2. If adequate, no treatment

*HBIG dose 0.06 ml/kg IM.
†HB vaccine dose—see table, Recommended Doses and Schedules of Currently Licensed HB Vaccines, page 110.
‡Adequate anti-HBs is ≥10 SRU by RIA or positive by EIA see Table 6-2, page 108, and the diagnostic table.

HEPATITIS B VIRUS POSTEXPOSURE RECOMMENDATIONS

Exposure	HBIG		Vaccine	
	Dose	Recommended timing	Dose	Recommended timing
Perinatal	0.5 ml IM	Within 12 hours of birth	0.5 ml IM*	Within 12 hours of birth†
Sexual	0.06 ml/kg IM	Single dose within 14 days of last sexual contact	1.0 ml IM*	First dose at time of HBIG treatment†

*For appropriate age-specific doses of each vaccine, see table, Recommended Doses and Schedules of Currently Licensed HB Vaccines, page 110.
†The first dose can be given the same time as the HBIG dose but in a different site; subsequent doses should be given as recommended for specific vaccine.

PT-NANB POSTEXPOSURE PROPHYLAXIS—IG (0.06 ml/kg) IM as soon as possible after exposure

References: 41.

1 ASSESS

ASSESSMENT	OBSERVATIONS
History	Sexual contact with multiple or unknown partners; homosexual contact; household contact with person with hepatitis; IV drug abuse; unimmunized for HB
Disease onset	Within 2-7 wks of exposure for HA; within 6 wks to 6 months for HB

Preicteric phase (3-10 days)

Subjective symptoms	Malaise, weakness, dull headache, anorexia, intermittent nausea and vomiting, myalgias, chills; right, upper quadrant abdominal pain
Body temperature	38°-40° C (100°-104° F) for hepatitis A; low-grade fever or normal for hepatitis B and non-A, non-B
Skin	For hepatitis B and non-A, non-B: urticarial pruritic hives, maculopapular lesions, or fleeting, irregular patches of erythema in some patients; multiple forearm pricks in drug users; exacerbation of acne; excoriations with severe pruritus
Musculoskeletal concerns	For hepatitis B and non-A, non-B: mild to moderate nondeforming polyarticular arthritis (migratory, affecting elbows, wrists, knees, and small joints of hands)
Abdomen	Bowel sounds normal; slightly enlarged, tender liver (9-13 cm), edges smooth, regular, and firm

Icteric phase (bilirubin > 2.5 mg/dl; lasts 1-3 wks)

Subjective symptoms	Nausea and vomiting frequently abate and appetite returns, but symptoms may worsen; malaise continues
Skin	Jaundice with or without pruritus may be present or absent; can be observed under the tongue
Eyes	Scleral icterus
Urine	Dark
Stools	May be clay-colored
Vital signs	Normal, although there may be a bradycardia with severe hyperbilirubinemia
Temperature	Normal or low-grade

Complications: Fulminant Hepatitis with Encephalopathy

Level of consciousness	Patient becomes lethargic and somnolent with personality changes; may show mild confusion, sexual or aggressive activity, loss of usual inhibitions Lethargy may alternate with excitability, euphoria, or unruly behavior Worsening of the condition leads to stupor and eventual coma An early sign is asterixis (the irregular flapping of forcibly dorsiflexed, outstretched hands)
Circulatory system	Prothrombin time is prolonged: abdominal bleeding; epistaxis; prolonged bleeding from puncture sites; blood in vomitus, stool, or urine; easy bruising

2   DIAGNOSE

NURSING DIAGNOSIS	SUPPORTIVE ASSESSMENT FINDINGS
Potential for infection (patient contacts) related to presence of HAV in feces and HBV and NANB in blood, semen, and saliva	History of contact with infected person or performance of behaviors at high risk for transmission; stool specimen positive for HAV; serologic tests indicate acute infection with HBV or HAV
Activity intolerance related to decreased energy metabolism by liver	Altered serum enzymes and bilirubin; malaise, weakness; musculoskeletal pain; fever
Altered nutrition: less than body requirements related to anorexia, nausea and vomiting, and altered digestion of food	Anorexia, nausea and vomiting; clay-colored stools; diarrhea
Potential fluid volume deficit related to vomiting and diarrhea	Persistent vomiting and diarrhea; inadequate urine output; decrease in skin turgor
Knowledge deficit related to disease transmission, prevention, and potential chronicity	Person engages in high-risk behavior and is unimmunized against HBV
Potential patient problem: hemorrhage related to complications of hepatitis	Bruising; epistaxis; blood in vomitus, stool, or urine
Potential patient problem: encephalopathy related to complications of hepatitis	CNS findings: lethargy and confusion, leading to stupor and/or coma; behavioral lability.

3   PLAN

Patient goals

1. Infection will not be transmitted to patient contacts.
2. Patient will achieve adequate rest to conserve energy during active disease and will return to preillness level of activity during convalescence.
3. Adequate calorie intake and nutritional status will be maintained; weight will be stable.
4. Fluid and electrolyte balance will be maintained.
5. Patient will have information to prevent future infections with hepatitis caused by other viruses. Patient describes measures to minimize complications of hepatitis.
6. Infection will resolve without complications.

4   IMPLEMENT

NURSING DIAGNOSIS	NURSING INTERVENTIONS	RATIONALE
Potential for infection (patient contacts) related to presence of HAV in feces and HBV and NANB in blood, semen, and saliva	Collect fecal or blood specimens as required.	Specimens must be handled correctly so as not to destroy or transmit the virus.
	Employ enteric precautions for 7 days after onset of jaundice for hepatitis A. Employ universal precautions for all patients.	Viable virus can be transmitted in these excretions and secretions.

➡ ➡ ➡

NURSING DIAGNOSIS	NURSING INTERVENTIONS	RATIONALE
	Ensure that all patient contacts, including health care personnel, are protected against hepatitis.	HB vaccine is a safe and effective preventive measure.
Activity intolerance related to decreased energy metabolism by liver	Maintain bed rest during acute symptoms. (Patients need not be limited in their activity during convalescence.)	To conserve energy and avoid unneccessary stress to the liver.
	Do necessary tests and procedures at one time.	To allow for uninterrupted rest.
Altered nutrition: less than body requirements related to anorexia, nausea and vomiting, and altered digestion of food	Encourage frequent small feedings as patient tolerates; largest meal in AM.	Anorexia frequently worsens as day progresses.
	Provide high-carbohydrate, low-fat feedings.	To provide easily digested meals.
	Administer nasogastric tube feedings for patients with hepatic encephalopathy and coma; administer IV fluids for patients with persistent vomiting or for those with hepatic encephalopathy, as ordered.	To avoid aspiration while ensuring adequate intake of food and fluids.
	Offer hard candy.	To soothe nausea.
Fluid volume deficit	Monitor fluid intake and output and lab values.	To detect fluid and electrolyte imbalance.
	Provide frequent high-carbohydrate fluids as tolerated during acute symptoms.	To compensate for fluid loss with vomiting and diarrhea.
Potential patient problem: hemorrhage related to complications of hepatitis	Monitor and report signs of bleeding. Provide care as warranted by bleeding.	For early detection and intervention for coagulation and bleeding problems.
Knowledge deficit	See Patient Teaching guidelines.	
Potential patient problem: encephalopathy related to complications of hepatitis	Monitor and report signs of encephalopathy as were described under NURSING ASSESSMENT. Monitor and report progression of icterus. Provide care as warranted by patient's level of consiousness.	These are severe signs of the progression of the disease; these patients require protection from injury and may require life support.

5 EVALUATE

PATIENT OUTCOME	DATA INDICATING THAT OUTCOME IS ACHIEVED
Infection is not transmitted	Patient returns for examination to determine when serum HBsAg and HBeAg tests are negative. Close, personal contacts of hepatitis B patients have received HBIG and HB vaccine or IG vaccine for hepatitis A.

PATIENT OUTCOME	DATA INDICATING THAT OUTCOME IS ACHIEVED
Patient achieves adequate rest during active disease and returns to pre-illness level of activity during convalescence	Extended periods of uninterrupted sleep are experienced. Patient has gradually increasing amounts of energy without relapses of extreme fatigue.
Adequate calorie intake and nutritional status are maintained; weight is stable	Patient has full appetite and energy. Weight is at preillness state. RBCs are normal.
Fluid and electrolyte balance is maintained	Fluid intake equals output. Urine is straw-colored. Specific gravity, sodium, and albumin levels are within normal limits. Skin turgor is normal; no ascites or edema.
Patient is knowledgeable about need for follow-up, means of preventing transmission to others, and convalescent self-care	Items listed in Patient Teaching are met.
Infection resolves without complications	There is no icterus. Patient has full appetite and energy and has no right upper quadrant abdominal pain. Urine and stool are normal-colored. There are no changes in personality or level of consciousness. SGPT (ALT), SGOT (AST), alkaline phosphatase, LDH, serum bilirubin, and prothrombin time are all within normal limits.

PATIENT TEACHING

1. Educate patient about disease and disease transmission. Emphasize the self-limited nature of most episodes of hepatitis but the need for follow-up of liver function tests and serum HBsAg.
2. Follow-up serology in 1 or 2 months is necessary for all hepatitis B patients to determine the presence or absence of HBsAg.
3. Patients should follow precautions with blood and secretions until they are determined to be free of HBsAg. Close personal contacts should be examined and receive HBIG or HB vaccine.
4. HBV carriers should be aware that their blood and secretions are infectious. Close contacts of HBV carriers should receive HB vaccine. Carriers should not share razors or toothbrushes and must be cautious in handling cuts and lacerations. HBV carriers and patients with a history of NANB should not donate blood.
5. Patients caring for themselves at home during the acute stage of the disease should avoid alcohol and any nonprescribed medications, particularly sedatives and aspirin.
6. Severity of symptoms can determine patterns for bed rest and diet. Frequent, small feedings of low-fat, high-carbohydrate foods may be better tolerated, but it is not necessary to limit the diet in any way.
7. Liver function tests should be monitored until normal.
8. Hepatitis A patients must wash hands thoroughly following toileting, must disinfect articles soiled with feces (boil 1 min), and must not prepare foods for others during symptomatic disease. They should avoid sharing eating utensils, toothbrushes, toys, etc.
9. Sexual activity should be avoided during acute stage of hepatitis B and non-A, non-B. Ideally hepatitis B patients should not resume sexual activity until tests for HBsAg are negative or until partner has received HB vaccine or HBIG if HB vaccine is unavailable.

Hematolymphatic Infectious Diseases

The infectious diseases grouped here produce either primary pathologic findings in the lymphatic system or disseminated infection with lymphadenopathy as part of the clinical picture (Table 6-3).

MONONUCLEOSIS

Mononucleosis is an acute viral infectious disease that produces a generalized lymph node hyperplasia and is characterized by fever, exudative pharyngitis, lymphadenopathy, and splenomegaly.

PATHOPHYSIOLOGY

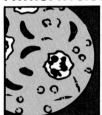

The Epstein-Barr virus (EBV) is transmitted in saliva by prolonged direct contact, probably through kissing with salivary exchange. The pathogen invades B lymphocytes in lymphatic tissue and stimulates the development of a surface membrane antigen on the infected lymphocytes. T lymphocytes actively proliferate in response to the antigen and produce a generalized lymph node hyperplasia. Atypical T lymphocytes infiltrate the spleen, tonsils, lungs, heart, liver, kidneys, adrenal glands, central nervous system, and skin. The circulating T cells are not infective and therefore do not produce necrosis in these systems. Their infiltration causes enlargement, particularly of the spleen, and disturbs functioning of those organs.

The severity of the disease varies from asymptomatic disease (usually in children) to severe systemic and localized organ involvement. Lymphadenopathy, splenomegaly, and exudative pharyngitis are characteristic. More serious manifestations of the disease include hepatitis, pneumonitis, and central nervous system involvement.

Saliva remains infective for 18 months despite the development of EBV-specific antibodies early in the disease. The virus can be cultured from the throats of 10% to 20% of normal, healthy adults, suggesting that the disease may be contracted from asymptomatic viral shedders.

COMPLICATIONS

Splenic rupture	Pericarditis
Hemolytic anemia	Orchitis
Agranulocytosis	Encephalitis
Thrombocytopenic purpura	Hepatitis

NURSING CARE

See pages 122 to 127.

Table 6-3

OVERVIEW OF HEMATOLYMPHATIC INFECTIOUS DISEASES

	Mononucleosis	Cytomegalovirus infections	Toxoplasmosis
Occurrence	Worldwide; highest in adolescents and young adults in developed countries; asymptomatic infection in children	Worldwide; many asymptomatic infections; congenital infection may be severe	Worldwide; common in humans, mammals, and birds; many asymptomatic infections; congenital infection may be severe
Etiologic agent	Epstein-Barr virus (EBV), one of the herpesviruses	Cytomegalovirus (CMV)—one of the herpesviruses	*Toxoplasma gondii*, a protozoan
Reservoir	Humans and possibly primates	Humans	Cats; other mammals and birds are intermediate hosts
Transmission	Direct contact with saliva; through blood transfusions	Direct contact with secretions and excretions; through blood transfusions, breast milk, and cervical secretions, and transplacentally	Transplacental if mother has active infection; eating infective meat; water contaminated with cat feces

DIAGNOSTIC STUDIES AND FINDINGS

Diagnostic Test	Findings
Differential white blood count	Lymphocytes and monocytes >50%, with more than 10% being atypical lymphocytes
Leukocyte count	Normal early in disease; rises to 12,000 to 20,000/mm^3 in second week; occasionally rises to 50,000/mm^3
Serology: heterophil agglutination antibody tests (rapid forms of this test are Monospot, Monoscreen, and Monotest—all commercially prepared kits)	Heterophil antibody titer >1:40 to 1:128 (depending on laboratory), usually by end of first week; usually disappears by fourth week, although disappearance may be delayed May be false negative reactions to this test If the heterophil antibody test is negative but there is strong clinical evidence for mononucleosis, the EBV-specific antibody tests may be performed (both IgM antibodies and IgG antibodies are present early in the disease)
EBV-specific antibody tests: immunofluorescence	Elevated EBV-IgM antibody titers of 1:80 to 1:160; may be false positive reactions; titers drop rapidly after clinical disease Elevated EBV-IgG antibody: 1:80 is suggestive; persists for life; titer >1:5 suggests immunity
Liver function tests	
Serum transaminases (AST [SGOT], ALT [SGPT])	All elevated in hepatic involvement; two to three times upper normal limits
Bilirubin	Elevated with hepatic involvement
Throat culture	Positive for group A hemolytic streptococci in 10% of patients; EBV may be cultured from oropharyngeal secretions; cultures are not routinely available
Platelet count (in complications)	<140,000/mm^3 occurs frequently; <1,000/mm^3 in severe complications

Table 6-3

OVERVIEW OF HEMATOLYMPHATIC INFECTIOUS DISEASES—cont'd

	Mononucleosis	Cytomegalovirus infections	Toxoplasmosis
Incubation period	4-6 wks	Unknown; 3-8 wks following transfusion; in neonate, 3-12 wks following delivery-produced infection	Unknown; probably between 5-23 days
Period of communicability	Prolonged; pharyngeal excretion may persist for years; 15%-20% of adults are carriers	Virus excreted in saliva and urine for months to years	Not directly transmitted except transplacentally; cysts in infected meat remain infective as long as meat is edible and uncooked
Susceptibility and resistance	General; infection confers a high degree of resistance	General; fetuses, immunosuppressed individuals, and those with other chronic disease have more severe symptoms	General, but risk for infection increases with age; immunity after infection persists indefinitely
Report to local health authority	No	No	In some states

Data from Benenson.[3]

MEDICAL MANAGEMENT

DRUG THERAPY

Corticosteroids:
 Prednisone (Deltasone, others), 30 mg/day in divided doses, decreasing for 5 days, for severe neurologic complications, airway obstruction, thrombocytopenic purpura, or hemolytic anemia

GENERAL MANAGEMENT

Bed rest during acute stage
Saline throat gargle
Aspirin or acetaminophen for sore throat and fever

SURGERY

For splenic rupture: surgical removal of the spleen

Reference: 129.

CYTOMEGALOVIRUS INFECTIONS

Cytomegalovirus infections are extremely common viral infections that are ordinarily asymptomatic. Clinical disease in the adult resembles mononucleosis. Congenital and perinatal acquired infections are serious in the neonate and lead to irreversible CNS damage.

PATHOPHYSIOLOGY

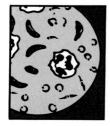

The cytomegalovirus (CMV), with several antigenically related strains, is a member of the herpesvirus group and has characteristics common to other herpesviruses. Like the Epstein-Barr herpesvirus, CMV produces a frequently asymptomatic mononucleosis-type infection in children and adults. CMV is similar to herpes types 1 and 2 in that it remains latent in body tissue and has the potential for producing recurrent infection. CMV, like herpes types 1 and 2, also crosses the placental barrier and is shed in cervical secretions. Therefore it has the potential for producing congenital infection with severe congenital anomalies and perinatal infection acquired during vaginal delivery. Like herpes type 2, the CMV is suspected of having oncogenic properties.

CMV can be found in all body secretions, including saliva, blood, urine, semen, cervical secretions, and breast milk, even in the presence of CMV-specific antibodies. Transmission requires prolonged direct contact with secretions. Although the exact mechanism for postnatal transmission is not known, sexual, oral, and blood transfusion transmission is suspected in postnatal-acquired infections.

Regardless of the mode of transmission, CMV may invade the cells of most tissues in the body. An inflammatory response with focal tissue destruction, areas of calcification, and hyperplasia of the reticuloendothelial system develops. Typical cellular lesions are characterized by enlarged cells containing intranuclear and cytoplasmic inclusion bodies. These lesions are disseminated widely, particularly in the brain, liver, lungs, kidney, and spleen.

A humoral and cell-mediated anti-CMV antibody response occurs. The response does not appear to alter the course of the spread of the virus from cell to cell or alter the presence of the virus in body secretions. Nor do circulating maternal antibodies in the fetus appear to impede the infectious process or the development of congenital anomalies.

Dependent on the mode of transmission, three different forms of the infection have been

See Table 6-3, pages 116-117, for an overview of cytomegalovirus infections.

identified: congenital-, perinatal-, and postnatal-acquired. All three forms can either be asymptomatic or occur as a mild or severe clinical disease.

Congenital CMV infection is acquired by transplacental transmission, usually resulting from a primary infection the mother acquired during pregnancy. Of infants with congenital infections, 95% are asymptomatic at birth. Maternal antibodies are present in cord blood at birth, and the virus can be detected in the infant's urine until age 15 months. In utero viral invasion is most destructive to the developing fetal central nervous system, particularly the cerebellum and cerebral cortex, leading to microcephaly and/or severe motor or mental retardation. The infant born with symptomatic CMV infection has evidence of a severe generalized infection plus symptoms of organ involvement of the liver, lung, kidney, or eye. This extraneural organ involvement is usually self-limited. If the child lives, there are invariably neurologic sequelae. Congenital CMV infections need to be differentiated diagnostically from toxoplasmosis, rubella, herpes, hemolytic anemias, and bacterial sepsis.

Perinatal infection is acquired at delivery from a serologic positive mother who had either a primary infection during pregnancy or a reactivation of a latent infection. Cervical secretions of CMV are high during the last trimester, having increased as the pregnancy progressed. Perinatally infected infants develop signs of infection (virus in urine and an antibody response with or without clinical evidence of organ involvement) 4 to 8 weeks following birth. The long-term effects on neurologic development are unknown.

Postnatal acquired infection requires close contact with body secretions containing the virus, usually from an asymptomatic person. Blood transfusions and renal and bone marrow transplants (possibly because of immunosuppression) have been linked with CMV transmission. Sexual transmission and kissing are also suspected as modes of transmission. The disease may be asymptomatic, or there may be symptoms of liver and lung involvement or a mononucleosis-like syndrome. There is no evidence of chronic organ impairment in acquired CMV infections. Primary or reactivation infection can be severe and life-threatening in the immunosuppressed individual.

COMPLICATIONS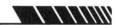

To immunocompromised: Progressive pneumonitis, hemolytic anemia, purpura, GI ulceration, hepatitis, and pericarditis

To neonate infected in utero: Neurologic defects (e.g., microcephaly, psychomotor retardation, and severe mental retardation)

DIAGNOSTIC STUDIES AND FINDINGS

Diagnostic Test	Findings
Cell culture of urine specimen, oral secretions, cervical secretions, or biopsy tissue	Positive for specific cytopathic effect of CMV
	Presence of CMV in infant's urine at birth suggests congenital infection
Biopsy of liver tissue	Histologic evidence of typical inclusion bodies
Complement fixation	Presence of IgG antibody in infant blood during first 6 months represents maternal antibodies; levels persisting after 6 months suggest congenital CMV infection
	Fourfold rise in titer in adult or child suggests current infection
	Very specific test with few false positive results
Indirect fluorescent antibody, immunofluorescence, anticomplement immunofluorescent test	Presence of IgM in cord blood at birth suggests congenital CMV infection
	Elevated titer in adult or child suggests current infection
	These tests are more sensitive and detect antibodies earlier in infection
Serum transaminase (AST)	Elevated in CMV hepatitis but rarely >800 U
Platelets	May be as few as 5,000/mm^3
Differential WBC count	Increase in lymphocytes, many atypical
Differential diagnosis: heterophil agglutination	Negative in CMV (positive in mononucleosis)

MEDICAL MANAGEMENT

DRUG THERAPY

Results of clinical trials using antiviral drugs, corticosteroids, or immune globulins in treating CMV infections are equivocal

GENERAL MANAGEMENT

Transfusion of sedimented RBCs for anemia
Transfusion of platelet-rich plasma for thrombocytopenia
Antipyretics for fever in CMV mononucleosis-like syndrome
Experimental live CMV vaccines currently being evaluated for prevention
Infants born of antibody-free mothers should not receive breast milk from a woman serologically positive for CMV antibodies, since the virus may be in the milk

References: 89, 94, 100.

NURSING CARE

See pages 122 to 127.

TOXOPLASMOSIS

Toxoplasmosis is a systemic protozoan infection, ranging from subclinical to severe to chronic. Four different clinical syndromes can be identified, depending on where the pathogen localizes in the body. Transplacental transmission results in cogenital toxoplasmosis, which may be fatal to the fetus or neonate.

PATHOPHYSIOLOGY

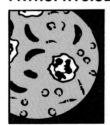

Toxoplasmosis, like the cytomegalovirus (CMV) infections, may be congenital or acquired. Unlike CMV, there is not a risk for perinatal acquired toxoplasmosis. Both forms of toxoplasmosis may be present, with clinical patterns ranging from subclinical infection to severe generalized infection (with neurologic and sensory sequelae) to death. Both may occur in latent or recurring forms under conditions of reduced host defenses.

The pathogen producing toxoplasmosis, *Toxoplasma gondii,* is a protozoan that is pathogenic to animals and humans. The pathogen can multiply only in living cells. This parasite exists in three forms: trophozoites, tissue cysts, and oocysts. Trophozoites are capable of invading, multiplying in, and necrotizing all host cells. Trophozoites can remain viable extracellularly in body secretions such as peritoneal fluid, breast milk, urine, saliva, or tears for a few hours to days. They cannot survive drying, heating, freezing, or contact with digestive juices.

Tissue cysts are formed within host cells. A surrounding membrane produced by the pathogen encapsulates up to 3,000 organisms. This enables the parasites to maintain their viability for the life of the host in spite of circulating host antibodies. Tissue cysts are responsible for recurrent infection in humans and for transmission of the pathogen from animal reservoirs. Tissue cysts also cannot survive freezing, drying, or heating.

Oocysts are a form in the life cycle of *T. gondii* that occur only in cats. Oocysts, a noninfectious form, are discharged in the feces of infected cats. Oocysts sporulate in 1 to 21 days in environmental temperatures of 4° to 37° C (39° to 99° F). They can remain infectious in the soil for 1 year, given favorable environmental conditions.

Transmission of *T. gondii* can occur by one of two modes: by ingestion of tissue cysts in uncooked meat or ingestion of sporulated oocysts by hands or food contaminated with cat feces, or by transplacental transmission of trophozoites in maternal circulation during acute infection acquired by the mother during the pregnancy.

See Table 6-3, pages 116-117, for an overview of Toxoplasmosis.

In ingestion-acquired toxoplasmosis the capsule surrounding ingested cysts is digested by gastric juices. This permits viable trophozoites to invade intestinal mucosa and to disseminate throughout the body by way of blood and the lymphatics. Organ cell invasion produces foci of necrosis surrounded by intense inflammatory reaction with mononuclear cell infiltration. The spleen, liver, brain, lung, myocardium, and eye are most frequently involved. The development of cysts and tissue calcifications may impair organ functioning.

An early antibody response destroys many parasites before they form tissue cysts and supports cyst formation by the remainder. Thus the infection is limited to its mild or subclinical form for the majority of infected persons. Failure of an immune response, as is the case with immunosuppressed patients or those with debilitating disease, is more likely to result in progressive, life-threatening infection with multiple organ involvement and extensive damage.

Transplacentally transmitted *T. gondii* is disseminated to every organ in the developing fetus, particularly to the brain, heart, lungs, adrenal glands, striated muscle, and eye. Focal necrotic and inflammatory lesions are produced with cyst formation and calcification. Extensive destruction may occur in the central nervous system, affecting the cortex, subcortical white matter, caudate and lenticular nuclei, midbrain, pons, medulla, and spinal cord. Obstruction of the foramina of Monro or the aqueduct of Sylvius may result in an internal hydrocephalus.

Infection in the eye produces edema and necrosis of the retina, necrosis and disruption of the pigmented layer of the rods and cones, and infiltration of the retina and choroid with inflammatory cells. Granulation tissue and exudate may spread to the vitreous. This chorioretinitis may be manifested within weeks after birth or at some time later in life when the latent infection becomes reactivated.

Maternal infection early in the pregnancy is usually associated with fetal death or severe disease at birth. Infection later in pregnancy results in less severe or no manifestations at birth. Only 11% of maternal infections result in infants damaged at birth. The majority, 60% of infants, are not affected; 29% have subclinical infections that are manifest as neurologic or sensory defects as the infant develops.

COMPLICATIONS

Spontaneous abortion
Microcephalus, hydrocephalus, or other CNS impairment in neonate
Chorioretinitis
Multiple organ involvement in immunocompromised patients
Encephalitis

NURSING CARE

See pages 122 to 127.

DIAGNOSTIC STUDIES AND FINDINGS

Diagnostic Test	Findings
Inoculation of mice with specimens from blood, spinal fluid, lymph nodes, muscle tissue; morphologic examination of mouse tissue after 4 weeks	Identification of *T. gondii* cysts or trophozoites in mouse tissue is presumptive evidence of present infection
Electron microscopic examination of tissue sections or smears	Identification of trophozoites present during acute infection; identification of cysts does not differentiate between acute or chronic infection
Indirect fluorescent antibody test or Sabin-Feldman dye test*	IgG antibodies (1:4) appear within 1 to 2 wks after acute infection; reach high titers (> 1:1,000) in 6-8 wks and then gradually decline over months or years to titers of 1:4-1:64
	False positive results may follow blood transfusions. Fourfold rise in titers or slow decline after the peak is diagnostic. A rapid decline in these antibodies in the neonate suggests the presence of maternal antibodies and the absence of infant infection. A titer of 1:256 at 4 months suggests congenital infection
Indirect hemagglutination test*	Becomes positive for IgG antibodies (1:16) in 2-4 weeks; reaches peak (1:1,000) in 8-16 wks and stays positive longer (1:16 to 1:64). There are many false negative results in congenital toxoplasmosis. Fourfold rise in titer is diagnostic
IgM fluorescent antibody test*	Detects IgM antibodies (1:10) in 5 days, which peak (1:80) in 2-4 wks. These antibodies decrease (1:10 to 1:40) during convalescence and are negative in 3 wks-4 months.
	Test is useful for diagnosing acute infection.
	Persistent IgM antibodies in neonate suggest active infection; a rapid drop suggests maternal antibodies
RIA, agglutination tests, and ELISA*	Detects both IgG and IgM antibodies
	Detects antigen in human sera
Cerebrospinal fluid	Congenital: protein: 2,000 mg/dl; increase in RBC and WBC counts
	Acquired: glucose and protein normal

*These tests may show false negative results in immunosuppressed hosts.

MEDICAL MANAGEMENT

DRUG THERAPY

Sulfadiazine (or sulfamerazine and sulfamethazine) in combination with pyrimethamine synergistically affects trophozoites but not cysts. Treatment does not prevent recurrence of chorioretinitis. It is indicated for severe, protracted disease, for those with chorioretinitis, for immunosuppressed individuals, and for active infections in newborns. Pyrimethamine is contraindicated for pregnant women.

Antiinfective agents: Sulfadiazine (Suladyne), or triple sulfonamides orally for 4 wks, initial dose of 50-75 mg/kg followed by 75-100 mg/day in 2-4 equal doses; **infants:** initial dose of 75-100 mg/kg followed by 100-150 mg/kg/day in four equal doses.
Pyrimethamine (Daraprim), for 4 wk, initial dose 100-200 mg/day in 2 divided doses for 2 days, followed by 1 mg/kg/day in two divided doses (maximum: 25-50 mg/day or every other day); **children:** first 2-3 days: 2 mg/kg/day in two divided doses, followed by 1 mg/kg/day in two divided doses.

Vitamins: Folinic acid (calcium leucovorin), IM or orally, 2-10 mg/day to prevent bone marrow suppression; 6-10 mg/day if platelets are less than 100,000/mm.^{3}
Baker's yeast, three or four cakes/day.

GENERAL MANAGEMENT

To prevent spread, reject leukocyte or organ donors who are antibody positive.

References: 68, 100, 106.

1 ASSESS

	OBSERVATIONS		
ASSESSMENT	MONONUCLEOSIS	CYTOMEGALOVIRUS INFECTION	TOXOPLASMOSIS
History	Contact with person with mononucleosis	Immunosuppression	Exposure to cat feces; immunosuppression
Subjective symptoms	Fatigue, anorexia, chills, retroorbital headache, photophobia, dysphagia	Fatigue, nausea, myalgia, headache, photophobia	Fatigue and malaise 6-10 days preceding other symptoms; headache; photophobia
Body temperature	Marked elevation (1-2 wks) 38° to 41°C (100° to 105°F), peaks in afternoon	Low-grade fever lasting 2-5 wks	Fever up to 41°C (106°F)
Eye	Periorbital edema	Retinitis	Chorioretinitis: blurred vision, pain, loss of central vision

ASSESSMENT	OBSERVATIONS		
	MONONUCLEOSIS	CYTOMEGALOVIRUS INFECTION	TOXOPLASMOSIS
Throat	Painful, exudative tonsillitis (white or greenish gray), pasty membrane with bad odor; inflammation and tonsillar edema may be severe	No involvement	No involvement
Oral cavity	Bleeding gums, palatine petechiae	No involvement	No involvement
Lymph nodes	Cervical, submandibular, and axillary node discrete enlargement and tenderness	No involvement	Generalized lymphadenopathy: firm, smooth, discrete, movable enlarged nodes; tenderness, or may be painless
Abdomen	Splenomegaly; hepatomegaly	Splenomegaly; hepatomegaly	Splenomegaly
Skin	Jaundice, macular rash, or purpura	Rubelliform rash	Generalized bright red or pink maculopapular rash, blanching on pressure
Respiratory	Symptoms of pneumonia	Cough or symptoms of pneumonia	Coarse rales, cough, dyspnea, cyanosis
Neurologic	Meningitis or encephalitis	Sensory and motor weakness, pyramidal tract signs	Encephalitis: convulsions, ataxia, vomiting, confusion
Other		Myocarditis	Symptoms of myocarditis
Congenital		Jaundice, petechial rash; hepatosplenomegaly; lethargy; microcephaly; respiratory distress; retardation; chorioretinitis; seizures	Hydrocephalus or microcephalus; convulsions; pneumonitis; jaundice, purpura, petechial or maculopapular rash; bilateral chorioretinitis; hepatomegaly, splenomegaly

2 DIAGNOSE

NURSING DIAGNOSIS	SUPPORTIVE ASSESSMENT FINDINGS
Potential for infection (patient contacts) related to methods of transmission of EBV and CMV	Laboratory findings positive for organism
Hyperthermia related to infection	Chills, malaise, headache; fever
Pain related to inflammation and fever	Headache, tender lymph nodes, dysphagia (mono); pharyngeal inflammation and edema (mono)

→ > >

NURSING DIAGNOSIS	SUPPORTIVE ASSESSMENT FINDINGS
Activity intolerance related to fatigue	Fatigue, malaise; fever; altered laboratory values
Ineffective breathing pattern related to pneumonitis	Dyspnea, cough, rales, cyanosis
Potential for injury related to splenomegaly and to antiinfective agents prescribed for toxoplasmosis	Splenomegaly; thrombocytopenia; administration of pyrimethamine
Sensory-perceptual alterations (visual) related to chorioretinitis of CMV and toxoplasmosis	Blurred vision, photophobia, loss of central vision in toxoplasmosis

Other related nursing diagnoses
Additional nursing diagnoses are related to congenital CMV and toxoplasmosis. Care of the neonate is beyond the scope of this book.
For care of patients with encephalitis, see Chapter 4.

3 PLAN

Patient goals

1. Infection with EBV or CMV will not be transmitted to patient contacts.
2. Body temperature will be maintained within the normal range. Comfort and safety will be maintained for patients experiencing fever.
3. Patient will obtain relief from pain.
4. Patient will achieve adequate rest to conserve energy during active disease and will return to preillness level of activity during convalescence.
5. Patient will demonstrate normal respiratory pattern, oxygen intake, and blood gas levels.
6. Patient will not experience injury from splenic rupture.
7. Patient will not be confused or frightened by environmental stimuli during time of alteration in vision; visual function will return to normal.
8. Patient with toxoplasmosis will be able to self-administer antiinfective agents as prescribed.

4 IMPLEMENT

NURSING DIAGNOSIS	NURSING INTERVENTIONS	RATIONALE
Potential for infection (patient contacts) related to methods of transmission of CMV	Employ secretion precautions for hospitalized infants known to be shedding CMV.	To prevent transmission of CMV or mono.
	Women of childbearing age or who are pregnant should wash hands thoroughly after handling diapers of neonates with congenital CMV.	To prevent acquiring CMV infection.
Hyperthermia related to infection	See inside back cover, Interventions 1-15.	
Pain related to inflammation and fever	Administer analgesics per order or saline gargle for sore throat.	To relieve pain.

NURSING DIAGNOSIS	NURSING INTERVENTIONS	RATIONALE
Activity intolerance related to fatigue	Encourage bed rest during acute symptomatic disease.	To conserve energy.
	Assist patient in developing a realistic plan for returning to work or school during convalescence following mono.	Prolonged malaise accompanying these diseases may be unanticipated.
Ineffective breathing pattern related to pneumonitis	Assess ventilation to include evaluation of breathing rate, rhythm, and depth; chest expansion; presence of respiratory distress (e.g., dyspnea, shortness of breath, nasal flaring, pursed-lip breathing, prolonged expiratory phase, use of accessory muscles, or adventitious sounds.)	To detect pneumonitis, which is a potential complication of these infections, particularly in the immunocompromised.
	Maintain patient in position that facilitates ventilation (head of bed in semi-Fowler's position or patient sitting and leaning forward on overbed table).	To facilitate lung expansion for improved air exchange.
	Instruct patient in proper pulmonary hygiene routines.	To promote easy effective breathing, facilitate removal of secretions from tracheobronchial tree, and minimize pulmonary congestion, which could lead to superinfections.
	Assess patient for tiring in relation to attempts to breathe. Assist ventilation if necessary. Administer O_2.	To provide adequate intake of O_2.
	Protect patient from known sources of secondary infection.	Secondary bacterial infections are common with these patients.
	Administer antiinfectives as prescribed.	To control progression of the pneumonitis.
Potential for injury related to splenomegaly and to antiinfective agents prescribed for toxoplasmosis	Monitor for signs of neurologic or purpuric complications.	To detect splenic rupture.
	Protect patient from activity.	To reduce risk of splenic rupture.
Sensory-perceptual alterations (visual) related to chorioretinitis of CMV and toxoplasmosis	Provide a safe environment for patients with chorioretinitis. Assist patient with interpreting the environment, personal care, and ambulation as needed. Refer for rehabilitation for vision loss.	To prevent injury.

→ › ›

5   EVALUATE

PATIENT OUTCOME	DATA INDICATING THAT OUTCOME IS REACHED
Infection will not be transmitted	Patient demonstrates behavior to prevent transmission of pathogens to others. Health care team washes hands after providing care to each patient and follows universal blood and body secretion procedures with all patients. Health care staff remain free of signs of infection.
Body temperature is maintained within normal range. Patient comfort and safety are maintained.	See inside back cover.
Patient obtains relief from pain	Patient swallows without pain. Patient's sleep is uninterrupted by pain. Patient rests in bed without overt signs of pain.
Patient achieves adequate rest to conserve energy during active disease and returns to preillness level of activity during convalescence	Patient maintains bed rest during acute disease, with gradual return of activity. No fatigue with exertion during convalescence.
Patient demonstrates normal respiratory pattern, oxygen intake, and blood gas levels	Bronchovesicular breath sounds are heard throughout lungs. There are no areas of decreased breath sounds or consolidation. Respiratory rate is normal. CO_2, Po_2, and Pco_2 are normal.
Patient does not experience injury	Spleen is nonpalpable and nontender. Leukocyte, lymphocyte, and platelet counts, bilirubin level, and serum transaminase (SGOT, SGPT) levels are normal.
Patient is not confused or frightened by environmental stimuli during time of alteration in vision; visual function returns to normal	Persons with vision loss are aware of counseling, support, or rehabilitation resources and have phone numbers and names of people to contact at those services.
Patient self-administers antiinfective agents as prescribed	Patient completes full course of antiinfective therapy. No preventable drug interactions or allergic reactions are experienced. If untoward reactions are experienced, the patient discontinues the drug and contacts the physician immediately.

PATIENT TEACHING

Instruct patients with infectious mononucleosis or CMV:

1. Although complete bed rest is usually unnecessary during acute disease or convalescence, the patient caring for himself or herself at home should be encouraged to rest as symptoms dictate. Convalescence may be as long as 3 to 4 weeks.
2. The patient with splenomegaly should avoid heavy lifting, contact sports, or any activity that may increase the risk of injury to the spleen. Active children must be protected from injury.
3. Report to physician any jaundice, excess bruising or bleeding, or symptoms of abnormal central nervous system functioning.
4. EB virus is transmitted by contact with saliva; CMV is transmitted by contact with all body secretions and excretions.

Instruct patients with toxoplasmosis:

1. Patients treated with pyrimethamine (which depresses bone marrow) should have peripheral blood cell and platelet counts twice a week during therapy. Explain medication regimen, particularly the use of folinic acid and/or baker's yeast to counteract effects of pyrimethamine.
2. Immunocompromised persons and pregnant women can avoid exposure by cooking all meat to 60°C (140°F), washing fruits and vegetables, washing hands thoroughly after handling uncooked meat, wearing gloves while working in soil, and avoiding cat feces. Children's sandboxes should be kept free of cat feces.
3. Infants born with asymptomatic toxoplasmosis should be evaluated periodically for visual problems and developmental delays.
4. Refer families of infants with congenital toxoplasmosis to counseling, support, or rehabilitation resources as needed. Provide information about the resource and its services and how to access the resource.
5. The congenital anomalies do not represent a hereditary defect.
6. There is not a risk for congenital toxoplasmosis in subsequent pregnancies. The risk is only present when toxoplasmosis is acquired during the pregnancy.

CHAPTER 7

Respiratory Infectious Diseases

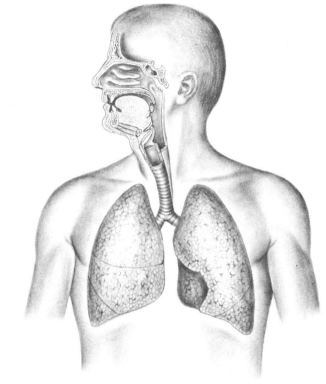

The respiratory infectious diseases discussed in this chapter are those acute and chronic respiratory pathologic conditions that are caused by a specific pathogenic agent that is transmitted by inhalation or by direct contact with infectious respiratory secretions. Although diphtheria, pertussis, polio, and measles fit this definition, they are discussed in this chapter under vaccine-preventable infectious diseases. Rheumatic fever and scarlet fever are discussed here because their etiologic agent, the group A streptococcus, which causes streptococcal throat infection, is transmitted through respiratory secretions (Table 7-1).

Streptococcal Throat, Scarlet Fever, Rheumatic Fever

Streptococcal throat is an acute exudative tonsillitis or pharyngitis caused by group A beta-hemolytic streptococci. Coincident or subsequent otitis media or peritonsillar abscess may be present. Rheumatic fever, chorea, and acute glomerulonephritis are possible sequelae.

Scarlet fever is a group A beta-hemolytic streptococcal disease characterized by a skin rash. It occurs when the infecting strain of streptococcus produces a toxin, causing a sensitivity reaction in the infected host.

Clinical characteristics may include those of streptococcal sore throat plus enanthem, strawberry tongue, and exanthem.

Rheumatic fever is a sequela of group A streptococcal infection of the upper respiratory tract, occurring in about 2.8% of those having a streptococcal throat infection. The condition is thought to result from an altered immune reaction to the streptococcus organism. Rheumatic heart disease is a potential complication.

Table 7-1

OVERVIEW OF STREPTOCOCCAL THROAT, SCARLET FEVER, AND RHEUMATIC FEVER

	Streptococcal throat	Scarlet fever (SF)	Rheumatic fever (RF)
Occurrence	More common in temperate zones; may be endemic, epidemic, or sporadic in occurrence; highest in late winter or spring; ages 3-15 years most often affected; no sex or racial difference		Increase in outbreaks since 1984
Etiologic agent	*Streptococcus pyogenes* (group A streptococcus of approximately 70 serologically distinct types)	Three erythrogenic toxins	Group A beta-hemolytic streptococcus (GABHS)
Reservoir	Humans	Humans	Humans
Transmission	Direct or intimate contact with patient or carrier; may follow ingestion of contaminated food	Contact with respiratory secretions containing *Streptococcus*	Contact with respiratory secretions containing *Streptococcus*
Incubation period	1-3 days	2-4 days (range: 1-7 days)	3-35 days after clinical strep throat (average: 19 days)
Period of communicability	Untreated, uncomplicated cases: 10-21 days; complicated: weeks to months; antibiotic treated: 24-48 h	Not communicable	Not communicable
Susceptibility and resistance	General; many develop antitoxic or antibacterial immunity to one of the types of streptococci through inapparent infection	Permanent acquired immunity from active disease with type of toxin; second attacks due to different toxin	Persons who have suffered one attack are predisposed to a recurrent episode following group A streptococcal upper respiratory infections
Report to local health authority	Epidemics only	Epidemics only	Case report in some states

Data from Benenson.[3]

PATHOPHYSIOLOGY

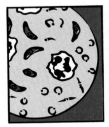

Infection with group A streptococci results in a number of related clinical disease entities, such as streptococcal throat, scarlet fever, and erysipelas, and nonsuppurative complications, such as nephritis and rheumatic fever. The type of disease resulting from group A streptococci depends on the site of tissue invasion, the antigenic characteristics of the infecting strain of streptococcus, and the immune status of the host. There are approximately 75 serologically distinct strains of group A streptococci, producing a variety of different enzymes and at least three different erythrogenic toxins. These antigenic characteristics determine the type of enzyme-specific and toxin-specific antibodies produced by the host. A host with adequate antibodies against a particular serotype with or without antitoxic immunity may develop no clinical disease if reinfected with the same serotype. A person with antitoxic immunity resulting from previous group A infections but with no antibodies against a particular invading serotype may develop a clinical streptococcal throat. A person with no antitoxic immunity and no antibodies against an invading toxigenic group A streptococcus may develop clinical scarlet fever. In all clinical streptococcal disease a leukocytosis is present.

Streptococcal Throat

Streptococcal throat (septic sore throat) results when the streptococcus invades and remains in the lymphoid tissue of the oropharynx, rapidly producing inflammation with edema, erythema, and infiltration with polymorphonuclear leukocytes. The mucosal surfaces, particularly over the tonsils, become ulcerated, releasing a mucopurulent exudate. Cervical lymphade-

For picture of streptococcal throat, see color plates 32 and 33, page xv.

nopathy is present. Severity of symptoms increases with age. Untreated, uncomplicated disease lasts a few days to a week. The streptococcus may invade surrounding tissue producing suppurative complications (see Complications).

Scarlet Fever

For picture of scarlet fever rash, see color plate 34, page xv.

Scarlet fever results if the invading streptococcus releases an erythrogenic toxin stimulating a sensitivity reaction in the host. Dilation of small capillaries and toxic injury of the vascular epithelium may be widespread in the body, particularly in the liver, myocardium, and kidneys. The pathologic changes are most visible on the skin, with an erythematous rash and desquamation, and in the oral cavity, with the strawberry tongue and an enanthem. Hepatocellular damage and destruction of red cells may result in jaundice, increase in bilirubin, mild anemia, and an increase in reticulocytes. In rare situations, toxins may be disseminated in the bloodstream, producing a severe toxic illness. Streptococcus may invade adjacent tissue and the bloodstream, producing a severe septic scarlet fever.

In severe cases of scarlet fever, septic scarlet fever or toxic scarlet fever (also known as fulminating scarlet fever) may result. In septic scarlet fever the body temperature is elevated to 40° to 42°C (104° to 108°F), and the pulse becomes rapid and weak. Throat manifestations are more severe, with ulceration and perforation on the uvula, soft palate, and tonsils. Other findings include seropurulent or mucopurulent nasal discharge and excoriations on the lips, mouth, and nares. Breathing is labored because of swelling and occlusion.

In toxic scarlet fever the body temperature is 41° to 42°C (105° to 108°F) and the pulse is rapid. A bright punctate or erythematous hemorrhagic rash appears on the skin. Capillary fragility is evidenced by hematuria, epistaxis, and hematemesis. The oropharynx becomes edematous but without exudate. Other manifestations include intense headache and vomiting, symptoms of toxic myocarditis, and altered mental state (e.g., delirium, irrationality, or coma).

Rheumatic Fever

Rheumatic fever is a delayed complication of upper respiratory infection with group A streptococci, producing nonsuppurative inflammatory lesions in connective tissue of the heart, joints, subcutaneous tissues, and central nervous system. Symptoms may be present in all or some of those systems. The exact causal mechanism is not known. The following have been hypothesized: (1) there is direct tissue invasion by group A streptococci or by cell wall antigens of the microorganism; (2) strep-

tococcal enzymes, particularly streptolysins S or O, induce tissue injury; (3) antigen-humoral antibody reactions localize in affected tissue; and (4) an autoimmune reaction is operative. The autoimmune theory is supported by the detection of heart-reactive antibodies (HRAs) in the sera of patients with rheumatic heart disease. A genetic predisposition to this disease is suggested by the fact that rheumatic fever consistently affects only 0.3% (3.0% during epidemics)[81] of those with a clinical upper respiratory streptococcal infection. Additionally, 38% of persons with rheumatic fever have a positive family history for the disease.[21]

Cardiac connective tissue lesions show early fragmentation of collagen fibers, cellular lymphocytic infiltration, and fibrin deposits. These changes are followed by the development of the Aschoff nodule, a perivascular locus of inflammation with an area of central necrosis surrounded by large mononuclear and polymorphonuclear leukocytes. Cardiac findings include pericarditis, myocarditis, and left-sided endocarditis. Valvular lesions begin with edema and cellular infiltration of the leaflets and chordae with small verrucae forming along the closure lines. With healing the valves become thickened and deformed, the valve commissures become fused, and the chordae become shortened. These changes result in valvular stenosis and insufficiency, varying in extensiveness and severity. Carditis may result in long-term disability or death.

Joint lesions are characterized by a fibrinous exudate over the synovial membrane and a serous effusion without joint destruction. Subcutaneous nodules form that resemble the Aschoff nodules described above.

A later neurologic sequela of rheumatic fever is Sydenham's chorea. The latent period for this condition may be so long as to occur in the absence of laboratory changes associated with rheumatic fever.

COMPLICATIONS

Streptococcal throat	Scarlet fever
Peritonsillar cellulitis and abscess	Severe disseminated toxic illness
Retropharyngeal abscess	Septicemia
Sinus empyema	Hepatic damage
Otitis media	**Rheumatic fever**
Mastoiditis	Valvular heart disease
Meningitis	Congestive heart failure
Cervical lymphadenitis	Persistent arthritis
Pneumonia	
Periorbital abscess	
Toxin dissemination leading to rheumatic fever or nephritis	

DIAGNOSTIC STUDIES AND FINDINGS

Diagnostic Test	Findings
Streptococcal throat	
Culture of throat exudate	Positive for group A hemolytic streptococci (GABHS) (10 or more colonies) in 24-72 h
Rapid antigen tests	Positive for GABHS in 1-2 h
Scarlet fever	
Schultz-Charlton reaction skin test	Rash blanches at site of intradermal injection of antitoxin
Dick skin test for susceptibility	Erythema and induration >3 mm within 24 h of intradermal injection of 0.1 ml exotoxin; reaction is compared with control site, where 0.1 ml of a control substance is injected intradermally
Rheumatic fever	
Antistreptolysin O (ASO)	Increase in ASO suggests recent infection with *Streptococcus;* ASO peaks 2-5 wks after streptococcal infection and decreases thereafter; 80%-85% of patients with rheumatic fever develop ASO titers of 200 Todd U/ml or greater; ASO titers >1:85 in adults may be diagnostic
Anti-DNAse B (ADN-B) test	ADN-B develops later and persists longer than ASO; titers >1:85 in adults are diagnostic
Streptozyme test (a slide hemagglutination test)	Measures five different streptococcal enzymes; titers of 100-200 are equivocal; titers of 300 indicate recent streptococcal infection
C-reactive protein (CRP)	Normally not present in serum; presence of CRP in serum is diagnostic
Erythrocyte sedimentation rate	Elevated
ECG	Elongation of PR interval

MEDICAL MANAGEMENT

DRUG THERAPY

Antiinfective agents: Benzathine penicillin G (Bicillin), 1,200,000 U IM one time for adults.
Oral penicillin, 125-250 mg bid q 10 days, *or*
Procaine penicillin (Wycillin), 600,000 U IM q 10 days for severe scarlet fever.
Erythromycin (Erythrocin, others), 250 mg PO qid q 10 days for patients allergic to penicillin.

Antipyretic agents: Aspirin, 90-100 mg/kg/day q 2 wks; 60-70 mg/kg/day for subsequent 6 wks for treatment of polyarthritis of rheumatic fever.
Antipyretics for management of fever.

Corticosteroids: Prednisone (Deltasone, others), 40-60 mg/day q 2-3 wks for treatment of carditis, *or*
Methyl prednisone sodium succinate (Solu-Medrol), IV, in severe cases; decrease to complete withdrawal in 3 wks.

Antiinfective agents (to prevent recurrent streptococcal infections in postrheumatic fever patients): Benzathine penicillin G (Bicillin), 1,200,000 U IM q 4 wks during and following convalescence for life (recommended duration is controversial), *or*
Erythromycin (Erythrocin, others), 250 mg bid PO for those allergic to penicillin.

GENERAL MANAGEMENT

Bed rest during febrile stage of all streptococcal diseases; bed rest for 3 wks for patients without carditis; for an additional month after carditis is detected.
Nonstimulating environment and sedation for patients with chorea.
Fluid therapy as indicated.
Treatment of heart failure with O_2, salt restriction, diuretics, and digitalis.
To prevent transmission to others: secretion precautions of hospitalized patients with an upper respiratory streptococcal infection for 24 h following initiation of antibiotic therapy.

References: 76, 100, 150.

1 ASSESS

ASSESSMENT	OBSERVATIONS		
	STREPTOCOCCAL THROAT	SCARLET FEVER (SF)	RHEUMATIC FEVER (RF)
History	Contact with person with sore throat	Contact with person with sore throat	Untreated sore throat within past month; previous episode or family history of RF
Subjective symptoms	Pain on swallowing, headache, anorexia, malaise, chills; abdominal pain in children	Pain on swallowing, headache, anorexia, malaise, chills; abdominal pain in children	Malaise, abdominal pain
Body temperature	38°-39°C (100°-103°F)	38°-39°C (100°-103°F)	Low-grade fever: 38°C (100°F)
Cardiovascular	Rapid pulse	Rapid pulse	Insidious onset of symptoms of carditis within 3 wks: cardiac enlargement, pericardial friction rubs, congestive heart failure, signs of effusion, tachycardia, gallop rhythm, and diastolic and possibly systolic murmurs Three types of murmurs associated with acute carditis: (1) high-pitched blowing holosystolic apical murmur of mitral regurgitation, (2) low-pitched apical middiastolic flow murmur, (3) high-pitched decrescendo diastolic murmur of aortic regurgitation heard at the secondary and primary aortic areas Mitral and aortic stenotic murmurs associated with chronic rheumatic valvular disease
Head and neck	Enlarged, tender cervical lymph nodes; suppurative complications (mastoiditis, otitis media, periorbital abscess, sinus empyema)	Enlarged, tender cervical lymph nodes; suppurative complications (mastoiditis, otitis media, periorbital abscess, sinus empyema)	

ASSESSMENT	OBSERVATIONS		
	STREPTOCOCCAL THROAT	SCARLET FEVER (SF)	RHEUMATIC FEVER (RF)
Oropharynx	Edema, erythema (fiery red to dull red), and petechiae of uvula, tonsils, and posterior oropharynx Confluent, easily removable mucopurulent exudate May be suppurative complications	Edema, erythema (fiery red to dull red), and petechiae of uvula, tonsils, and posterior oropharynx Confluent, easily removable mucopurulent exudate May be suppurative complications	
Oral cavity		Tongue is inflamed and heavily coated at first; after the rash appears, the papillae become swollen and appear as red bumps on a gray background (strawberry tongue); within a few days the tongue peels, first at the tip and margins; by day 6 the tongue is completely denuded, beefy red, moist, and glistening (raspberry tongue); tongue returns to normal by the end of the second week Enanthem: for a few days around the time of rash, appearance on the skin there may be a hemorrhagic rash on the soft palate and anterior pillars of the fossae	
Respiratory	Complications: symptoms of pneumonia	Complications: symptoms of pneumonia	
Skin		Erythematous and punctate rash appearing within 2 days of streptococcal throat, becoming generalized rapidly; appearing first on upper chest and back and then on the lower back, upper extremities, abdomen, and lower extremities Extensiveness of rash is variable; it may be better felt (like sandpaper) than seen Petechiae may precede the rash on the lower extremities; more common in skin folds	One to two dozen firm, painless, variable in size (3 mm-2 cm), subcutaneous nodules; usually over bony prominences and tendons; lasting 1-2 wks Nonpruritic, erythematous macular eruption on the trunk or proximal extremities (erythema marginatum); lesions appear to be a vasomotor phenomenon, moving over the skin with a tendency to advance at the margins and clear at the center; individual lesions clear within hours, but the process persists intermittently for weeks or months

	OBSERVATIONS		
ASSESSMENT	STREPTOCOCCAL THROAT	SCARLET FEVER (SF)	RHEUMATIC FEVER (RF)
		Desquamation may develop between 5 days-4 wks after appearance of the rash, starting on the neck, upper chest, back, fingertips, or toes; skin peels in large sections, particularly on the palms and soles Flushing of cheeks with circumoral pallor	
Neurologic	Complications: symptoms of meningitis	Complications: symptoms of meningitis	Symptoms of chorea: involuntary, purposeless, rapid motions; irritability; emotional lability; weakness; restlessness/fretfulness, gradually increasing in intensity over 2 wks, reaching a plateau, and gradually subsiding
Musculoskeletal		Tender, slightly inflamed; edematous joints possible	Acute onset of mild to severe symptoms of polyarthritis: heat, swelling, redness, and severe tenderness affecting mainly the knees, ankles, elbows, and wrists; migratory, with multiple joint involvement at one time; inflammation subsides in each joint in 1-2 wks; entire episode subsides in 4 wks
Abdomen		Liver may be slightly enlarged and tender	

2 DIAGNOSE

NURSING DIAGNOSIS	SUPPORTIVE ASSESSMENT FINDINGS
Potential for infection (patient contacts) related to GABHS in pharyngeal exudate	History of contact with infected person; pharyngeal specimen positive for GABHS
Hyperthermia related to infectious process	Fever, chills, malaise, rapid pulse
Activity intolerance related to cardiovascular complications of RF and SF	Malaise and pain in joints; symptoms of carditis, sepsis, CNS involvement, or chorea; edema and erythema of joints; limited movement

NURSING DIAGNOSIS	SUPPORTIVE ASSESSMENT FINDINGS
Altered oral mucous membrane related to exudative infectious process of GABHS and inflammatory response to toxin in SF	Pain on swallowing; edema, erythema (fiery red to dull red), and petechiae of uvula, tonsils, and posterior oropharynx; mucopurulent exudate in oropharynx; inflamed, denuded tongue; hemorrhagic rash on soft palate

Other related nursing diagnoses

Severe or complicated disease: Decreased cardiac output, Impaired physical mobility, Impaired swallowing, Potential for injury, and Fluid volume deficit

3   PLAN

Patient goals

1. Infection will not be transmitted to patient's contacts.
2. Body temperature will be maintained within the normal range; comfort and safety will be maintained for patients experiencing fever.
3. Patient will achieve adequate rest to conserve energy during active disease and will return to preillness level of activity during convalescence.
4. Mucous membranes will return to prepathogenic state.
5. Patient will self-administer antiinfective agents as prescribed.
6. Complications will be prevented.

4   IMPLEMENT

NURSING DIAGNOSIS	NURSING INTERVENTIONS	RATIONALE
Potential for infection related to complications of streptococcal throat	Collect pharyngeal secretions for culture.	For diagnosis of *Streptococcus* organisms and proper interventions.
	Administer antibiotics as prescribed.	To prevent progression to SF or RF.
Potential for infection (patient contacts) related to GABHS in pharyngeal exudate	Maintain respiratory secretion precautions of hospitalized patients for 24 h after antibiotic therapy is initiated.	To prevent transmission to others.
Hyperthermia related to infectious process	See inside back cover.	
Activity intolerance related to cardiovascular complications of RF and SF	Maintain complete bed rest for SF and RF patients. Provide all care, including hygiene and feeding.	To conserve patient energy and prevent complications by relieving stress on the cardiovascular system.
Altered oral mucous membrane related to exudative infectious process of GABHS and inflammatory response to toxin in SF	Assess pharyngeal area	To detect hyperemia and exudate.
	Provide frequent oral fluids and oral hygiene. Provide high humidity in room. Lubricate lips and nares.	To promote comfort for patient.

→ > >

5 EVALUATE

PATIENT OUTCOME	DATA INDICATING THAT OUTCOME IS REACHED
Infection is not transmitted	All patient contacts are examined and treated for infection.
Body temperature is maintained within the normal range; comfort and safety are maintained	Body temperature is between 36°-38°C (96.8°-100°F). Pulse and respiration are normal. Skin is cool to touch and free of excess perspiration. Patient's clothing and bedding are dry. Patient is free of headache and malaise associated with the fever.
Patient achieves adequate rest during active disease and returns to preillness level of activity during convalescence	Patient maintains bed rest during acute disease with gradual return of activity. Patient does not experience fatigue on exertion.
Mucous membranes return to prepathogenic state	Mucous membranes are moist, with natural color. There is no edema, inflammation, or exudate in oropharynx. Exanthem and enanthem of scarlet fever are not present.
Patient self-administers antiinfective agents as prescribed	Patient completes full course of antiinfective therapy. No preventable drug interactions or allergic reactions are experienced. If untoward reactions are experienced, patient discontinues drug and contacts physician immediately.
Complications are prevented	Pulse rate is normal. ECG is normal. No murmurs are auscultated. There is no limitation of joint movement. Patient can move all joints without pain. Patient exhibits purposeful movement, indicating no signs of chorea.

PATIENT TEACHING

1. Oral antibiotics must be taken for prescribed length of time. Follow-up throat cultures may be necessary.
2. Compliance with prescribed long-term antibiotic therapy is necessary to minimize risk for recurrence of rheumatic fever with subsequent streptococcal infections.
3. Upper respiratory infections should be diagnosed and treated promptly in postrheumatic fever patients.
4. Continued rest during convalescence is necessary for postrheumatic fever patients.
5. Medical monitoring for cardiac complications is necessary after rheumatic fever.
6. Persons with residual rheumatic valvular disease must follow an antimicrobial regimen whenever they undergo dental or surgical procedures that would increase their risk for bacteremia.

Histoplasmosis

Histoplasmosis is a pulmonary and systemic infection, similar to tuberculosis, resulting from inhalation of the spores of *Histoplasma capsulatum*, which are frequently found in the soil. Infection is common, but overt clinical disease is rare. Five clinical forms of the disease have been recognized.

PATHOPHYSIOLOGY

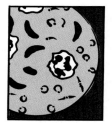

Spores of *H. capsulatum*, a fungus, are inhaled when soil containing them is disturbed. A lesion is formed within the lung parenchyma where the spores convert to a yeast phase and are phagocytosed by macrophages. Lesions may also be formed in the hilar or mediastinal lymph nodes as a result of migration of yeast-laden macrophages to those areas. Dissemination and lesion formation may also occur in the spleen and liver. These primary lesions become necrotic at the center, build up a fibrotic capsule, and frequently calcify. In most cases where calcification occurs there is no reactivation of the infection and the host manifests no symptoms except an immune response to histoplasmin.

Four other clinical forms of the disease are possible: acute benign respiratory disease, acute disseminated disease, chronic disseminated disease, and chronic pulmonary disease. In acute benign respiratory disease the primary pulmonary lesion remains active, resulting in a spreading infiltration pneumonia. In acute disseminated disease, inflammatory and necrotic lesions may result in septic-type fever, hepatosplenomegaly, severe prostration, and death. Chronic disseminated histoplasmosis results when there is extensive invasion by yeast-laden macrophages via the reticuloendothelial system to bone marrow, spleen, liver, and lungs. The inflammatory and necrotic reaction in those tissues is subacute but progressive and may eventually result in death. Chronic pulmonary histoplasmosis is manifest as a progressive emphysema. Fluid-filled cysts surrounded by chronic inflammation progress through stages of caseation necrosis and cavitation, continuing to disseminate the yeast through pulmonary tissue.

The clinical symptoms are quite varied but are generally more severe in infants, immunosuppressed persons, and chronically debilitated persons.

HISTOPLASMOSIS

Occurrence: Worldwide; higher in eastern and central United States; increases with age to 30 years; no differences by sex; outbreaks in groups with common exposure

Etiologic agent: *Histoplasma capsulatum* (a fungus)

Reservoir: Soil around chicken houses, caves harboring bats, and around starling roosts and decaying trees

Transmission: Inhalation of airborne spores

Incubation period: 5 to 18 days after exposure, commonly 10 days

Period of communicability: Not transmitted from person to person

Susceptibility and resistance: General; inapparent infections are common and result in increasing resistance

Report to local authority in some states

COMPLICATIONS

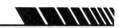

Pneumonia
Progressive emphysema
Septic type of fever
Hepatosplenomegaly
Severe prostation
Death

SIGNS AND SYMPTOMS OF PROGRESSIVE HISTOPLASMOSIS

- **Acute pulmonary histoplasmosis**
    Pleural and substernal chest pain
    Dry or productive cough with metallic tone, suggesting tracheobronchial obstruction
    Low-grade fever
    Erythema multiforme, erythema nodosum
    May have complicating symptoms of pericarditis
- **Chronic pulmonary histoplasmosis**
    Purulent sputum; hemoptysis; increasing signs of pulmonary insufficiency
    Chronic low-grade fever
    Erythema multiforme, erythema nodosum
    May have complicating symptoms of pericarditis
- **Acute disseminated histoplasmosis**
    High fever
    Enlarged liver or spleen
- **Chronic disseminated histoplasmosis**
    Symptoms of pneumonia
    Purpura
    Symptoms of endocarditis
    Symptoms of GI ulcer, hepatitis, and peritonitis
    Ulcerated lesions resembling epidermoid cancer in larynx, mouth, nose, or pharynx

DIAGNOSTIC STUDIES AND FINDINGS

Diagnostic Test	Findings
Sabouraud's agar culture; Giemsa- or Wright-stained smears of respiratory exudate, blood, or exudate from ulcerated lesions	Positive for *H. capsulatum* Results are frequently erratic, necessitating the culture of many specimens
Precipitation and complement fixation tests	Increase in antibodies within 3 to 4 weeks; fourfold increase suggests disease progression
Agglutination test	Agglutinins >1:8 or 1:16 have suggestive diagnostic value
Skin test	Induration >5 mm in 24 h indicates past or present infections; not routinely used for diagnosis
Chest x-ray	Acute: transient parenchymal pulmonary infiltrates resembling lobar pneumonia Chronic: progressively enlarging areas of necrosis with or without cavitation

---

MEDICAL MANAGEMENT

DRUG THERAPY

Antiinfective agents: Amphotericin B (Fungizone), 5-10 mg initial dose, increasing 10 mg/day until 50 mg is attained; then 50 mg 3 times/wk until a total of 2.5 g has been administered; give IV in 500 ml 5% dextrose and water.

Corticosteroids: Corticosteroids, 10-20 mg may be mixed with the infusion to minimize the side effects of amphotericin B.

Antihistamines: Diphenhydramine (Benadryl), 25-50 mg added to IV to control side effects.

Reference: 79.

1 ASSESS

ASSESSMENT	OBSERVATIONS
History	Outdoor exposure to fungus; immunosuppression
Subjective symptoms	Malaise, weakness; anorexia

2 DIAGNOSE

NURSING DIAGNOSIS	SUPPORTIVE ASSESSMENT FINDINGS
Potential for injury related to chemotherapeutic agent	Amphotericin, the antiinfective of choice, is potentially toxic
Knowledge deficit related to environmental risk factor	Patient history of exposure

Other related nursing diagnoses
Progressive disease: Ineffective breathing pattern, Hyperthermia, Decreased cardiac output, Activity intolerance, Altered oral mucous membranes

3 PLAN

Patient goals

1. Patient will be free of signs of infection and complications of treatment.

2. Patient will not experience reinfection.

4 IMPLEMENT

NURSING DIAGNOSIS	NURSING INTERVENTIONS	RATIONALE
Potential for injury related to chemotherapeutic agent	Monitor for cyanosis, changes in pulse, respiratory rate, and signs of renal dysfunction.	To detect signs of amphotericin toxicity.
	Administer antihistamines and corticosteroids as prescribed.	To prevent and control allergic reaction to amphotericin.
	Encourage fluids high in potassium if nausea and vomiting persist.	To replace lost potassium.
	Use small-gauge needle for IV line. Agitate IV bag every 15-20 min while chemotherapeutic agent is administered to evenly distribute drug and fluid in bag and in IV line. Give infusion over 5-6 h.	To prevent phlebitis associated with amphotericin.
	Frequently reposition patient during prolonged, painful IV infusions. Provide diversional activities.	To promote patient comfort.
	Administer analgesics before IV administration as prescribed.	To decrease pain from drug therapy.

5   EVALUATE

PATIENT OUTCOME	DATA INDICATING THAT OUTCOME IS REACHED
Patient is free of signs of infection and complications of treatment.	Sputum cultures are negative. Body temperature is normal. There is no cough, dyspnea, sputum, or hemoptysis. There are no lesions in mouth, larynx, pharynx, or nose. There is no purpura, erythema multiforme, or erythema nodosum. Patient has energy to carry out all daily activities. Patient does not have abdominal pain, is able to eat all desired foods, and is not jaundiced. There are no signs of phlebitis, renal dysfunction, electrolyte imbalance, pain, or neuritis.
Patient does not experience reinfection.	Patient states intent to see physician on a regular basis for 1 year after hospitalization. Patient states methods to use to avoid reexposure.

PATIENT TEACHING

1. Inform the patient that medical follow-up for 1 year after treatment to prevent relapses is necessary.
2. Inform the patient that reinfection can be prevented by avoiding infected sites, wearing a protective mask, or sterilizing the site with 3% formalin solution.

Influenza

Influenza is a generalized, acute, febrile disease associated with upper and lower respiratory infection; it is characterized by a severe and protracted cough, fever, headache, myalgia, prostration, coryza, and mild sore throat. The disease may be indistinguishable clinically from the common cold.

PATHOPHYSIOLOGY

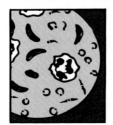

Influenza viruses A, B, or C, each with many mutagenic strains, are inhaled in aerosolized mucous droplets shed from infected persons. The viruses are deposited on and penetrate the surface of upper respiratory tract mucosal cells, producing cell lysis and destruction of the ciliated epithelium. Viral neuraminidase decreases the viscosity of the mucosa, thus facilitating the spread of virus-containing exudate to the lower respiratory tract. An interstitial inflammation and necrosis of the bronchiolar and alveolar epithelium result, filling the alveoli with an exudate containing leukocytes, erythrocytes, and hyaline membrane.

Regeneration of epithelium, following necrosis and desquamation, slowly begins after the fifth day of illness. Regeneration reaches a maximum within 9 to 15 days, at which time mucus production and cilia begin to appear. Before complete regeneration the compromised epithelium is prone to secondary bacterial invasion, resulting in bacterial pneumonia usually caused by *S. aureus*.

The initial invasion of the virus can be aborted at the portal of entry if virus-specific secretory antibodies (IgA) are present in mucous secretions and if virus-specific serum antibodies are adequate.

The disease is usually self-limited. Acute symptoms last 2 to 7 days and are followed by a convalescent period of about a week. The disease is important because of its cyclic epidemic and pandemic nature and because of the high mortality associated with pulmonary complications resulting from secondary bacterial pneumonia. This risk is highest in elderly and chronically diseased persons.

COMPLICATIONS

Primary viral pneumonia
Secondary bacterial pneumonia

INFLUENZA

Occurrence: Worldwide in pandemics, epidemics, localized outbreaks, and sporadic cases; highest in winter in temperate zones

Etiologic agent: Three types of viruses (A, B, and C), each with many strains

Reservoir: Humans; some mammals suspected as sources of new strains of viruses

Transmission: Direct transmission by inhalation of virus in airborne mucous discharge

Incubation period: 24-72 h

Period of communicability: 3 days from onset of symptoms

Susceptibility and resistance: Universal; infection produces immunity to a specific strain of virus, but duration of immunity depends on antigenic drift in strain

Mandatory case report to local health authority

DIAGNOSTIC STUDIES AND FINDINGS

Diagnostic Test	Findings
Tissue culture of nasal or pharyngeal secretions	Positive for influenza virus
Sputum culture	Positive for bacteria in secondary infections
Fluorescent antibody staining of secretions	Positive for influenza virus
Hemagglutination inhibition or complement fixation tests	Fourfold increase in antibody titer between acute and convalescent stages

MEDICAL MANAGEMENT

DRUG THERAPY

Antiinfective agents: Amantadine, 100 mg PO q day or bid for duration of epidemic (3-6 wks) for prevention of high-risk persons over age of 9 yrs; 100 mg/day PO for persons over the age of 65 yrs (dosage to be reduced further for persons with impaired renal function); reduced dosage for children. Amantadine is given as therapy within 24-48 h of symptoms until 48 h after symptoms resolve.

Agent-specific antiinfective agents for bacterial complications or for patients with chronic pulmonary disease.

Antipyretics: ASA, 600 mg orally q 4 h for adults; aceteminophen for children.

Adrenergic agents: Phenylephrine (Neo-Synephrine), 0.25%, 2 drops in each nostril for nasal congestion.

Antitussive agents: Terpin hydrate with codeine, 5-10 ml PO q 3-4 h for adults for cough.

Active immunization: Vaccine must be repeated yearly in the fall for viral strain expected in the winter; recommended for any person over 6 months who, because of age or medical condition, is at risk for complications of influenza. This includes residents of nursing homes and chronic care facilities and health care providers in contact with high-risk patients.

Children under 12 years should only receive split virus vaccine.

Age group	Dosage	No. of doses	Route
6-35 months	0.25 ml	1 or 2	IM
3-8 yrs	0.5 ml	1 or 2	IM
>12 yrs	0.5 ml	1	IM
9-12 yrs	0.5 ml	1	IM

GENERAL MANAGEMENT

Oxygen and IV fluid and electrolytes for complications.

References: 47, 52.

1 ASSESS

ASSESSMENT	OBSERVATIONS
History	Failure to receive influenza vaccine within the present season; exposure to person with influenza
Subjective symptoms	Prostration; myalgia (particularly in back and legs), anorexia and malaise, headache, photophobia, and retrobulbar aching
Body temperature	Sudden-onset fever (38° to 39°C [102° to 103°F]) that gradually falls and rises again on the third day
Head and neck	Conjunctivitis and anterior cervical lymphadenopathy may be present; flushed face
Respiratory concerns	Initial (mild at first): sore throat, substernal burning; nonproductive cough; coryza Advanced: severe and productive cough; erythema of soft palate, posterior hard palate, tonsillar pillars, and posterior pharynx; increased respiratory rate Complicating viral pneumonia: Dyspnea, cyanosis, hemoptysis, crepitant and subcrepitant rales Complicating bacterial pneumonia: Same as for viral pneumonia plus purulent or bloody sputum

2 DIAGNOSE

NURSING DIAGNOSIS	SUPPORTIVE ASSESSMENT FINDINGS
Potential for infection (patient) related to risk status	Patient is unimmunized and in high-risk group for complications
Potential for infection (patient contacts) related to presence of virus in nasopharyngeal secretions	Specimen is positive for influenza virus
Hyperthermia related to infection	Sudden-onset fever (38° to 39°C) [102° to 103°F]) that gradually falls and rises again on the third day
Ineffective breathing pattern related to infectious process in respiratory epithelium	Severe and productive cough, increased respiratory rate; signs of complications (e.g., dyspnea, cyanosis, hemoptysis, and rales)

3 PLAN

Patient goals

1. Infection will be prevented in persons experiencing risk factors.
2. Infection will not be transmitted to patient's contacts.
3. Body temperature will be maintained within the normal range; comfort and safety will be maintained for patients experiencing fever.
4. Patient will demonstrate normal respiratory pattern, oxygen intake, and blood gas levels.

4   IMPLEMENT

NURSING DIAGNOSIS	NURSING INTERVENTIONS	RATIONALE
Potential for infection (patient and patient contacts) related to presence of virus in nasopharyngeal secretions	Collect pharyngeal specimen (as described in Chapter 3).	Incorrect collection and handling of specimens may destroy the pathogen or contaminate the specimen with environmental organisms, interfering with accurate diagnosis and treatment. Improper handling can also contaminate the health care worker.
	Administer vaccine or antiviral agent as prescribed.	Antiviral agents decrease severity of influenza.
	Protect patient from exposure to bacteria. Monitor for a subsequent increase in temperature accompanied by chest pain, dyspnea, hemoptysis, purulent sputum, or ear pain; report findings.	Early detection of secondary infection and treatment with antiinfective agents may prevent dissemination of the pathogen, severe disease, and death.
	Initiate universal blood and body secretion precautions.	To prevent transmission to health care workers, other patients, and patient contacts.
	Utilize protective isolation procedures as indicated. Prevent patient exposure to infected visitors/staff. Limit visitors, if necessary.	To limit the exposure of patients to additional pathogens.
	Participate in follow-up of high-risk patient contacts.	To ensure that they receive flu vaccine or antiviral agent.
Hyperthermia related to infection	See inside back cover.	
Ineffective breathing pattern related to infectious process in respiratory epithelium	Administer decongestants as prescribed.	To reduce edema in air passages.
	Provide cool, humidified air.	To liquify secretions.
	Suction if necessary.	To remove secretions.
	Monitor for signs of viral or bacterial pneumonia.	To intervene early with antiinfectives.
	Provide oxygen as prescribed.	To ensure an adequate supply of oxygen.
	Encourage fluids as much as patient can tolerate (3,000 ml for adult).	To liquify secretions.
	Administer IV fluids as prescribed.	To provide additional fluids required during infection.
	Encourage bed rest.	To decrease demands on respiratory system.

→ > >

5   EVALUATE

PATIENT OUTCOME	DATA INDICATING THAT OUTCOME IS REACHED
Infection is prevented in persons experiencing risk factors	High-risk persons are vaccinated or are receiving antiviral agent. Sputum cultures are negative. Body temperature is normal. Leukocyte count and sedimentation rate are normal.
Infection is not transmitted	All patient contacts are adequately immunized or examined and treated with antiviral agent.
Body temperature is maintained within the normal range; comfort and safety are maintained	Body temperature is between 36° and 38°C (96.8° and 100°F) orally. Pulse and respirations are between normal limits. Skin is cool to touch and free of excess perspiration. Patient's clothing and bedding are dry.
Patient demonstrates normal respiratory pattern and blood gas levels	Breathing patterns are normal. Blood levels (O_2 saturation, CO_2, and P_{O_2}) are normal. Skin is warm and normal colored. No signs of pneumonia. Secretions are clear and thin. There is no cough.

PATIENT TEACHING ■■■■■■■■■■■■■■■■■■■■■■■■■■■■■■■■■■■■■■

1. Maintain bed rest for 2 or 3 days after temperature returns to normal.
2. Force fluids.
3. Continue to take antibiotics for duration as prescribed for bacterial complications.
4. Report symptoms of secondary infection (e.g., ear pain, purulent or bloody sputum; chest pain, increase in temperature) to physician.

5. High-risk persons should be encouraged to receive influenza vaccine before the start of the flu season.
6. Side effects of amantadine prophylaxis include nausea, dizziness, nervousness, insomnia, and impaired concentration. These disappear when the drug is stopped. These and other side effects, particularly in persons at risk for impaired renal function, should be reported to a physician.

Legionellosis (Legionnaires' disease)

Legionellosis (**Legionnaires' disease**) is an acute bacterial infection so named because it caused an outbreak of pneumonia at a convention of American Legionnaires at a Philadelphia hotel. The acute disease is a patchy pulmonary infiltrate and consolidation, with a high fever, malaise, myalgia and headache, nonproductive cough, and a high risk for respiratory failure and death.

PATHOPHYSIOLOGY

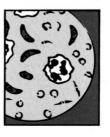

Inhalation of *Legionella pneumophila* causes two distinct clinical syndromes: Pontiac fever, which resembles influenza, and Legionnaires' disease, with pathologic changes characteristic of lobar pneumonia. In the latter there is a cellular exudate consisting of polymorphonuclear leukocytes and macrophages with extensive necrosis of the exudate and alveolar septa. Bronchi are clear of the necrotic process. Rarely is a purulent sputum produced. The disease progresses rapidly during the first 4 to 6 days of clinical illness.

COMPLICATIONS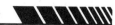

Renal failure, bacteremic shock, and respiratory failure resulting in death to 15% of patients

LEGIONELLOSIS (LEGIONNAIRES' DISEASE)

Occurrence: Europe, United States, and Canada; first recognized in 1977; sporadic cases and outbreaks in summer and autumn; increases with age
Etiologic agent: *Legionella pneumophila* (a bacteria with subgroups)
Reservoir: Unknown but probably environmental; organism survives in hot and cold tap water and distilled water for months
Transmission: Common source, airborne transmission suspected
Incubation period: 2-10 days, commonly 5-6 days
Period of communicability: No documented person-to-person transmission
Susceptibility and resistance: General; rare in those less than 20 years; greatest in males, smokers, and immunosuppressed persons
Report to local health authority in some states

DIAGNOSTIC STUDIES AND FINDINGS

Diagnostic Test	Findings
Culture of blood, sputum, pleural fluid, and lung tissue	Positive for *L. pneumophila*
Direct immunoflurescent stain of respiratory secretions	Positive for *L. pneumophila*
ELISA on urine	Positive for *L. pneumophila* antigen
Indirect immunofluorescence	Fourfold or greater rise in antibody titer to 1:128 within 21 days of onset of illness
Chest x-ray	Shows patchy pattern of pneumonia and small pleural effusions
WBC	Slightly elevated
Sedimentation rate	Markedly elevated
Others	Hematuria, proteinuria, and laboratory evidence of liver dysfunction

MEDICAL MANAGEMENT

DRUG THERAPY

Antiinfective agents: Erythromycin (Robimycin), 0.5-1 g/6 h for adults (15 mg/kg/6 h for children) IV or oral, for 14 days.
Rifampin (Rifomycin, others) as adjunct therapy.

GENERAL MANAGEMENT

Assisted ventilation, oxygen therapy, temporary renal dialysis, and IV fluids and electrolytes.

Reference: 3.

1   ASSESS

ASSESSMENT	OBSERVATION
Body temperature	38° to 41° C (102° to 105° F) within a day
Subjective symptoms	Anorexia, malaise, myalgia, chills, abdominal pain
Respiratory concerns	Nonproductive cough, dyspnea, tachypnea, pluritic chest pain, rales or rhonchi
Cardiovascular concerns	Tachycardia, symptoms of shock
Digestive concerns	Diarrhea, sometimes vomiting
Neurologic concerns	Confusion, slurring of speech, and falling; infrequent symptoms
Elimination	Renal insufficiency; hematuria

2   DIAGNOSE

NURSING DIAGNOSIS	SUPPORTIVE ASSESSMENT FINDINGS
Hyperthermia related to infection	Rapid onset fever 39° to 41°C (102° to 105°F), chills, malaise
Ineffective breathing pattern related to pneumonia	Nonproductive cough, dyspnea, tachypnea, pleuritic chest pain, rales or rhonchi

Other related nursing diagnoses: Progressive disease: Altered tissue perfusion (generalized) related to septicemia and shock

3   PLAN

Patient goals

1. Patient's body temperature will be maintained within the normal range; comfort and safety will be maintained for patients experiencing fever.

2. Patient will demonstrate normal respiratory pattern, oxygen intake, and blood gas levels.

4 IMPLEMENT

NURSING DIAGNOSIS	NURSING INTERVENTIONS	RATIONALE
Hyperthermia related to infection	See inside back cover, interventions 1-15.	
Ineffective breathing pattern related to pneumonia	Assess ventilation to include evaluation of breathing rate, rhythm, and depth: chest expansion; presence of respiratory distress, such as dyspnea, nasal flaring, pursed-lip breathing, prolonged expiratory phase, use of accessory muscles.	To detect signs of respiratory failure for immediate intervention.
	Assess patient for tiring from exertion in relation to attempts to breathe; assist ventilation, if necessary. Administer oxygen.	To maintain circulating oxygen.
	Maintain patient in position with head of bed in semi-Fowler's position or patient sitting and leaning forward overbed table.	These positions facilitate respiration by decreasing abdominal pressure on diaphragm.
	Instruct patient in proper pulmonary hygiene routines such as postural drainage.	These will promote easy, effective breathing and facilitate removal of secretions from tracheobronchial tree and minimize pulmonary congestion, which could lead to superinfections.

5 EVALUATE

PATIENT OUTCOME	DATA INDICATING THAT OUTCOME IS REACHED
Body temperature is maintained within the normal range; comfort and safety are maintained	Body temperature is between 36° and 38°C (96.8° and 100°F) orally. Pulse and respirations are between normal limits. Skin is cool to touch and free of excess perspiration. Patient's clothing and bedding are dry. Patient is free of headache and malaise associated with the fever.
	Patient experiences no injury associated with seizures. Body fluids are adequate. Serum electrolytes are within normal limits. Urine output and specific gravity are normal.
Patient demonstrates normal respiratory pattern, oxygen intake, and blood gas levels	Bronchovesicular breath sounds are heard throughout lungs. There are no areas of decreased breath sounds or consolidation. Respiratory rate is normal. CO_2, P_{O_2}, and P_{CO_2} are normal.

PATIENT TEACHING

To prevent reinfection:

1. Decontaminate implicated sources of infection by chlorination and/or super-heating of water supply.

2. Cooling water towers, misters, etc. should be drained and cleaned when not in use.

Tuberculosis

Tuberculosis (TB) is a chronic pulmonary and extrapulmonary infectious disease acquired by inhalation of a dried-droplet nucleus containing a tubercle bacillus into the alveolar structure of the lung; it is characterized by stages of early infection (frequently asymptomatic), latency, and a potential for recurrent postprimary disease.

PATHOPHYSIOLOGY

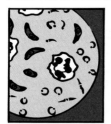 Tuberculosis infection is different from tuberculosis disease. **Tuberculosis infection** is characterized by the presence of mycobacteria in the tissue of a host who is free of clinical symptoms and who demonstrates the presence of antibodies against the mycobacteria. **Tuberculosis disease** is manifest as pathologic and functional symptoms indicating destructive activity of mycobacteria in host tissue. Both infection and disease result from tissue invasion by *Mycobacterium tuberculosis*, *M. bovis*, or a variety of atypical mycobacteria. All are spore formers capable of remaining viable and virulent for long periods inside or outside host tissue. *M. tuberculosis*, the tubercle bacillus, is the most frequent etiologic agent in human tuberculosis. Transmission is primarily by inhalation of minute dried-droplet nuclei (each containing a single tubercle bacillus), coughed or sneezed into the air by a person whose sputum contains virulent tubercle bacilli. Less commonly, transmission may occur by ingestion or by invasion of the skin or mucous membranes.

The pathologic condition of the infection and disease occurs in three stages: initial (primary infection), latency, and postprimary disease. In the initial infection the bacilli invade the tissue at the portal of entry, usually the middle or lower zones of the lungs, multiply there over 3 weeks, and create a small inflammatory lesion. Bacilli immediately enter the lymphatic system and are carried to the nearest group of lymph nodes, where they also produce inflammatory lesions. In addition, hematogenous dissemination of bacilli results in a subclinical bacteremia and the production of inflammatory lesions throughout the body. The sites and the extensiveness of the systemic lesions depend on the numbers of disseminated bacilli and the speed with which the host produces an immune response. These early lesions at the portal of entry and in the lymph nodes and hematogenously disseminated lesions are referred to as the **primary complex.**

The extent of inflammatory response at the sites of tissue invasion increases with the number of invading bacilli. Nonspecific cellular resistance permits some phagocytosis of tubercle bacilli, producing suppuration and necrosis in the central portion of the lesion. Bacilli continue to replicate at the periphery of the lesion. This initial or primary infection stage is generally symptomless.

Within 3 to 12 weeks a cellular and humoral immune response can be detected by a skin test. *Mycobacterium*-specific lymphocytes and antibodies stimulate a fibroblastic response at the periphery of the lesion, resulting in a dense connective tissue enclosure and the formation of a noncaseating granuloma. The focal lesions continue to harbor viable tubercle bacilli, with the potential for reactivation under conditions of decreased host resistance.

The specific immune response results in successful encapsulation of all lesions in 85% to 95%, depending on age, of those persons infected. These people enter the latent stage of the disease and remain disease free for variable periods of time, depending on their ability to maintain specific and nonspecific resistance. The specific immune response does not preclude reinfection with subsequent exposure.

For 5% to 15% of infected persons, host responses are inadequate to contain the infection, and active disease progresses in the portal of entry lesion or in all lesions in the body. Necrosis and cavitation continue in the lesions, forming caseation. The lesions may rupture, spreading necrotic residue and bacilli throughout the tissue and throughout the body. Disseminated bacilli establish new focal lesions that progress through stages of inflammation, noncaseating granulomas, and caseating necrosis.

The disease symptoms vary with the body tissue affected. Extrapulmonary tuberculosis in the meninges, blood vessels, kidneys, bones, joints, larynx, skin, intestines, lymph nodes, peritoneum, or eyes is much less common than pulmonary tuberculosis.

Reactivated disease following latency accounts for most of the active tuberculosis diagnosed today. It occurs most frequently in aged persons and persons with chronic and debilitating disease. Although reactivation may occur in any of the focal lesions, it most commonly occurs in those in the upper lobes or at the apex of the lower lobes of the lungs, forming abscesses and tuberculous cavities at those sites. Untreated reactivated disease has a variable course with many exacerbations and remissions. Complications caused by excessive cavitation are common.

COMPLICATIONS

Extrapulmonary disease
Cavitation and destruction of lungs

TUBERCULOSIS

Occurrence: Worldwide; after a period of decline, incidence is increasing; outbreaks among homeless, migrants, persons with AIDS, and in correctional facilities

Etiologic agent: *Mycobacterium tuberculosis* and *M. bovis;* drug-resistant organisms have been isolated

Reservoir: Humans; *M. bovis* in diseased cattle

Transmission: Inhalation of bacilli in airborne mucous droplets from sputum of persons with active disease; less frequent: ingestion or skin penetration

Incubation period: 4-12 wks after exposure or anytime when disease is in latent stage

Period of communicability: As long as bacilli are in sputum; some are intermittently communicable for years

Susceptibility and resistance: General; highest in children less than 3 yrs, those greater than 65 yrs, chronically ill, silicone and asbestos workers, and malnourished and immunosuppressed individuals

Mandatory case report to local health authority

DIAGNOSTIC STUDIES AND FINDINGS

Diagnostic Test	Findings
Sputum culture	Positive for *M. tuberculosis* within 2-3 wks of active disease; will not be positive during latency
Acid-fast with Ziehl-Neelsen stain smear of sputum (CSF or blood in extrapulmonary disease)	Positive for acid-fast vacilli
Histolytic examination or culture of tissue in extrapulmonary disease	Positive for *M. tuberculosis*
Skin tests: intradermal injection of antigen (Mantoux test: five tuberculin units of purified protein derivative (PPD) injected intradermally)	Test is read in 48-72 h. A positive reaction* indicates past infection and presence of antibodies; does not indicate active disease; nonspecific reactions during first 48 h can be overlooked. If reaction is questionable, a second test may be done 1 wk later; if the second test is < significant, the patient is considered not infected; increase in size of induration >6 mm to a diameter of 10 mm indicates recent tuberculin infection.
Pleural needle biopsy	Positive for granulomas of tuberculosis; giant cells indicating caseation necrosis
Chest x-ray	Findings may show calcification at the original site, enlargement of hilar lymph nodes, parenchymal infiltrate representing extension of the original site of infection, or the appearance of pleural effusion or cavitation; not diagnostically definitive of TB

---

*Positive reaction is indicated by (1) induration >5 mm in persons positive for HIV, close contacts of person diagnosed with TB, or persons with x-ray changes consistent with TB; or (2) induration >10 mm in IV drug abusers, persons with medical conditions that increase risk for TB, the homeless, persons in correctional facilities, migrants from high-prevalence areas, and other high-risk groups; or (3) induration >15 mm in low-risk persons.

MEDICAL MANAGEMENT

DRUG THERAPY   A combination of antiinfective agents is recommended: two primary drugs or a primary plus a secondary drug; initial dosages are higher, followed by prolonged therapy at reduced dosages; the combination of drugs used, the dosage, and duration of administration depend on the stage of the infection or disease, the presence of extrapulmonary disease, and the sensitivity of the patient to certain chemotherapeutic agents.

Antiinfective agents:
  Primary drugs—
    Isoniazid (INH), 10-20 mg/kg/day (up to 300 mg/day) orally for 1-2 yrs.
    Ethambutol (Myambutol), 15 mg/kg/day orally for 1-2 yrs; initial dose: 25 mg/kg/day for 2 months.
    Rifampin (Rifomycin, others), 20 mg/kg/day orally for 6 months to 2 yrs.
    Streptomycin, 30 mg/kg/day IM for 2-3 mo
  Secondary drugs—
    Pyrazinamide (Aldinamide), 20-30 mg/kg/day
    Ethionamide (Trecator), 10-30 mg/kg/day
    Para-amino salicylic acid (PAS), 0.2 mg/kg/day orally for 1-2 yr
    Cycloserine (Seromycin), 0.5-1 g/day orally in divided doses
    Capreomycin (Capastat), 0.75-1 g/day IM for 30 days; twice weekly thereafter
    Kanamycin (Kantrex), 1 g/day IM
    Viomycin (Viocin), 1 g/day IM
  An example of recommended treatment plans—
    Primary pulmonary tuberculosis
    Isoniazid, 300 mg/day orally for 9 months plus
    Rifampin, 600 mg/day orally for 9 months *or*
    Isoniazid, 300 mg/day orally for 18-24 months plus
    Ethambutol, 15-18 mg/kg/day orally for 18-24 months
  Chronic pulmonary tuberculosis—
    Isoniazid, 10-20 mg/kg/day for 18 months or more, plus
    Rifampin, 20 mg/kg/day for 18 months or more, or
    PAS, 0.2 mg/kg/day for 18 months or more, or
    Ethambutol, 15 mg/kg/day for 18 months or more

Corticosteroids: May be used in conjunction with the antiinfective agents for overwhelming and life-threatening disease

GENERAL MANAGEMENT

After stabilization most patients can be effectively managed on an outpatient basis with monitoring for compliance with drug taking, drug side effects, and patient response to the drug therapy.

AFB isolation until antimicrobial therapy is successfully initiated for sputum-positive patients to prevent spread to others (Chapter 13).

Secretion precautions until wounds stop draining for patients with external TB lesions (Chapter 13).

Skin testing: identify recent converters to TB skin tests; trace their contacts to identify persons with active disease; isoniazid therapy for 1 yr for recent converters and for close household contacts of persons with active disease (not routine for those over 35 yrs); TB skin testing is recommended for children at school entry and again at age 14 yrs.

BCG vaccine for children and infants who are at high risk for contact with active cases, who are skin test negative, and who are not immunosuppressed (benefits of BCG vaccine are controversial); receiving the vaccine results in a positive skin test.

SURGERY

Intervention for complications.

Resectional procedures for persisting cavitary lesions (less common since antimicrobial therapy).

Surgical intervention for massive hemoptysis, spontaneous pneumothorax, abscess drainage, intestinal obstruction, or ureteral stricture.

References 3, 31, 48, 49, 62.

1 ASSESS

ASSESSMENT	OBSERVATIONS
History	Close contact with a person with TB or previous positive TB skin test; immunosuppression or chronic disease
Subjective symptoms	History of weight loss, anorexia, generalized weakness and fatigue
Body temperature	Slight continued elevation with chills and night sweats
Respiratory	**Initial:** a nonproductive cough; later mucopurulent secretions **Advanced:** hemoptysis; dyspnea on exertion and at rest; rales over apex of lung; chest pain with respiratory movement if pleura is involved; hoarseness with involvement of larynx; dysphagia with pharyngeal involvement; sibilant and sonorous rhonchi
Cardiovascular	Tachycardia

Extrapulmonary TB: depends on the system involved. The onset of symptoms is generally insidious, as is the onset of pulmonary TB:

Cardiovascular	**TB pericarditis:** Precordial chest pain, fever, and pericardial friction rubs; jugular venous distention, hepatic congestion, ascites, and peripheral edema
GI	**TB peritonitis:** Abdominal pain simulating that of appendicitis; abdominal distention; anorexia, vomiting, and weight loss; night sweats; abdominal tenderness when palpated; ascites
	TB of GI tract: Symptoms depend on area involved; may have GI bleeding, pain, constipation, or diarrhea; partial or complete obstruction
Systemic	**Miliary TB:** More severe symptoms of respiratory involvement: dyspnea, hyperventilation, and cough; hypoxemia; spontaneous unilateral or bilateral pneumothorax (manifested by sudden chest pain and breathlessness) and fever; painful, nodular cutaneous lesions (which may ulcerate) may be present
Neurologic	**TB meningitis:** Headache, vomiting, fever, and anorexia; alterations in intellectual function, diminishing levels of consciousness, and neurologic deficits; CSF leukocytes of 100 to 400 cells/mm^3 and increase in protein
Lymphatic	**TB lymphadenitis:** Palpable enlargement of supraclavicular and cervical lymph nodes
Musculoskeletal	**Osteoarticular TB:** Pain in joints, aggravated by movement; swelling, minimal erythema, and tenderness to palpation; limitation of motion and gross deformities (most common in vertebral column, hip, and knee joints)
GU	**TB of GU organs:** Urgency, frequency, dysuria, hematuria, and pyuria; salpingitis with lower abdominal pain and infertility; amenorrhea; abnormal vaginal discharge or bleeding

→ > >

2 DIAGNOSE

NURSING DIAGNOSIS	SUPPORTIVE ASSESSMENT FINDINGS
Potential for infection (patient contacts) related to viable *M. tuberculosis* in respiratory secretions	Sputum or tissue specimen positive for *M. tuberculosis* **Signs of infection:** fever with night sweats, history of weight loss, anorexia, generalized weakness and fatigue
Potential for infection (chronic in patient) related to noncompliance with therapy	Patient does not return for checkups and medication renewal on a regular basis.
Ineffective breathing pattern related to necrosis of lung tissue	**Initial:** Nonproductive cough; later mucopurulent secretions **Advanced:** hemoptysis; dyspnea on exertion and at rest; rales over apex of lung; chest pain with respiratory movement if pleura is involved; hoarseness with involvement of larynx; dysphagia with pharyngeal involvement; sibilant and sonorous rhonchi

Other related nursing diagnoses: Extrapulmonary TB: Potential for injury related to perforation; altered tissue perfusion (CNS, cardiovascular, hepatic, renal, or GI) related to infectious process

3 PLAN

Patient goals

1. Patient will be free of infection and complications of TB.
2. Patient will self-administer antiinfective agents as prescribed.

3. Infection will not be transmitted to patient's contacts.
4. Patient will demonstrate normal respiratory pattern, oxygen intake, and blood gas levels.

4 IMPLEMENT

NURSING DIAGNOSIS	NURSING INTERVENTIONS	RATIONALE
Potential for infection (patient contacts) related to viable *M. tuberculosis* in respiratory secretions	Obtain specimen for culture (as described in Chapter 3).	Incorrect collection and handling of specimen may destroy or contaminate specimen, thus interfering with diagnostic results.
	Employ AFB isolation until antimicrobial therapy is successfully initiated for sputum-positive patients.	To prevent transmission of organism.
	Employ secretion precautions until wounds stop draining for patients with external TB lesions.	To prevent transmission of organism.
	Teach hospitalized patient to cough and sneeze into paper tissues and to dispose of tissues properly.	To prevent transmission of organism.

NURSING DIAGNOSIS	NURSING INTERVENTIONS	RATIONALE
Potential for infection (chronic in patient) related to noncompliance with therapy	Instruct patient regarding the prescribed therapy; see Patient Teaching.	To ensure patient takes medication as prescribed.
Ineffective breathing pattern related to necrosis of lung tissue	Monitor breathing.	To detect dyspnea and signs of pneumothorax.
	Initiate respiratory assistance as needed. Observe sputum for hemoptysis.	To detect signs of complications.
	Assist immobile patient to turn, cough, and deep breathe every 2-4 h.	To prevent pooling of secretions.
Knowledge deficit	See Patient Teaching.	

5 EVALUATE

PATIENT OUTCOME	DATA INDICATING THAT OUTCOME IS REACHED
Patient is free of infection and complications of TB.	Sputum cultures are consistently negative. Chest x-rays show a reduction in the size of cavities and decrease in the thickness of cavity walls. Body temperature is normal. Patient does not experience chills or night sweats. Serum alkaline phosphatase levels, hematocrit, hemoglobin, and leukocyte count are normal. Urine does not contain erythrocytes. Patient does not manifest the extrapulmonary symptoms described under "Nursing Assessment."
Patient self-administers antiinfective agents as prescribed.	Patient completes full course of antiinfective therapy. No preventable drug interactions or allergic reactions are experienced. If untoward reactions are experienced, the patient discontinues the drug and contacts the physician immediately.
Infection is not transmitted to patient's contacts.	Contacts do not convert to a positive skin test. Patient demonstrates behavior to prevent transmission of pathogens to others or to prevent contamination of the environment.
Patient demonstrates normal respiratory pattern, oxygen intake and blood gas levels.	Patient does not experience dyspnea, cough, or pain on breathing.

PATIENT TEACHING

1. Teach care of sputum if discharged patient still has positive sputum cultures.
2. Teach handwashing and good hygiene.
3. Drug therapy must be continued uninterrupted for the designated time period. Explain dosage, frequency of administration, and purpose for prolonged treatment.
4. Explain medication's toxic and side effects:
   - INH: infrequent toxic effects—peripheral neuropathy, convulsions, ataxia, dizziness, optic neuritis; older patients may experience a drug-related hepatitis with fatigue, malaise, and anorexia.
   - Ethambutol: reduced visual acuity with inability to perceive the color green.
   - Streptomycin: skin rash, fever, malaise, vertigo, and deafness; gastrointestinal disturbances and central nervous system symptoms.
   - PAS: toxic reactions more common with this drug and include symptoms of hypersensitivity, hepatic damage, gastrointestinal disturbances, and renal failure.
   - Rifampin: red-orange colored urine common, jaundice, nausea, anorexia, vomiting, diarrhea, cramps, occasional central nervous system disturbances, and hypersensitivity reactions; may interfere with actions of oral contraceptives.
   - Ethionamide: gastrointestinal irritation and symptoms of hepatotoxicity.
   - Pyrazinamide: hepatoxicity.
   - Cycloserine: central nervous system effects, including seizures, somnolence, and muscle twitching.
5. Report side effects to physician immediately.
6. Emphasize need for periodic reculturing of sputum during period of therapy—monthly until cultures are negative, then every 3 months for duration of therapy.
7. Report to physician: hemoptysis, chest pain, difficulty in breathing, hearing loss, or vertigo.
8. Maintain adequate fluid and caloric intake.
9. Household and close contacts should be examined at time of treatment of patient and again in 2 to 3 months.

CHAPTER 8

Acquired Immune Deficiency Syndrome (AIDS) and HIV Infection

AIDS virus

T-helper cell

AIDS is an acronym for the term **acquired immune deficiency syndrome.** This syndrome is a set of defined clinical conditions that are the final result of infection with **human immunodeficiency virus (HIV).**

Infection with HIV initiates a process of gradual and accelerating destruction of the body's immune system. This process can be described as having five phases (Table 8-1). *Transmission of the virus is possible during all five phases.* The **first phase** of the infection is not detectable by present laboratory technology. This phase may be as short as 4 weeks or as long as 6 months and is sometimes referred to as the **window period.**

The **second phase** of the infection is a short, symptomatic period early in the infection. Symptoms are flu-like, with fever, lymphadenopathy, skin rash, and malaise. It is believed that the symptoms coincide with the body's production of sufficient detectable antibodies. Ideally, HIV-infected persons should be identified during this phase so that they can take precautions to prevent further transmission. This phase of the infection can be termed **acute primary HIV infection.**

The **third phase** of the disease is a prolonged asymptomatic period following the brief flu-like illness. The infected person continues to demonstrate serum

antibodies against HIV. These antibodies, however, are not protective. This phase of the disease may last from 1 year to as long as 15 to 20 years, depending on the state of the person's immune system at the time of infection, behaviors to maintain health, and therapeutic interventions. During this period the infected individual experiences a decline in immune function that can be documented by laboratory analysis. However, because of the asymptomatic nature of this phase, few infected persons actually have their immune status evaluated. Recent developments in antiviral therapy have been shown to extend this phase. Therefore it is considered extremely important to identify HIV-infected persons during this asymptomatic period if they have not been diagnosed earlier. This third phase is called **asymptomatic HIV infection.**

The **fourth phase** of the infection is when the infected person begins to have symptoms of immune suppression but does not have one of the AIDS-defining conditions described below. The symptoms result from two pathologic processes: (1) failure of the immune system to defend against pathogens, and (2) the virus' direct attack on nerve cells. Symptoms vary but may include persistent low-grade fever, night sweats, continu-

Table 8-1
PHASES OF HIV INFECTION AND AIDS

Phase	Length of phase	Antibodies detectable	Symptoms	Can be transmitted
1. Window period	4 wks to 6 months after infection	No	None	Yes
2. Acute primary HIV infection	1-2 wks	Possible	Flu-like illness	Yes
3. Asymptomatic infection	1-15 or more yrs	Yes	None	Yes
4. Symptomomatic immune suppression	Up to 3 yrs	Yes	Fever, night sweats, weight loss, diarrhea, neuropathy, fatigue, rashes, lymphadenopathy, cognitive slowing, oral lesions	Yes
5. AIDS	Variable: 1-5 yrs from first AIDS-defining condition	Yes	Severe opportunistic infections and tumors in any body system; neurologic manifestations	Yes

1987 REVISION OF CASE DEFINITION FOR AIDS FOR SURVEILLANCE PURPOSES

I. Without laboratory evidence regarding HIV infection

- Candidiasis of the esophagus, trachea, bronchi, or lungs
- Cryptococcosis, extrapulmonary
- Cryptosporidiosis, with diarrhea persisting >1 month
- Cytomegalovirus disease of an organ other than the liver, spleen, or lymph nodes in a patient >1 month of age
- Herpes simplex virus infection causing a mucocutaneous ulcer that persists >1 month; or bronchitis, pneumonitis, or esophagitis for any duration affecting a patient >1 month of age
- Kaposi's sarcoma affecting a patient <60 years of age
- Lymphoma of the brain (primary) affecting a patient <60 years of age
- Lymphoid interstitial pneumonia and/or pulmonary lymphoid hyperplasia affecting a child <13 years of age
- *Mycobacterium avium* complex or *M. kansasii* disease, disseminated (at a site other than or in addition to lungs, skin, or cervical or hilar lymph nodes)
- *Pneumocystis carinii* pneumonia
- Progressive multifocal leukoencephalopathy
- Toxoplasmosis of the brain, affecting a patient >1 month of age

II. With laboratory evidence for HIV infection

- Bacterial infections, multiple or recurrent, affecting a child <13 years of age
- Septicemia, pneumonia, meningitis, bone or joint infection, or abscess of an internal organ or body cavity caused by *Haemophilus* or *Streptococcus* organisms or other pyogenic bacteria
- Coccidioidomycosis, disseminated (at a site other than or in addition to lungs, or cervical or hilar lymph nodes)
- Isosporiasis with diarrhea persisting >1 month
- Kaposi's sarcoma at any age
- Lymphoma of the brain (primary) at any age
- Non-Hodgkin's lymphoma of B-cell or unknown immunologic phenotypes and small noncleaved lymphoma (Burkitt's) and immunoblastic sarcoma histologic types
- Mycobacterioses, including tuberculosis, disseminated or miliary, at a site other than or in addition to lungs, skin, or cervical or hilar lymph nodes
- *Salmonella* (nontyphoid) septicemia, recurrent HIV wasting syndrome ("slim" disease)

III. Diagnosed presumptively

- Candidiasis of the esophagus
- Cytomegalovirus retinitis with loss of vision
- Kaposi's sarcoma
- Lymphoid interstitial pneumonia and/or pulmonary lymphoid hyperplasia affecting a child <13 years of age
- Mycobacterioses, disseminated
- *Pneumocystis carinii* pneumonia
- Toxoplasmosis of the brain affecting a patient >1 month of age

Centers for Disease Control, 1987.[22]

ous or intermittent diarrhea, lymphadenopathy, unintended weight loss, oral lesions, fatigue, rashes, cognitive slowing, and peripheral neuropathy. Any of these symptoms are indicators that the disease is likely to progress to diagnosable AIDS within the next 2 to 3 years.

The **fifth phase** of the infection is AIDS. This means that the patient has acquired a condition that meets the criteria for a diagnosis of AIDS, as specified by the Centers for Disease Control (CDC). The criteria for diagnosing AIDS were established to assure uniformity in reporting of AIDS cases. Therefore a diagnosis of AIDS should be considered an assistive diagnosis in determining the extent of HIV-related disease rather than a diagnosis for clinical management of patients. This is illustrated in the box on the opposite page, which reproduces a portion of the CDC Case Definition for AIDS. The list contains one constitutional syndrome, two forms of cancer, neurologic dysfunction, and infectious diseases caused by over a dozen different organisms that can attack any of several body sites. While a poor term for clinical management, an AIDS diagnosis has important prognostic value. Of persons who receive an AIDS-defining diagnosis, 80% to 90% die within 3 years of the diagnosis.

EPIDEMIOLOGY

The epidemic of AIDS is a reminder of the continuing vulnerability of humans to infectious disease. No disease of modern time has had the impact on society that AIDS has. From the documentation of the first case in 1981 to the end of 1990, approximately 150,000 cases have been reported in the United States. Sixty percent of these persons have died. It is estimated that 10 times the number AIDS-diagnosed cases (1,500,000 persons) are infected with the HIV virus. Given present medical knowledge, these persons will be diagnosed with AIDS during the next 5 to 20 years even if transmission of the virus ceases today. The epidemic nature of AIDS disease and HIV infection prevents the most current documentation of the extent of these conditions in a publication of this type. However, it must be noted that AIDS is everywhere, not just in large metropolitan areas. There are geographic differences as to the population groups infected. For example, a large portion of the AIDS cases are homosexual males in California and IV drug abusers in New York. The disease is increasing in women and children in the United States. A general overview of the epidemiology of AIDS is presented in Table 8-2.

Table 8-2

OVERVIEW OF THE EPIDEMIOLOGY OF AIDS

Occurrence	Worldwide and increasing everywhere. Highest in persons with identified risk factors: homosexual and bisexual males, heterosexual contact with persons with AIDS, IV drug abuse, transfusion recipients, hemophilia or coagulation disorder, infant born of HIV-positive mother.
Etiologic agent	Human immunodeficiency virus (HIV); two types of HIV virus have been identified: HIV-1 (prevalent in the United States) and HIV-2 (prevalent in West Africa and countries with epidemiologic links to West Africa).
Reservoir	Humans.
Transmission	The virus is present in blood and serum-derived body fluids; transmitted person to person through anal or vaginal intercourse, transplacentally, and by breastfeeding; transmitted indirectly by transfusion of contaminated blood or blood products, use of contaminated needles or syringes, or direct contact with infected blood or body fluids on mucous membranes or open wounds; theoretically possible to transmit by oral/genital contact and deep French kissing. There are no reports of transmission from saliva, tears, urine, bronchial secretions, biting insects or any type of casual contact.
Incubation period	Variable. The time from exposure to seroconversion is 4 wks to 6 months. The time to symptomatic immune suppression and to AIDS diagnosis can be up to 20 yrs.
Period of communicability	Lifelong; from presence of HIV in sera until death. The degree of contagiousness may vary during the course of HIV infection.
Susceptibility and resistance	Unknown; presumed to be general. Antibody response is not protective.
Report to local health authority	AIDS case report required. Report of HIV positive status varies by state.

Data from Benenson.[3]

PATHOPHYSIOLOGY

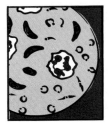

The virus causing HIV infection is called **human immunodeficiency virus (HIV)**. There are two known types of this virus: HIV-1 and HIV-2. HIV-1 is widespread throughout the world, whereas HIV-2 is mainly found in West Africa and, increasingly, in those countries that are commercially and epidemiologically linked to West Africa.

HIV belongs to a family of viruses called **retroviruses,** so named because they convert their genetic RNA (ribonucleic acid) to DNA (deoxyribonucleic acid) once they enter the host cell. HIV, like other retroviruses, infects a host target cell by binding to a receptor on the cell and then penetrating the cell. Once inside, the virus strips itself of its protective coating, exposing its core RNA to the target cell. The virus releases an enzyme, **reverse transcriptase,** which converts the viral RNA to DNA. The viral DNA then enters the target cell's genetic material and integrates with the cellular DNA. The alteration of the cell's genetic material into part virus−part cell (provirus) changes the cell's normal function in favor of the virus. One of the products of the altered cell is more virus. Thus the infected host cell produces more HIV. When sufficient quantities of the virus are produced, the host cell ruptures, destroying the cell and releasing the virus in the blood to seek new target cells with the appropriate receptor.

The cellular receptor sought by HIV is called CD4, found on the surface of T4 lymphocytes (T-helper cells, T4 cells) and certain nerve cells. Therefore HIV infection causes destruction of T4 cells and nerve cells. The destruction of the T4 cells deprives the body of an important agent in cellular immunity (see Chapter 1). It is interesting to note that the converted DNA, described above, can remain dormant until the cell is activated. T4 lymphocytes are activated by invasion of pathogens and other foreign antigens, such as cancer-inducing agents. In the case of HIV-infected T4 cells, activation results in replication of HIV rather than the T4 cells. Thus an important defender is not only denied to the immune system, but also adds to the infection burden by creating more HIV. Gradually, through repeated pathogenic invasions, T4 cells become depleted. The normal ratio of T4 helper to T8 suppressor cells is 2:1. However, as more and more T4 cells are destroyed, T8 cells predominate, thus changing the ratio. A T4 to T8 ratio that is 1:1 or less (i.e. 1:2) is an indicator of severe immune system compromise. T cell-mediated immunity is important for control of tumors and for defense against intracellular pathogens such as viruses, mycobacteria, fungi, and protozoa. Failure of cell-mediated immunity results in the pathologic processes associated with symptomatic HIV infection and AIDS.

Recent research has demonstrated that HIV does not limit its invasion to T4 cells, but the action in other cells is less clear. HIV invades monocytes and macrophages, which probably carry the virus throughout the body. HIV has been found in neurons and glial cells of the brain. Many of the CNS manifestations of HIV infection are attributed to the direct destruction of these cells by the virus. In addition, it is believed that HIV invades some B lymphocytes, the Langerhans' cells, progentin cells of bone marrow, follicular dendritic reticulum cells of lymph node germinal centers, and natural killer (NK) cells.

The pathophysiology resulting from HIV infection is incredibly complex and the resulting disease manifestations are extremely variable. The immunocompromised patient is at risk for invasion and serious infection by any pathogen, even those that are ubiquitous to the environment or part of the normal flora of the body. Organisms that are normally limited to one part of the body or organ system can become pathogenic in any system. To complicate matters, more than one infection is often present at any one time. The immunocompromised patient is also at risk for certain neoplasms, particularly Kaposi's sarcoma and lymphomas. These may be manifest in any body system concurrent with multiple infections. The box on pages 159 and 160 summarizes the major pathologic manifestations seen in persons with symptomatic HIV infection in phases 4 and 5. The box and the discussion that follows are organized according to body system. It must be emphasized that disease may be manifest in more than one body system at once. Some body systems are excluded from the box and the discussion that follows because of space considerations. The absence of discussion of an organ or body system disease does not indicate that the organ or system will not be affected. It merely means that the affect is likely to be secondary to the diseases being discussed.

Many of the infections listed in the box on pages 159 and 160 are discussed in depth elsewhere in this book. These infections and their location in the book are listed in the box on page 161.

The **oral cavity** is one of the first areas of the body to show the effect of immune suppression. Eventually, 80% to 90% of HIV-infected persons will experience some or all of the oral pathologies listed in the box on page 159. The appearance of unusual lesions in and around the mouth should cause one to be suspicious of HIV infection. These lesions are easily seen in the mouth in their early stages and, often, cause widespread ulcer-

For pictures of oral lesions of AIDS, see color plates 5 through 10, pages x and xi.

PATHOLOGIC MANIFESTATIONS OF AIDS

Oral manifestations

Possible causes

Lesions due to: *Candida*, herpes simplex, Kaposi's sarcoma; papillomavirus oral warts; HIV gingivitis or peridontits; oral leukoplakia

Possible effects

Oral pain leading to difficulty in chewing and swallowing, decreased fluid and nutritional intake, dehydration, weight loss and fatigue; disfigurement

Neurologic manifestations

Possible causes

AIDS dementia complex due to: direct attack of HIV in nerve cells

Possible effects

Personality changes; impaired cognition, concentration, and judgment; impaired motor ability; weakness; needs assistance with ADL or unable to perform ADL; unable to talk or comprehend; paresis and/or plegia; incontinence; caregiver burden; inability to comply with medical regimen; inability to work; social isolation

Acute encephalopathy due to: therapeutic drug reactions; drug overdose; hypoxia; hypoglycemia from drug-induced pancreatitis; electrolyte imbalance; meningitis or encephalitis resulting from *Cryptococcus,* herpes simplex virus, cytomegalovirus, *Mycobacterium tuberculosis,* syphilis, *Candida, toxoplasma gondii;* lymphoma; **Cerebral infarction** resulting from: vasculitis, meningovascular syphilis, systemic hypotension, and marantic endocarditis

Headache, malaise, fever; full or partial paralysis; loss of cognitive ability, memory, judgment, orientation or appropriate affect; sensory distortion; seizures, coma, death

Neuropathy due to: inflammatory demyelination resulting from direct HIV attack; drug reactions; Kaposi's sarcoma lesions

Loss of motor control; ataxia; peripheral numbness, tingling, burning sensation; depressed reflexes; inability to work; caregiver burden; social isolation

Gastrointestinal manifestations

Possible causes

Diarrhea due to: *Cryptosporidium, Isopora Belli, Microsporidium, Strongyloides stercoides,* cytomegalovirus, herpes simplex, enterovirusus, adenovirus, *Mycobacterium avium intracellulare, Salmonella, Shigella, Campylobacter, Vibrio parahaemolyticus, Candida, Histoplasma capsulatum, Giardia, Entamoeba histolytica,* normal flora overgrowth, lymphoma, and Kaposi's sarcoma

Possible effects

Weight loss, anorexia, fever; dehydration, malabsorption; malaise, weakness and fatigue; loss of ability to perform social functions due to inability to leave house; incontinence and caregiver burden

Hepatitis due to: *Mycobacterium avium intracellulare, Cryptococcus,* cytomegalovirus, *Histoplasma, Coccidiomycosis, Microsporidium,* Epstein-Barr virus, Hepatitis A, B, C, D (Delta agent) and E viruses, Lymphoma, Kaposi's sarcoma, illegal drug use, alcohol abuse, and prescribed drug use (particularily sulfa drugs)

Anorexia, nausea, vomiting, abdominal pain, jaundice; fever, malaise, rash, joint pain, fatigue; hepatomegaly, hepatic failure, death

Biliary dysfunction due to: Cholangitis from cytomegalovirus and *Cryptosporidium;* Lymphoma and Kaposi's sarcoma

Abdominal pain, anorexia, nausea, vomiting and jaundice.

Anorectal disease due to: perirectal abscesses and fistulas, perianal ulcers and inflammation resulting from infections with *Chlamydia, Lymphogranulum venereum,* Gonorrhea, Syphilis, *Shigella, Campylobacter, M. tuberculosis,* Herpes simplex, Cytomegalovirus, *Candida ablicans* obstruction from lymphoma; Kaposi's sarcoma and papillomovirus warts

Difficult and painful elimination; rectal pain, itching, diarrhea

Continued.

PATHOLOGIC MANIFESTATIONS OF AIDS—cont'd

Respiratory manifestations

Possible causes

Infection due to: *Pneumocystis carinii, M. avium intracellulare, M. tuberculosis, Candida, Chlamydia, Histoplasma capsulatum, Toxoplasma gondii, Coccidioides immitis, Cryptococcus neoforms,* cytomegalovirus, influenza viruses, *Pneumococcus, Strongyloides*

Lymphoma and Kaposi's sarcoma

Possible effects

Shortness of breath, cough, pain; hypoxia, activity intolerance, fatigue; respiratory failure and death

Same as above.

Dermatologic manifestations

Possible causes

Staphylococcal skin lesions (bullous impetigo, ecthyma, folliculitis); herpes simplex virus lesions (oral, facial, anal; vulvovaginal); herpes zoster; chronic mycobacterial lesions appearing over lymph nodes or as ulcerations or hemorrhagic macules; other lesions related to infection with *Pseudomonas aeruginosa, Molluscum contagiosum, Candida albicans,* ringworm, *Cryptococcus, Sporotrichosis; Xerosis*-induced dermatitis, seborrheic dermatitis; drug reactions, (particularly from sulfa-based drugs); lesions from parasites such as scabies or lice; Kaposi's sarcoma; decubiti and impairment in the integrity of the skin resulting from prolonged pressure and incontinence

Possible effects

Pain, itching, burning, secondary infection and sepsis; disfigurement and altered self-image

Sensory system

Possible causes

Vision: Kaposi's sarcoma on conjunctiva or eyelid; cytomegalovirus retinitis

Hearing: Acute external otitis and otitis media; hearing loss related to myelopathy, meningitis, cytomegalovirus, and drug reactions

Possible effects

Blindness

Pain and hearing loss

---

ation and disfigurement. With the exception of oral hairy leukoplakia, all will have varying degrees of pain associated with them. Sometimes the lesions will be continuously painful, whereas at other times the lesions will be sensitive to temperature or spicy foods. The lesions will interfere with the ability to eat, often to the point of severely compromising the person's nutritional needs.

The **neurologic system** is highly impacted by HIV. More than half of HIV-infected persons will eventually experience some neurologic manifestation. Some of these pathologies are, apparently, the result of HIV invasion of nerve cells. Others result from infections or neoplasms in the brain or elsewhere. Still other neurologic manifestations result from therapeutic drug interactions or are secondary to systemic problems such as dehydration, electrolyte imbalance, or malnutrition.

Many HIV-infected persons experience what is called **AIDS dementia complex (ADC).** Autopsy evidence suggests that HIV invades and damages nerve cells of the brain and elsewhere in the body. The person with ADC manifests impairment in cognition and motor skills. This ranges from mild to severe. In a mild state of impaired cognition the person experiences short-term memory loss and/or inability to find words when speaking. In advanced stages, persons may be close to a vegetative state. Impaired motor skills may start with loss of fine motor skills and/or loss of spatial orientation. At advanced stages, the person can experience paresis and/or paralysis, accompanied by painful neuropathies.

Cerebral and meningeal infection can be caused by a variety of opportunistic organisms that cause localized abscesses and necrotic areas or generalized inflammation. The extent of impairment in CNS function depends on the area and extent of the infection.

Cerebral circulation may be compromised by a range of systemic pathologies, such as infarction, sepsis, fever, hypotension, and circulatory collapse.

The impact of a damaged neurologic system can be profound. The person is at increased risk for injury and progressively loses ability to work, care for self, and follow medical directions. This places an extra burden on the professional and home caregiver.

Gastrointestinal disease affects over 90% of HIV-infected persons. Over 20 infectious agents, including normal flora organisms, have been implicated in causing diarrhea in these persons. The diarrhea is characteristically secretory, with some persons excreting up to 15 liters per day. Rapid dehydration, electrolyte imbalance, and circulatory collapse are potential risks. Sometimes the diarrhea lasts for months, causing malabsorption of nutrients and further weakening of the immune system.

Impaired liver function is common in HIV-infected persons. This may result from a primary infection with hepatitis viruses, infection secondary to infection with other organisms, prescribed drugs that are hepatotoxic, or alcohol or drug abuse. Biliary ducts may become blocked with neoplasms, particularly Kaposi's sarcoma.

Anorectal disease is common in HIV-infected persons, particularly in those with infections sexually transmitted to the anus. These anorectal manifestations take the form of ulcers, abscesses, fistulas, masses, and tumors, all which have the potential to cause painful or difficult defecation.

***Pneumocystis carinii* pneumonia (PCP)** is the condition that allows the diagnosis of AIDS to be made in about 60% of AIDS-infected people. Many of the remaining 40% will experience one or more bouts of PCP after being diagnosed with AIDS. *Pneumocystis carinii* is a protozoa that is ubiquitous in the environment. It is part of the normal flora in most healthy persons but becomes an aggressive pathogen in the immunocompromised host. The pathogen invades the lungs bilaterally and multiplies extracellularly. As the infestation grows, more and more alveoli become filled with organisms and exudative material, resulting in impaired gas exchange. As the infection progresses, the alveoli hypertrophy and thicken, eventually showing extensive consolidation. The clinical picture is of insidious onset with increasing dyspnea on exertion and a nonproductive cough. Fever may or may not be present. Untreated PCP progresses to life-threatening pulmonary insufficiency.

PCP is just one of a dozen or more organisms that can cause pneumonia and other lung infection in the immunocompromised. Of particular concern is the degree to which TB is found in HIV-infected persons. This is true of both typical TB (*Mycobacterium tuber-*

INFECTIONS COMMON TO HIV AND WHERE DISCUSSED IN THIS BOOK

Meningitis and Encephalitis, pages 52-65
Campylobacter, pages 74-80
Entamoeba, pages 81-82, 84-86
Enterovirus, page 94-104
Giardia, pages 82-86
Salmonella, pages 86-93
Shigella, pages 74-80
Strongyloides stercoralis, pages 94-104
Vibrio parahaemolyticus, pages 67, 69-74
Cytomegalovirus, pages 118-120
Epstein-Barr virus (mononucleosis), page 116
Hepatitis A, B, C, D, E, pages 105-115
Toxoplasmosis, pages 120-127
Histoplasmosis, pages 137-140
Tuberculosis, pages 148-154
Candida (vulvovaginitis), pages 199-202
Chlamydia, pages 186-189
Gonorrhea, pages 186-189
Herpes simplex, pages 193-194
Lymphogranuloma venereum, page 195
Molluscum contagiosum, pages 198-199
Papillomavirus (Condylomata acuminata), pages 198-199
Syphilis, pages 189-192

culosis) and several atypical and rare species of tuberculosis-causing organisms. Aggressive identification of TB in HIV-infected persons is important so that they can be treated. This is necessary to prevent transmission to health care workers and close personal contacts. TB, unlike PCP, can be transmitted directly to others.

Dermatologic disorders are common. These include eruptions from systemic infections, such as herpes or staphylococcal infections. Other skin lesions result from drug reactions and parasitic infestations. Dry and irritated skin seems to accompany HIV infection from the start. Many other skin manifestations, particularly in the anogenital and axillary areas, result from problems with hygiene associated with chronic fever-induced diaphoresis and diarrhea. In addition, HIV-infected persons who are malnourished, dehydrated, or bedridden are at risk for decubiti. As in other chronically ill persons, bedsores are almost impossible to heal. Decubiti and other lesions are dangerous in immunocompromised persons because they easily become infected, leading to septicemia.

One manifestation of HIV infection that is commonly seen first on the skin is **Kaposi's sarcoma (KS)**. KS was one of the early manifestations, seen primarily in homosexual males, that heralded the begin-

For pictures of Kaposi's sarcoma lesion, see color plates 2 through 4, page x.

ning of the AIDS epidemic. KS is seldom seen in women, hemophiliacs, and children with AIDS. It is also one of the conditions that leads to an AIDS diagnosis. The frequency of this manifestation of HIV infection, however, is declining. KS was considered an extremely rare neoplasm until the advent of the AIDS epidemic. It was only found in Africans or elderly men of Mediterranean descent. In its classic form, KS was a slowly developing disease, usually limited to the skin, that was seldom life-threatening. The KS associated with HIV infection is very aggressive. Once it has appeared somewhere in the body, it is likely to be in the process of developing everywhere.

KS is a malignant tumor of the endothelium, the layer of epithelial cells that lines the blood vessels, heart cavity, lymphoid tissues, and serous cavities. Incompletely formed blood vessels proliferate, blood is extravasated from them, and lesions of varying shades in color and size are formed based on the amount of blood they contain. The first lesions often appear on the face and head and in the oral cavity. KS lesions can also be found in the lung, rectum, esophagus, viscera, nasopharynx, liver, biliary ducts, lymph nodes, kidneys, and brain. They are considered to be multicentric rather than metastatic, meaning that several primary lesions will arise at the same time in different places in the body.

Persons who contract KS as their first manifestation of immunosuppression once were considered to have a better prognosis. Recent data do not support that finding. KS is an important contributor to mortality among HIV-infected persons.

Understanding the **psychological reactions** to HIV infection is critical to caring for the infected person. The box on page 163 summarizes some of the common reactions. Unlike many of the other complications of HIV, these can be present early in the infection. However, like the physical manifestations, psychologic responses are also variable. Responses will vary, depending on cultural and socioeconomic factors, age, gender, and life condition of the infected person.

Fear and anxiety begin early. The decision to submit oneself to HIV testing provokes anxiety because of the long-term implications of a positive result. Anxiety soars during the time while one waits for the test results. Many high-risk persons prefer to not know their HIV antibody status because such information will create unbearable anxiety.

Once the HIV positive status is known, an infected person frequently uses the psychologic defense of denial to cope with the awful reality. Others seriously contemplate suicide. All have justifiable fears about the reaction of others to their infected status, and many respond to their fears by isolating themselves from others to avoid disclosure. Some express feelings of guilt over the life-style behaviors that exposed them to infection. Many become preoccupied with measures to maintain their present health status. These persons are particularly vulnerable to fads, experimental therapies, and frauds. For many asymptomatic HIV-infected persons, life becomes little more than a constant monitoring for symptoms, often to the point of hypochondria.

Some of the initial reactions may intensify when one becomes symptomatic. In addition, new reactions are likely to occur. Depending on the course of the symptoms and one's social situation, the HIV-infected person may experience job loss, impoverishment, decline in physical function, social isolation, and intractable physical pain. Even if the course of the disease process is not as bad as expected, there is always fear that it will be worse. Disease can no longer be denied. Frequently, the disease and its progress permeates the person's life. Emotional exhaustion (feeling that one cannot go on) and suicidal ideation are often present.

Preoccupations with pain relief and preparing for death frequently dominate later stages of the disease. Issues such as living wills and property wills must be decided. This is the time to complete the unfinished business of one's life—to reconcile with loved ones and to say good-bye. People at this stage of HIV disease are highly dependent on others to provide basic needs and comfort. They will frequently fear being abandoned in such a dependent state.

Throughout the course of the infection, HIV-infected persons are likely to feel and express anger—anger about pain, about dying prematurely, about their many losses, about the rejection and prejudice they experience, and about the reaction of society towards them and the disease. Often the anger is directed toward health care workers who are inflicting the painful and humiliating procedures and treatments without guaranteeing the hoped for cure. Health care workers should recognize that the anger is not directed to them personally but toward the situation. In addition, persons with CNS involvement or other affective disorders may have less control over their expressions of anger. Health care workers can help dissipate the anger by reassuring patients of their worth and acceptance.

PSYCHOLOGICAL REACTIONS TO HIV INFECTION

Reactions to learning that one is HIV positive

Denial

Affective numbing

Anger

Feeling of powerlessness

Persistent anxiety

Depression and suicidal ideation

Fear of loss of sex life

Fear of contaminating others

Fear of rejection by significant others

Fear of loss of job and health insurance

Fear of loss of financial independence

Feelings of guilt and self-blame

Fear of life-threatening infections

Hypochondria

Preoccupation with lifestyle changes and measures to protect immune system

Self-isolation and difficulty in interacting with others (resulting from fears of society's stigmatization)

Summary: HIV infection dominates the infected person's thinking process, often to the exclusion of other major life concerns. The person is frequently preoccupied with issues of confidentiality and fear of stigmatization.

Reactions to becoming symptomatic

In addition to the previous reactions:

Grief over losses: health, physical attractiveness, job, ability to care for self

Preoccupation with maintaining normalcy of life and meeting basic needs for food, shelter

Recognition of likely mortality

Hopelessness

Suicidal ideation

Emotional exhaustion

Stress reaction to dealing with demands of medical treatment, pain, and medical expenses

Embarrassment because of physical symptoms (e.g., lesions and diarrhea)

Loneliness

Uncontrollable expressions of anger related to neurologic effects of the disease

Summary: Symptom management during the course of the HIV infection continues to dominate the infected person's life. Medical treatment and maintaining basic activities of daily life are all consuming. Living with AIDS is a full-time job.

Reactions to dying

Concern with resolving the business of one's life (e.g., reconciliations, disposing of property, and preparing a will)

Preoccupation with pain and pain control

Preoccupation with other disease symptoms

Fear of abandonment before death

Concern with planning for death with care providers

Fear of dying

Fear of dying alone

Summary: Dying becomes a full-time job.

DIAGNOSTIC STUDIES AND FINDINGS

Diagnostic Test	Findings
Tests to diagnose HIV infection:	
ELISA	Positive for antibodies against HIV (because of the possibility for false-positive results, the test will be run twice)
Western blot	Positive result indicates presence of antibodies against HIV; test is performed to confirm a positive result obtained on the ELISA; negative result indicates no antibodies
P24 antigen test	Positive result indicates circulating HIV antigen
HIV culture	Positive based on a measure of the presence of reverse transcriptase activity in suspected T lymphocyte (may take up to 60 days to obtain results)

Tests to detect impairment of the immune system: change in the test results in the direction indicated is a sign of worsening immune status. Absolute values are less important with these tests.

Hematocrit	Decrease in the normal range of 37%-49%
Erythrocyte sedimentation rate	Elevation of the normal range of <15 mm/h
CD4 lymphocytes	Decrease in the normal range of 600-1200
CD4/CD8 lymphocyte ratio	The normal 2:1 ratio is lowered or reversed
Serum B2 microglobulin	Elevation of the normal value of <3.0 mg/L
Serum neopterin	Elevation above baseline
Hemoglobulin	Decrease in normal range of 12-18 g/dl

Tests of overall health status of HIV-infected person: the following tests would be ordered soon after the patient is found to be HIV positive. They would be periodically repeated to monitor general health and repeated in response to symptoms. While individual test results might indicate pathology, their purpose is to establish a baseline against which subsequent findings can be compared.

CBC, differential, platelet count	
SMA-12 or similar blood screening panel	
Serologic tests for syphilis, toxoplasma, cryptococcus and hepatitis	
Urinalysis; chest x-ray	
Pap smear and/or pregnancy test	
Tuberculin skin test	A weak reaction of 5 mm induration is positive for an immunocompromised person

Tests for oral diseases:
(See also Chapter 9)

Inspection	Observable oral lesions
Microscopic exam of KOH prepared sputum specimen	Positive for yeast cells of *Candida*
Herpes simplex viral culture	Positive for herpes simplex virus
Microscopic exam of tissue scrapings or biopsied tissue	Positive for multinucleated giant cells
Electron microscopy	Positive for viral particles
Exam of tissue biopsy	Positive for warts, Kaposi's sarcoma, and/or hairy cell leukoplakia

DIAGNOSTIC STUDIES AND FINDINGS—cont'd

Diagnostic Test	Findings
Tests for neurologic disease: (See also Chapter 4)	
Neurologic exam	Hyperreflexia, Babinski's sign, ataxia; inability to perform ADL
Mini-mental status exam	Decreasing mental function since baseline
CT scans or magnetic resonance imaging (MRI)	Abnormal cerebral lesions, atrophy, distortions of ventricles, infarctions
Electroencephalogram	Generalized slowing
Electromyelogram (EMG)	Abnormal electrical conduction
Analysis of CSF	Protein and blood are abnormal findings
Microscopic exam of CSF	Positive for pathogens
Tests for GI disease: (See also Chapter 5)	
Endoscopy	Visualization of GI lesions
Culture and microscopic examination of stool, GI fluids, or biopsied tissue	Positive for pathogens, KS lesions, or lymphoma
Serum electrolytes	Increased serum sodium; decreased serum potassium and chloride
Hepatic enzymes (AST, ALT) (ALP)	Elevated above baseline for patient
Bilirubin	Elevated above baseline for patient
CT scan or ultrasound of abdomen	Enlarged liver or other abnormalities
Sigmoidoscopy	Visualization of rectal disease
Inspection of anus	Visualization of lesions, KS, or exudates
Tests for respiratory disease: (See also Chapter 7)	
X-ray	Abnormal findings
Pulmonary function tests	Diminished function
Exam of tissue obtained by bronchoscopy or open lung biopsy	Characteristic organisms or neoplasms
Gallium citrate scan	Increased uptake is found in HIV-infected persons
Microscopic exam or culture of specimen of sputum or bronchial secretions obtained by lavage	Positive for characteristic pathogens
Blood gas levels	Results indicative of hypoxemia
Tests for dermatologic disease:	
Microscopic exam of lesion biopsy	Characteristic appearance of lesions, pathogens, or neoplasms
Tests for sensory system disease:	
Ophthalmic exam	Retinal damage consistent with CMV retinitis
Audiometry	Diminished hearing

MEDICAL MANAGEMENT OF HIV INFECTION

The goal of medical management of HIV infection is to maintain the body's immune status at the highest level to ward off opportunistic disease. This is approached in three ways. The first is to promote general health status (health promotion) and to improve or maintain immune function by treating preexisting disease and educating the patient toward behaviors that will improve resistance to opportunistic infections. The second is to prevent infections that may trigger T4 helper cell activation and consequent HIV replication. This is accomplished through immunization and prophylactic therapies. The third approach is to suppress HIV action in the body.

DRUG THERAPY

Prevention of infections: **Immunizations:** Live measles, mumps, and rubella (MMR); inactivated polio vaccine (IPV); pneumococcal vaccine and yearly influenza vaccine. Individuals at risk for hepatitis B should receive the hepatitis B vaccine.

Antiinfective therapy is used to suppress pathogen growth. Because antiinfective agents probably do not eradicate the organism in the immunocompromised, many patients are maintained on antiinfective agents even after symptoms of the infection are resolved.

Prophylaxis of pneumocystis carinii pneumonia: Aerosolized pentamidine isethionate (Pentam).

Prophylaxis of all pneumocystis carinii infections: Trimethoprim/sulfamethoxole (Bactrim).

Prophylactic protocols for other opportunistic infections are being investigated.

Suppression of HIV: This is an area of rapid drug development and testing through drug trials. The agents being tested primarily have an antiviral action. They either inhibit HIV replication, interfere with the virus's ability to attach to CD4 receptors, eliminate HIV reservoirs in cells, or activate antiviral defenses.

Zidovidine, also called AZT (Retrovir) is the only drug approved for HIV suppression at the time of this writing. AZT acts by interfering with DNA synthesis, thus inhibiting HIV replication. Decisions regarding dosages and time of administration during the infection are changing. AZT was originally utilized at high doses late in the infection. Recent research supports use earlier in the infection at lower, less toxic doses.

Two other drugs, which are **zidovidine analogs,** are not yet approved but are being used widely in drug trials. These are dideoxyctidine (DDC) and dideoxyinosine (DDI).

Recombinant human erythropoietin (r-HuEPO) stimulates RBC production and is used for treatment of AZT-induced anemia.

GENERAL MANAGEMENT FOR HEALTH PROMOTION

Treatment of existing health problems: In addition to their HIV status, infected persons are at risk for all of the health conditions that uninfected persons of their age and gender may experience. These include pregnancy and complications of pregnancy, chronic diseases such as diabetes or gastric ulcers, psychiatric disorders, and alcohol or drug abuse.

Mental health care: It is believed that clinical depression has negative effects on immune system function either directly or through influences on the depressed person's life-style and ability to comply with treatment. Therefore psychotherapy and antidepressant therapy are frequently employed.

Health education: See Patient Teaching in this chapter.

MEDICAL MANAGEMENT OF AIDS RELATED DISEASE:

The goal is to restore equilibrium as soon as possible once opportunistic disease has occurred. Disease is likely to affect one or more body systems with one or more concurrent disease processes. This requires rapid treatment with antiinfective drugs plus general management to support the body systems affected by the disease. Medical management is organized in this table by body system. Antiinfective drugs, which are generally prescribed according to the pathogen causing infection, are presented in Table 8-3. Specific dosages and routes of administration are not included in the table because therapeutic regimens vary greatly, depending on the intractability of the infection, potential for systemic dissemination of the pathogen, body site of the infection, whether the therapy is prophylactic or curative, other concurrent drug therapies, patient tolerance, and the patient's general health. It must be noted that knowledge of management of the patient with HIV infection and AIDS is still evolving. Consequently, controversy and variability in all therapies exists.

DRUG THERAPY

Oral manifestations: See Table 8-3; antimicrobial oral rinses; topical steroids; chemotherapy for KS lesions.

Neurologic manifestations: See Table 8-3; psychostimulants, antianxiety drugs, antidepressants, antipsychotics; analgesics for pain; chemotherapy and/or radiotherapy; radiotherapy for CNS lymphoma.

GI manifestations: See Table 8-3; topical ointments for ano-rectal disease; chemotherapy for KS lesions and lymphomas; antinausea and antidiarrheal agents.

Respiratory manifestations: See Table 8-3; chemotherapy for KS and lymphomas; radiotherapy for KS lesions.

Dermatologic manifestations: See Table 8-3; lindane for scabies; topical steroids to promote healing; topical lotions for dry skin; chemotherapy for KS lesions.

Sensory system manifestations: See Table 8-3; chemotherapy for ocular and eyelid KS lesions (if lesions are also widespread elsewhere in body); ophthalmic ointments for nonopportunistic bacterial infections; systemic antimicrobials for otitis media; radiotherapy for KS lesions.

GENERAL MANAGEMENT

Oral manifestations: Plaque removal; teach oral hygiene.

Neurologic manifestations: Psychiatric consultation; assessment of medication use to rule out effects from polypharmacy; teach patient techniques for living with cognitive impairment. Refer patient to support groups, family counseling, and social services to provide for unmet needs that are causing anxiety, psychiatric hospitalization, and/or drug and alcohol treatment.

GI manifestations: Diet therapy, enteral supplementation or hyperalimentation; fluids and electrolytes.

Respiratory manifestations: Oxygen, hydration, humidified air; assisted respiration.

Dermatologic manifestations: Egg crate or water mattress to relieve pressure; monitoring of drugs to prevent dermatologic reactions.

Sensory system manifestations: Vision and hearing aids.

SURGERY

Oral manifestations: Debridement of periodontitis; excision of warts and KS lesions; radiotherapy and laser surgery for KS.

GI manifestations: Removal of neoplasms and warts; draining of abscesses, debridement of anorectal lesions.

Dermatologic manifestations: Electrosurgery; laser surgery; excision of lesions, currettage; cryotherapy.

Table 8-3

ANTIINFECTIVE DRUG THERAPY FOR AIDS-RELATED INFECTIONS

Organism (disease name)	Body system	Antiinfective agents (generic name only)
Bacteria:		
Mycobacterium tuberculosis (Tuberculosis)*	Respiratory, bone marrow	Isoniazid, rifampin, cycloserine, ethionamide, ethambutal, clofazamine, rifabutin
Mycobacterium avium intracellulare (MAI, atypical tuberculosis)	Systemic	Rifabutin, ethambutol, cycloserine, ethionamide, clofazimine
Salmonella species (Salmonellosis)*	GI, gallbladder, systemic	Ampicillin, amoxicillin, chloramphenicol
Shigella (Shigellosis)*	GI	Ampicillin, cotrimoxazole, quinolones
Chylamydia trachomatis (Chylamydia)*	GU, respiratory	Erythromycin, tetracycline
Viruses:		
Herpes simplex (Herpes)*	Oral, genital and rectal mucosa, skin, conjuctiva, CNS	Acyclovir
Herpes zoster (Shingles)	Peripheral nerves, skin	Acyclovir
Cytomegalovirus (CMV infection)*	Retina, GI, CNS, respiratory	Gancyclovir (DHPG)
Helminths:		
Strongyloides stercoralis (Strongyloidiasis)*	Intestinal tract	Thiabendazole, albendazole
Fungi:		
Cryptococcus neoformans (Cryptococcosis)	CNS, respiratory, bone marrow, skin	5-Flucytosine with amphotericin B or amphotericin B alone
Histoplasma capsulatum (Histoplasmosis)*	Systemic, bone marrow, skin, respiratory, GI	Amphotericin B, ketoconazole
Candida albicans (Candidiasis)*	GI, mouth, skin, respiratory, anorectal-genital area	Ketoconazole, nystatin, clotrimoxazole, amphotericin B
Protozoa:		
Pneumocystis carinii (PCP)	Respiratory	Cotrimoxazole, pentamidine, trimetrexate with leucovorin, sulfamethoxazole/trimethoprim
Toxoplasma gondii (Toxoplasmosis)*	CNS, lymph nodes, respiratory	Pyrimethamine and sulfadiazine (together)
Microsporum species (Microsporosis)	Skin, GI tract	Griseofulvin, topical antifungals
Giardia lamblia (Giardiasis)*	GI tract	Metronidazole, quinacrine
Entamoeba histolytica (Amebiasis)*	GI, CNS, liver, respiratory	Metronidazole followed by iodoquinol

*Treatment of these infections is also discussed in other chapters in this book. See the box on page 161 for chapter locations.

NURSING CARE FOR THE HIV-INFECTED PATIENT

Nursing care of HIV-infected persons differs little from care of persons with other acute and chronic health problems. People with HIV, for example, have the same nursing diagnoses as other patients and require the same nursing interventions. The major difference is that those with HIV infection experience almost all of the diagnoses at some time during the course of the infection. There is also great variation in the course of the infection between those infected. No two patients have the same constellation of problems at the same time. Nursing care must be holistic and flexible to meet the complex needs of patients with HIV infection.

__1__ ASSESS

ASSESSMENT	OBSERVATIONS
History	HIV positive test or possible exposure to the virus; history of engaging in high-risk behaviors; diagnosis of STD, hepatitis B, persistent lymphadenopathy or other infectious disease; Reports use of multiple drugs, including prescribed, OTC, recreational, and unapproved drugs
General appearance	Cachectic, pale
Subjective symptoms	Chronic fever, with or without chills; recurrent night sweats; malaise, weakness, severe fatigue; anorexia, weight loss; pain; difficulty sleeping
Psychosocial	Anxious appearance; history of recent loss of job and health insurance; alienation from significant others, changed living situation, and multiple life changes; expresses feelings of guilt, grief, or fear
Mental status	Behavior changes, expressions of anger or hopelessness; depressed affect, suicidal ideation, apathy, withdrawal, loss of interest in surroundings; reports selling or giving away possessions; disturbances in thought processes; impaired judgment; cognitive "slowing," memory loss, confusion; altered attention and concentration; impaired communication, aphasia, difficulty finding words; slurred speech; hallucinations, delusions
Head, ears, eyes, nose, and throat (HEENT)	Periorbital pain, photophobia, blurred or double vision, total loss of vision; diffuse hemorrhaging, exudates; headache; facial edema; tinnitus or hearing loss; white or red raised lesion(s) in oral cavity; ulcers on lips or in mouth, bleeding in mouth; dry mouth, voice changes; dysphagia; palpable lymph nodes; epistaxis
Neurologic	Altered pupillary reflexes, nystagmus; peripheral neuropathy; vertigo, imbalance, ataxia; neuromuscular incoordination; nuchal rigidity, severe headache; seizures, loss of consciousness; paraplegia, quadraplegia
Musculoskeletal	Muscle wasting; focal motor deficits; weakness and inability to perform ADLs
Cardiovascular	Tachycardia related to fever; hypotension related to dehydration; irregular heart rate, dizziness related to electrolyte imbalance; absent peripheral pulses and peripheral edema
Respiratory	Dyspnea, tachypnea, cyanosis; shortness of breath upon exertion; uses accessory muscles; positions self to facilitate respiration; productive or nonproductive cough; distant or decreased breath sounds upon auscultation
GI	Decreased food or fluid intake; reports oral pain (causing difficulty in eating); anorexia, nausea, vomiting, weight loss; diarrhea, incontinence; abdominal tenderness, cramping; hepatomegaly, splenomegaly, jaundice; bowel sounds (absent or hyperactive); anal lesions, rectal bleeding
GU	Lesions or exudate on genitalia; female reports pelvic pain; decreased urine output related to dehydration; incontinence
Integumentary	Reports dryness and pruritis, night sweats; rash or lesions anywhere on body; red-violet, raised lesions, petechiae; palpable lymph nodes; jaundice; poor skin turgor related to dehydration; skin warm and very moist to touch; markings from IV drug use

➤ ➤ ➤

2 DIAGNOSE

NURSING DIAGNOSIS	SUPPORTIVE ASSESSMENT FINDINGS
Potential for infection related to immunosuppression, effects of chemotherapy or radiation, frequent venipuncture, malnutrition, and high-risk life-style	History of high-risk life-style; laboratory findings of HIV infection and immunosuppression; reports recurrent fevers and night sweats, weight loss, fatigue; cachexia; pale skin color and poor skin turgor
Potential for infection (patient contacts) related to HIV infection, lifestyle, and presence of nonopportunistic infections that can be transmitted	History of exposure to HIV; body secretions, excretions, or exudates contain viable pathogens; fever; lymphadenopathy; lesions

The following nursing diagnoses are not in order of importance. All are important at different phases of HIV infection.

NURSING DIAGNOSIS	SUPPORTIVE ASSESSMENT FINDINGS
Altered thought processes related to CNS infection with HIV or other pathogens, malignancies, hypoxemia, drug reactions, depression	Reports forgetfulness, slowness in thinking and solving problems; demonstrates confusion, altered judgment, disorientation, personality change, memory loss; delusions and hallucinations; signs of meningitis; signs of self-neglect (e.g., failure to eat or pay bills); laboratory or diagnostic findings of CNS infection or malignancy
Potential for injury related to CNS disease, mental status changes, generalized weakness and neuromuscular impairment	Reports forgetfulness, unrealistic expectations of self, weakness, poor vision, altered feeling in extremities; falls; demonstrates impaired balance, gait, and muscle strength; confusions; has seizures
Potential for poisoning related to toxic effects of drug therapy	Findings depend on drug; often mimic influence with CNS disease, dizziness, sensory disturbances, hypertension or hypotension, rashes, edema, hair loss; disturbance in mood; sedation, loss of consciousness
Activity intolerance related to weakness, CNS and neurologic involvement, altered O_2 exchange, malnutrition, fluid and electrolyte imbalance, fatigue	Reports fatigue, weakness, shortness of breath and tremors upon exertion; unable to perform ADLs; muscle atrophy; paralysis of limbs; exertional dyspnea and tachycardia; psychomotor incoordination
Sensory-perceptual alterations (visual, auditory, and kinesthetic) related to CMV retinitis, otic infections and HIV damage to CNS	Reports photophobia, loss of vision, impaired hearing; ataxia, apraxia
Impaired verbal communication related to CNS disease	Demonstrates inability to recognize or understand written/spoken word; difficulty articulating words; unable to recall familiar words
Chronic pain related to neurologic disease, pressure of KS lesions on nerves, and lymphadenopathy	Reports burning pain in extremities, severe headache or tenderness in areas of enlarged lymph nodes
Sleep pattern disturbance related to anxiety, night sweats, chills, and schedule of treatments	Reports inability to sleep, changing sleep patterns, and daytime fatigue
Social isolation related to others' fear of AIDS, family rejection, society's stigmatization, patient's withdrawal from people and activities	Reports loss of job, living alone; withdrawn behavior; no visitors in the hospital; expresses loneliness

NURSING DIAGNOSIS	SUPPORTIVE ASSESSMENT FINDINGS
Self-care deficit in all ADLs related to deterioration of condition, exertional dyspnea, mental changes, neurologic impairment, depression, impoverishment	Reports being too tired to take care of self; stays in bed; decreases participation in self-care activities; appears to have neglected appearance
Impaired home maintenance management related to activity intolerance, inadequate finances, and lack of knowledge about sources of help	Reports living alone with limited or no help; limited finances; reports and demonstrates inability to care for self
Anxiety related to diagnosis; fear of treatment, hospitalization, pain, dying, and death; multiple losses associated with diagnosis of HIV	Expressions of helplessness, anger, regretfulness, fear, denial; demonstrates restlessness, agitation, pacing, inability to sleep
Powerlessness related to poor prognosis of disease and perceived lack of control over disease outcome and health care decisions	Verbalizes having no control over life, future or treatment; expresses anger, apathy, or passivity; increases dependence on others; demonstrates noncompliance with medical regimen
Grieving/hopelessness related to multiple losses (health, attractiveness, job, insurance, relationships (family), and lack of personal future	Has depressed affect; decreases communication; increases sleeping or staying in bed; sells or gives away all possession; expresses anger, sorrow, suicidal ideation; demonstrates self-neglect
Impaired gas exchange related to pulmonary infections or malignancies	Reports progressive shortness of breath, productive or nonproductive cough, fatigue; exertional dyspnea; tachypnea; use of accessory muscles for respiration; distant or decreased breath sounds; circumoral cyanosis; laboratory and radiographic findings of respiratory disease
Altered nutrition: less than body requirements related to decreased intake (associated with oral pain, dysphagia, anorexia, and nausea), increased metabolic needs (caused by infections) and decreased absorption of nutrients (caused by GI disease)	Reports inability to eat, decreased appetite, nausea, vomiting, diarrhea; weight loss of more than 20% of normal body weight; cachectic, pale; abdominal tenderness, abnormal bowel sounds, enlarged liver or spleen; laboratory findings indicate anemia, intestinal parasites, or malignancies
Diarrhea related to GI infection or malignancy, chemotherapy, radiation or drug reactions	Up to 20 liquid stools/day; abdominal tenderness; hyperactive bowel sounds; incontinence of stool; laboratory and diagnostic findings indicate intestinal infections or malignancies
Fluid volume deficit related to nausea, vomiting, diarrhea, fever, and diaphoresis	Reports vomiting, diarrhea, decreased fluid intake, weight loss, dry mouth and skin, postural dizziness, and profuse diaphoresis; poor skin turgor, hypotension, oligura/anuria; laboratory findings of electrolyte and fluid imbalance
Hyperthermia related to infections	Elevated temperature; hot, flushed skin; tachycardia; diaphoresis
Impaired skin integrity related to multiple skin infections, KS lesions, malnutrition, immobility, incontinence, radiation therapy	Reports itching, burning; rash, lesions, or decubiti anywhere on body; excoriated genital or perianal area; edema of extremities

→ > >

NURSING DIAGNOSIS	SUPPORTIVE ASSESSMENT FINDINGS
Altered oral mucous membrane related to oral, pharyngeal, or esophageal infections or lesions; malnutrition	Reports soreness of mouth or throat, dysphagia, changes in taste; inflammation, ulceration, or lesions of oral and pharyngeal mucosa; bleeding of gums or nose
Alteration in sexual patterns related to fear of transmission of HIV; alteration in self-concept; severed relationships; activity intolerance	Reports changes in life-style and sexual activities, loss of significant persons
Ineffective family coping related to anxiety about loved one's condition, fear of infection or stigmatization, long-term dysfunctional relationships, and demands of providing care for the patient	Family/significant others demonstrate anxious or hostile behaviors, do not visit patient; patient expresses concern about how family/significant others are coping; patient is discharged home to care of family/significant others

3 PLAN

Patient goals

1. Patient will be free of opportunistic infections and their complications.
2. HIV infection will not be transmitted to patient contacts; health care workers observe blood and body fluid precautions; patient observes methods to prevent transmission of HIV or other pathogens.
3. Effects of altered thought process on patient's life will be minimized.
4. Patient will not experience accidental injury or falls.
5. Preventable drug interactions or allergic reactions will be avoided; patient will self-administer drugs as prescribed.
6. Patient will participate in energy-sparing activities as tolerated; will be free of dyspnea and tachycardia during activity.
7. Patient will not be confused or frightened by environmental stimuli; injury will not result from impaired vision, hearing, or kinesthetic sense.
8. Communication with patient will be maximized; patient will communicate needs by nonspeech methods if necessary.
9. Patient will obtain relief from pain.
10. Patient will obtain adequate and uninterrupted rest and sleep.
11. Patient will maintain significant relationships or adapt to changes in relationships; patient will be introduced to other sources of social support.
12. Patient will have daily needs met by others during episodes of acute illness and will participate in self-care as tolerated.
13. Patient and significant others will be knowledgable about community resources and services to facilitate home management.
14. Patient will verbalize anxiety.
15. Patient will identify factors that he or she can control and will make informed decisions regarding personal, legal, and health care needs; patient will participate in decisions regarding treatment.
16. Patient will demonstrate beginning progress through the grieving process.
17. Patient will demonstrate normal respiratory pattern, blood gas levels, and cellular oxygenation; patient will demonstrate ability to self-administer oxygen and will experience relief from symptoms of dyspnea and air hunger.
18. Patient will have adequate calorie and protein intake to meet metabolic needs; weight will stabilize or increase toward preillness levels.
19. Patient will experience maximum comfort and control of diarrhea; complications of diarrhea will be minimized.
20. Fluid and electrolyte balance will be maintained.
21. Body temperature will be maintained within the normal range; comfort and safety will be maintained for patient experiencing fever.
22. Patient will be free of preventable and treatable skin lesions; further skin breakdown will be prevented.
23. Damage to mucous membranes will be minimized; patient will experience maximum oral comfort.
24. Patient/couple will be provided with support and counseling to enable resumption of safe sexual activity or alternative means of sexual satisfaction.
25. Family/significant others will strengthen and maintain mutual support system and adapt to changing demands on them.

4   IMPLEMENT

NURSING DIAGNOSIS	NURSING INTERVENTIONS	RATIONALE
Potential for infection related to immunosuppression, effects of chemotherapy or radiation, frequent venipuncture, malnutrition, and high-risk life-style	Monitor for signs of new infection.	For early treatment.
	Use strict aseptic technique for any invasive procedure. Wash hands before giving care.	To avoid exposing patient to hospital-acquired pathogens.
	Instruct patient in methods to avoid exposure to environmental pathogens (see Patient Teaching).	To prevent added infection burden.
	Obtain specimens for laboratory analysis as ordered.	To ensure accurate diagnosis and treatment.
	Administer antiinfectives as prescribed.	To maintain therapeutic blood levels of drugs.
Potential for infection (patient contacts) related to HIV infection, life-style, and presence of nonopportunistic infections that can be transmitted	Instruct patient/significant others on methods of preventing transmission of HIV and other pathogens (see Patient Teaching).	Patient wants and needs this information.
	Use blood and body fluid precautions when caring for patient. Use other barriers, such as masks, as necessary.	Although the risk of transmitting HIV to health care workers is very small, it is real. The risk for exposure to hepatitis B or TB is greater.
Altered thought processes related to CNS infection with HIV or other pathogens, malignancies, hypoxemia, drug reactions, depression	Assess mental and neurologic processes.	To establish baseline data.
	Monitor for infections, electrolyte imbalance, drug interactions, depression, hypoxemia; administer therapy as prescribed.	These conditions are treatable.
	Structure the environment; maintain comfortable and familiar stimuli.	To minimize disorienting stimuli.
	Encourage patient to have familiar objects nearby. Encourage presence of familiar people. Reorient patient to new occurrences in the environment. Provide clues for orientation (clocks, calendars).	Tangible reminders aid memory and orientation.
	Encourage patient to handle tasks in incremental steps; speak slowly and give simple, short instructions.	Requires less use of memory.
	Help patient to obtain a power of attorney.	To handle legal and financial matters.

➤ ➤ ➤

NURSING DIAGNOSIS	NURSING INTERVENTIONS	RATIONALE
Potential for injury related to CNS disease, mental status changes, generalized weakness, and neuromuscular impairment	Structure environment for patient safety (e.g., provide safety bars and adequate lighting and eliminate clutter); instruct patient/significant other on home safety (see Patient Teaching); counsel patient about driving a car; refer for alternative transportation; supervise disoriented patient; initiate seizure precautions for seizing patient; supervise while patient smokes; keep patient's belongings within reach; encourage patient to ask for help when getting out of bed or ambulating.	To prevent accidents and injury.
	Refer for physical therapy evaluation.	Physical therapist will consult with patient about environmental aids and prosthetics to aid in mobility.
Potential for poisoning related to toxic effects of drug therapy	Instruct patient/other on all prescribed medications: their dosage, route of administration, action, side effects, and untoward reactions and under what conditions to discontinue the drug and call a physician. Have patient keep list of medications and time of administration.	Patients with HIV are frequently taking multiple drugs with increased risk for drug reactions; patients with memory loss have increased risk for medication errors.
	Teach maintenance of IV line for patient receiving IV therapy at home.	To prevent complications.
Activity intolerance related to weakness, CNS and neurologic involvement, altered O_2 intake, malnutrition, fluid and electrolyte imbalance, fatigue	Monitor physiologic response to activity.	Tolerance varies from day to day.
	Structure the environment to conserve patient energy; instruct on measures to use at home to conserve energy and also protect from injury (e.g., ambulation aids, grab bars).	To decrease energy demands.
	Provide care that patient cannot provide for self.	Debilitation sometimes interferes with patient's ability to perform ADLs.
	Structure nursing care to provide for uninterrupted rest.	Extra rest is necessary because of increased metabolic demands.
	Assist patient to develop a manageable schedule that balances activity with adequate rest periods.	Patient's quality of life will be improved if patient can continue with some activity.
Sensory-perceptual alterations (visual, auditory, kinesthetic) related to CMV retinitis, otic infections and HIV damage to CNS	Assess amount of sensory impairment.	To establish baseline data for care.
	Orient patient to the environment; encourage significant others to stay with patient.	To decrease fear and anxiety.
	Speak to and touch patient often.	To provide sensory stimulation.

NURSING DIAGNOSIS	NURSING INTERVENTIONS	RATIONALE
Impaired verbal communication related to CNS disease	Assess patient's verbal ability.	To establish baseline data for care.
	Provide alternative methods of communicating (e.g., picture boards).	To provide a means for patient to communicate needs.
Chronic pain related to neurologic disease, pressure of KS lesions on nerves, and lymphadenopathy	Assess patient's pain. Encourage patient to describe pain and measures used to relieve it.	To establish baseline data. To plan interventions for pain that are individualized.
	Implement palliative measures (e.g., relaxation, backrubs). Instruct patient in alternative therapies or refer patient for instruction (e.g., guided imagery, relaxation, affirmation). Provide distracting activities.	Promotes relaxation and sense of control over pain.
	Administer analgesics as prescribed.	To provide relief from pain.
Sleep pattern disturbance related to anxiety, night sweats, chills, and schedule of treatments	Assess sleep patterns; assist patient in maintaining bedtime rituals.	To plan care based on individual needs.
	Maintain quiet, calm environment; schedule nursing care to avoid interrupting sleep; administer medication as ordered.	To induce uninterrupted sleep.
Social isolation related to others' fear of AIDS, family rejection, society's stigmatization, and client's withdrawal from people and activities	Identify the important relationships in patient's life. Involve these people in patient's care, if patient desires. Encourage visitors and telephone calls.	Encouraging interaction in the health care environment may stimulate continued interaction at home.
	Talk with patient frequently. Avoid wearing mask when there is no risk for splashes.	Mask is usually not required and adds an unnecessary barrier to communication.
	Instruct patient and significant others on transmission.	To provide assurance that HIV is not transmitted casually.
	Refer to support groups and community AIDS resources.	To increase contact with people.
Self-care deficit in all ADLs related to deterioration of condition, exertional dyspnea, mental changes, neurologic impairment, depression, impoverishment	Assess patient's needs for help with ADLs. Provide help with the activities that patient cannot do for self.	Patient's needs change with changes in patient's condition.
	Refer patient to occupational therapy for assistive devices and home equipment.	To make it possible for patient to perform his or her own ADLs; this increases self-respect.
	Teach significant other to provide ADLs for patient.	So that care can be maintained at home.

→ › ›

NURSING DIAGNOSIS	NURSING INTERVENTIONS	RATIONALE
Impaired home maintenance management related to activity intolerance, inadequate finances, and lack of knowledge about sources of help	Assess availability of someone in the home to help patient with shopping, meal preparation, simple housekeeping, and transportation. Assess adequacy of income to support living.	Patient's condition hinders his or her ability to maintain home's comfort and safety.
	Refer patient/family/significant other to community resources for help (e.g., food stamps, food pantries, transportation for handicapped, housekeeping services).	Services are organized in most communities to help persons with HIV, low income, or special needs.
Anxiety related to diagnosis; fear of treatment, hospitalization, pain, dying, and death; multiple losses associated with diagnosis of HIV	Assess patient's coping skills. Be alert to signs of ineffective coping.	May be using defenses (e.g., denial).
	Provide accurate, consistent information about condition and treatment.	To minimize fear of unknown.
	Allow patient to verbalize fears and anger. Recognize that anger is not directed toward health care worker. Reassure patient that feelings are normal.	Anger is a natural reaction; expressing it helps to control it.
	Provide quiet, nonthreatening environment.	Minimizes anxiety-producing stimuli.
	Encourage interaction with support system.	Decreases feelings of isolation.
	Refer patient to mental health care or counseling.	To intervene if anxiety becomes dysfunctional.
Powerlessness related to poor prognosis of disease and perceived lack of control over disease outcome and health care decisions	Respect patient. Provide for patient control of activities pertaining to care. Encourage patient's independent activities to improve health status. Assist patient to identify his or her strengths in coping with the disease. Reinforce behavior that demonstrates the patient is planning for the future and taking control of his or her present situation.	Enhances feelings of self-worth and power over life.

NURSING DIAGNOSIS	NURSING INTERVENTIONS	RATIONALE
Grieving/ hopelessness related to multiple losses (health, attractiveness, job, insurance, relationships, family) and lack of a personal future	Encourage verbalization of feelings.	Shows recognition of importance of losses and grief process.
	Identify patient's lifetime coping mechanisms and reinforce the healthy ones; refer for alcohol or drug counseling if necessary.	Major coping mechanisms for some have been alcohol or drugs.
	Guide patient to think positively about what he or she can do to make life situation better.	Positive thinking is energy providing; allows constructive handling of grief.
	Refer to support groups.	To help with grieving, which will be long-term.
Impaired gas exchange related to pulmonary infections or malignancies	Monitor breathing patterns and breath sounds.	To detect respiratory complications.
	Position patient to facilitate breathing and coughing; teach use of incentive spirometer; teach relaxation techniques and breathing through pursed lips.	To improve lung expansion.
	Provide chest physiotherapy; suction if necessary.	To aid in removal of secretions.
	Administer humidified O_2.	To reduce risk of hypoxemia.
	Provide preprocedure care and teaching for patients undergoing bronchoscopy.	To reduce anxiety.
Altered nutrition: less than body requirements related to decreased intake (associated with oral pain, dysphagia, anorexia, and nausea), increased metabolic needs (caused by infections) and decreased absorption of nutrients (caused by GI disease)	Monitor patient's chewing and swallowing.	Decreased intake is often related to oral and throat pain.
	Monitor weight and intake and output.	To establish baseline data.
	Assess availability of food in home and of someone to prepare food.	Loss of job and income may be a problem.
	Eliminate noxious stimuli, such as odors or unpleasant sights, from the environment.	They stimulate the gag reflex.
	Administer antiemetics as prescribed.	To reduce vomiting.
	Plan diet with patient and significant others.	To ensure that foods are offered that patient likes.
	See Patient Teaching for nutrition suggestions. Consult with dietician.	For additional suggestions tailored to patient's needs.
	Maintain nasogastric tube feeding.	For patient who cannot tolerate swallowing.

➔ ❯ ❯

NURSING DIAGNOSIS	NURSING INTERVENTIONS	RATIONALE
Diarrhea related to GI infection or malignancy, chemotherapy, radiation, or drug reactions	Assess consistency and frequency of stools and presence of blood.	To establish baseline data.
	Auscultate bowel sounds.	Hypermotility is common with diarrhea.
	Administer antimotility agents and psyllium (Metamucil) as prescribed.	Slows intestinal motility; psyllium acts to absorb fluid and form a more solid mass.
	Assess perianal area for excoriation; provide cleansing after every stool; apply A & D Ointment, Vaseline, or zinc oxide.	To minimize burning of skin and decrease discomfort; heavy ointments act as a barrier to keep moisture off skin.
Fluid volume deficit related to nausea, vomiting, diarrhea, fever, and diaphoresis	Monitor for signs of dehydration (e.g., poor skin turgor, postural hypotension, tachycardia, oliguria).	Fluid volume depletion is a common complication and can be corrected.
	Monitor intake and output and weight.	To establish baseline data.
	Encourage intake of oral fluids.	To compensate for increased output.
	Administer IV and electrolytes as prescribed.	For patient that cannot tolerate oral fluids.
Hyperthermia related to infections	See inside back cover.	
Impaired skin integrity related to multiple skin infections, KS lesions, malnutrition, immobility, incontinence, radiation therapy	Monitor status of skin and lesions daily.	To establish baseline data.
	Help patient keep skin clean and dry; apply moisturizing lotions; care for perianal area as described above.	To prevent breakdown or cracking of skin.
	Change bed linen when soiled; reposition patient frequently; make use of air, water, or foam mattresses, sheep skin pads, and elbow and heel protectors.	To lessen pressure and shearing forces on skin to prevent pressure sores.
	Cover open areas with sterile dry or hydrocolloidal dressing.	To prevent entry of bacteria.
	Implement care of pressure sores as indicated.	To prevent further damage; it may be impossible to heal them.
	Elevate edematous extremities; elevate head of bed if face is edematous; apply cold cloths to face.	To help drain areas blocked by KS lesions.

NURSING DIAGNOSIS	NURSING INTERVENTIONS	RATIONALE
Altered oral mucous membrane related to oral, pharyngeal, or esophageal infection or lesions; malnutrition	Monitor status of oral cavity, throat, and lips.	To identify treatable conditions.
	Refer to dentist.	For care of periodontitis.
	Teach/provide oral hygiene (use of soft toothbrush, nonabrasive toothpaste, nonalcohol-based mouth wash). Encourage frequent rinsing of mouth with saline/hydrogen peroxide solution; apply lip balm.	Prevents spread of lesions and promotes comfort.
	Administer antiinfectives as prescribed.	To control opportunistic infections in mouth.
	Counsel patient to avoid spicy and salty foods and foods of extreme temperatures.	To prevent irritation.
	Encourage oral fluid intake of at least 2,500 ml.	To maintain hydration of mucous membranes.
Alteration in sexual patterns related to fear of transmission of HIV; alteration in self-concept; severed relationships; activity intolerance	Assess patient and partner's concerns about sexual activity; provide complete information on transmission of HIV and on safe, safer, and unsafe sexual practices (see Patient Teaching).	To decrease the risk of further transmission of HIV and to reduce chance of acquiring other STDs, which would further weaken the immune system.
	Provide information on support groups or counselors.	To obtain long-term help with adjustment to effects of HIV on sexuality.
	Offer support to patient's partner.	Partner is likely to be confused and devastated by patient's diagnosis.
Ineffective family coping related to anxiety about loved one's condition, fear of infection or stigmatization, long-term dysfunctional relationships, and demands of providing care for patient	Establish rapport with family/significant other; assess their strengths in coping with patient's illness and with caring for patient.	To begin a relationship for working constructively with the family.
	Allow them to verbalize their feelings (anger, withdrawal, blame)	They may have no one else that they can freely talk to.
	Refer to family support groups.	Families benefit from interacting with others in a similar situation.
	Teach family about disease and transmission.	To relieve anxiety about transmission by casual contact.
	Instruct on home care of patient; refer for respite care or for any other help they may need.	To enable family to provide care without excess stress.

→ › ›

5 EVALUATE

PATIENT OUTCOME	DATA INDICATING THAT OUTCOME IS REACHED
Patient is free of opportunistic infections and their complications	There are no new signs of infection; laboratory findings indicate absence of opportunistic infection; temperature, pulse and respirations are normal; absence of lesions or exudates.
HIV infection is not transmitted; health care workers observe blood and body fluid precautions	Patient contacts and health care workers are not exposed to HIV—they do not test positive; health care workers are not infected with other pathogens, such as *M. tuberculosis.*
Effects of altered thought processes on patient's life are minimized	Patient is able to participate in ADLs without evidence of frustration; has arranged for help with personal and legal affairs.
Patient does not experience accidental injury or falls	Patient is adequately supervised, does not fall or sustain injury; uses assistive devices safely; home environment is free of obstructions that could cause an injury; impaired person does not drive automobile.
Preventable drug interactions or allergic reactions are avoided; patient self-administers drugs as prescribed	Patient completes full course of prescribed medications. If untoward reactions occur, patient discontinues medication and calls physician. Patient informs health care provider of all drugs he or she is taking.
Patient participates in energy-sparing activities; is free of dyspnea and tachycardia during activity	Environment is modified to accomodate patient's modified activity level; patient uses energy-saving methods; patient rests between activities.
Patient is not confused or frightened by environmental stimuli; injury does not occur	Patient is oriented to the environment, does not express fear of stimuli, and does not experience an injury.
Communication with patient is maximized	Patient rests comfortably with needs met; communicates in nonverbal manner without excess frustration.
Patient obtains relief from pain	Patient sleeps, rests, and performs ADLs without apparent pain.
Patient obtains adequate rest and sleep	Patient describes sleeping 7-9 h/day and has energy upon awakening.

PATIENT OUTCOME	DATA INDICATING THAT OUTCOME IS REACHED
Patient maintains significant relationships or adapts to changes in relationships	Patient has visitors; can identify people with whom he or she is close; has names of people to call if help is needed.
Patient has daily needs met by others and participates in self-care as tolerated	Patient participates in ADLs with assistance and with help of devices; or patient is fed, bathed, clothed, and toileted by a caregiver.
Patient and significant others are knowledgeable about community resources and services	Patient/significant others describe services that are available to provide help and how to arrange for help in the home; patient completes plans for adequate living situation.
Patient verbalizes anxieties and fears; uses individual strategies to cope with anxiety	Patient demonstrates decreased anxiety about hospitalization or treatment; verbalizes understanding about condition and treatment; patient demonstrates methods to manage anxiety in productive ways.
Patient identifies factors that he or she can control and makes informed decisions regarding personal, legal, and health care needs	Patient participates actively in decisions about care; asks questions about treatment; verbalizes steps he or she will take to maintain present level of health and improve the quality of daily life.
Patient demonstrates beginning progression through the grieving process	Patient expresses grief and describes the meaning of his or her losses; participates in planning for the future.
Patient demonstrates normal respiratory pattern, blood gas levels, and cellular oxygenation; patient demonstrates ability to self-administer O_2	Patient is free of dyspnea, cough, cyanosis; bronchovesicular sounds are heard throughout lungs; CO_2, P_{O_2}, and P_{CO_2} levels are normal; patient engages in activity without shortness of breath.
Patient has adequate calorie and protein intake to meet metabolic needs	Nausea and vomiting are controlled; patient eats frequent meals of high-protein and high-calorie content; serum albumin and protein are within normal limits; weight is approaching preillness level.

→ → →

PATIENT OUTCOME	DATA INDICATING THAT OUTCOME IS REACHED
Patient experiences maximum comfort and control of diarrhea; complications are minimized	Abdomen is soft and nontender; stools are soft and normal colored and occur at preillness frequency; patient has relief from cramping; perianal area is free of tenderness.
Fluid and electrolyte balance are maintained	Fluid intake equals output; skin turgor is normal; mucous membranes are moist; urine specific gravity is normal; serum sodium and albumin levels are normal.
Body temperature is maintained within normal range; comfort and safety are maintained	Temperature is within normal limits; there are no chills, flushing, or diaphoresis; clothing and bedding are dry; patient is free of headache and malaise.
Patient is free of preventable and treatable skin lesions	Patient is free of decubiti and other skin breakdown or infection associated with patient's debilitated condition.
Damage to mucous membranes is minimized, patient experiences maximum oral comfort	Mucous membranes are moist, with natural color and without bleeding or lesions; mouth is clean and free of food debris and exudates; lesions, if present, are being treated.
Patient/couple are provided with support and counseling to enable resumption of safe sexual activity or alternative means of sexual satisfaction	Patient/couple describe methods for safe sexual expression; verbalize intent to use counseling resources as needed.
Family/significant others strengthen and maintain mutual support system and adapt to changing demands on them	Patient and family interact in constructive ways; family is supportive without denying patient power over decision making; family has information for obtaining help with home care of patient if needed.

PATIENT TEACHING

Pretest counseling

Persons who should be voluntarily tested: anyone being treated for STDs or IV drug abuse, male and female prostitutes, women whose sexual partners are bisexual or have used IV drugs, anyone who received a blood transfusion in the United States between 1978 and 1985, and anyone who considers themselves at risk.

Additional persons may be tested: persons planning marriage, those in correctional institutions, persons undergoing medical evaluation and treatment for infectious disease, and persons admitted to hospitals (CDC, 1987).

1. Discuss reasons patient wants the test.
2. Inform patient that if positive results are obtained with the ELISA test, they will be confirmed with a second test (Western Blot).
3. Assess the impact that the test results will have on the patient's life-style, risk behaviors, and psychological state.
4. Determine if patient has support system.
5. Discuss how patient plans to handle the waiting time until test results are available.
6. Counsel patient to return for test results (they should not be given over the phone).
7. Counsel patient on behaviors to prevent transmission, even if results are negative:

   ■ Risk can be prevented by: (safe)
   Abstaining from IV drugs
   Avoiding vaginal, anal, or oral intercourse and any exchange of body secretions
   ■ Risk can be lessened by: (less safe)
   Maintaining a mutually monogamous sexual relationship
   Using latex condoms with 5% non-oxynol-9 from start to finish with each sexual encounter
   Avoid passing or receiving body fluids (semen, vaginal secretions, blood) during sex
   Using own needles for drug use

8. Provide information on alcohol and drug treatment programs
9. Inform patient of reporting laws in state for positive results

Posttest counseling

A positive test does not indicate AIDS but does indicate a 30% to 50% chance of developing AIDS within 7 years after infection. However, if time of infection is unknown, patients should be prepared to experience symptoms at any time.

1. Instruct patient that the virus can be transmitted at all phases after infection. Repeat Instructions for reducing risk of transmission provided during pretesting. In addition, caution patient to avoid sharing personal items that may be contaminated with blood, such as razors or toothbrushes, and to avoid donating blood, tissue, or sperm.
2. Encourage patient to inform sexual and needle-sharing partners.
3. Counsel women to avoid pregnancy and breastfeeding.
4. Provide patient information on additional counseling and community support services.
5. Counsel patient to inform physician and dentist of HIV status when seeking care.
6. The person with a positive test is likely to hear nothing after hearing the results of the test. Schedule a repeat visit as soon as possible for follow-up counseling on maintaining the immune system and improving general health status.

Follow-up counseling

1. Instruct patient on the signs and symptoms of HIV-related illnesses.
2. Encourage the patient to keep a diary of illnesses, treatments, and medications used.
3. Counsel patient to obtain regular medical care and early treatment of all HIV-related diseases.
4. Remind patients to update their immunization status.
5. Review basic principles to maintain health status, such as diet, exercise, rest, avoidance of drugs and alcohol, cessation of smoking, and stress reduction.
6. Instruct patient on methods to prevent exposure to pathogens:

   ■ Safe and "safer" sexual practices
   ■ Avoidance of needle sharing
   ■ Avoidance of contact with people with infections
   ■ Avoidance of food-borne infections through proper cooking and handling of food, particularly poultry and shellfish

7. Reteach patient proper use of condom.
8. Respond to questions that patient may have about medical treatment to boost the immune system.
9. Instruct patient on balanced program of rest and activity.
10. Teach pursed lips and diaphragmatic breathing to decrease respiratory effort; teach use of incentive spirometer.

11. Instruct patient on prescribed medications, expected effects, dosages, routes of administration, side effects, and untoward reactions.
12. Instruct patient on hygiene and skin care: use mild soaps; rinse well; avoid powders or alcohol-based products that dry the skin; use lotions liberally; avoid scented products that may induce nausea.
13. Instruct patient that nutrition is important; to avoid fad diets (e.g., the antiyeast diet and macrobiotic diet), that are limited nutritionally, and to avoid megadosing with vitamins, herbs, or other unproven products.
14. Teach patient these methods to minimize effects of nausea: clean mouth before eating; avoid tepid foods; eat salty foods, which are sometimes less nauseating; avoid odors of food preparation area; eat small meals; eat dry foods in morning; and avoid drinking liquids with meal. Hard candy or mints between meals may help prevent nausea.
15. Teach patient these methods to manage sore throat and mouth: use a straw, begin meal with cold fluids or juices, avoid highly seasoned or acid foods, and rinse mouth frequently with water during meal.
16. Teach patient these methods to improve nutritional value of meals: fortify meals with high-protein skim milk powder; add milk instead of water in recipes; fortify vegetable and pasta dishes with cheese or ground meat; eat puddings and custards for desert; eat foods with a high-potassium content (e.g., bananas).
17. Teach patient to eat when well-rested to ensure completing the meal.
18. Instruct the patient to avoid cramping by avoiding foods that cause gas, eating small amounts of food often, and chewing with mouth closed to limit swallowing of air.
19. Teach patient to prevent heartburn by not lying down after eating or by elevating the head of bed.

HOME CARE

Home health care and hospice care are often preferred alternatives to hospitalization. Assessments of the desires of the patient and family/significant others and of the home environment are essential. Patient and home caregiver teaching includes:

- Maintenance of central lines for IV therapies
- Self-administration of aerolosized pentamidine therapy
- Instruction in how to maintain ADLs at the highest level (i.e., hygiene for the bedridden patient)
- Assistance with obtaining community resources for help. These include but are not limited to: income assistance, food stamps, home-delivered meals, transportation, support groups for patient and caregiver; legal assistance, housekeeping assistance, chore services, respite help for the caregiver, and help with shopping.
- Assistance with modification of the environment and obtaining equipment that will facilitate care in the home, conserve energy, and promote independence. Useful equipment includes tub seat, hand-held shower, bathtub and shower safety strips and rails; adaptive utensils for eating, dressing, and bathing; walker or wheelchair; hospital bed and bedside commode. Refer to an occupational therapist if accessible for additional guidance.

Persons with AIDS can care for pets if some precautions are followed. It is important to keep the animal well so that it cannot transmit zoonotic infections to the person with AIDS. Pets should be restricted to indoors or to walks on a leash, fed commercial pet foods, examined periodically by a veterinarian, and kept free of fleas. Cat litter should be discarded by a person who is not at risk. A person with AIDS who must handle the litter should wear gloves and a mask during the process.

CHAPTER 9

Sexually Transmitted Diseases

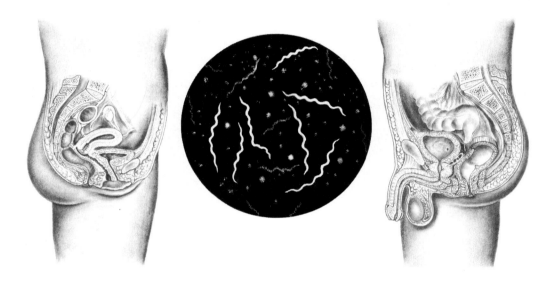

The term **sexually transmitted diseases (STDs)** refers to a large group of disease syndromes that can be transmitted sexually irrespective of whether the disease has genital pathologic manifestations. STD is more encompassing than the previously used "veneral disease" categorization. The STDs, similar to other infectious diseases, can be classified as to their etiologic agent or according to their disease manifestations. The following pathogens are known or thought to be sexually transmitted:

- **Bacteria:** *Neisseria gonorrhoeae; Chlamydia trachomatis; Mycoplasma hominis; Ureaplasma urealyticum; Treponema pallidum; Gardnerella vaginalis; Haemophilus ducreyi; Shigella; Calymmatobacterium granulomatis*
- **Viruses:** Herpes simplex virus; *Papillomavirus;* hepatitis A, B, and non-A, non-B viruses; molluscum contagiosum virus; cytomegalovirus; human immunodeficiency virus (HIV)
- **Protozoa:** *Trichomonas vaginalis: Entamoeba histolytica; Giardia lamblia*
- **Fungi:** *Candida albicans*
- **Ectoparasites:** *Pthirus pubis; Sarcoptes scabiei*

The list of disease syndromes produced by the above pathogens is equally extensive. Many pathogens produce multiple disease syndromes, and many of the disease syndromes may be caused by more than one pathogenic agent. The STDs are grouped in this section according to disease manifestations patients are most likely to present to health care providers (Table 9-1). It must be noted that patients with symptoms of a sexually transmitted disease frequently have multiple sexually transmitted diseases and should be evaluated accordingly.

Table 9-1

STD CATEGORIES ACCORDING TO DISEASE MANIFESTATIONS

Disease manifestations	STD
Urethritis, cervicitis with an inflammatory pyogenic exudate, salpingitis, and related sequelae; proctitis	Gonorrhea; nongonococcal urethritis (*Chlamydia*)
Ulcerative lesions with systemic dissemination of pathogen	Syphilis; lymphogranuloma venereum; herpes
Ulcerative lesions only	Chancroid; granuloma inguinale (donovanosis)
Nonulcerative lesions	Molluscum contagiosum; condylomata acuminata
Vulvovaginitis	Trichomoniasis; candidiasis; bacterial vaginosis (*Gardnerella vaginalis* vaginitis)
Systemic infections without lesions	Cytomegalovirus; hepatitis; Acquired Immunodeficiency Syndrome (AIDS)
Enteric infections	Giardiasis; *Campylobacter enteritis*; shigellosis; amebic dysentery; salmonellosis; *Mycobacterium avium intracellulare* (MAI); cryptosporidium; isospora
Pubic infestations	Scabies; pediculosis
Congenital and perinatal infections and anomalies	Syphilis; gonorrhea; *Chlamydia*; herpes; *Candida* infections; trichomoniasis; AIDS; cytomegalovirus (CMV); hepatitis B; genital warts; bacterial vaginosis

Data from the Centers for Disease Control, 1989.

Gonorrhea and Nongonococcal Urethritis

Gonorrhea (clap, strain, gleet, dose, jack) is an inflammation of the columnar and transitional epithelium caused by the sexually transmitted gonococcus. Symptoms, course of disease, and severity differ between males and females. Chronic and severe complications may result from untreated infections.

> For closeups of gonococcal infection, see color plates 11, 12, and 13, pages xi and xii.

Nongonococcal urethritis is a sexually transmitted urethritis in males (cervicitis and salpingitis in females) caused by an agent other than the gonococcus, most commonly *Chlamydia trachomatis.*

The diseases discussed in this section are manifest as urethritis or cervicitis with an inflammatory pyogenic exudate. Salpingitis and other related sequelae may be present (Table 9-2).

PATHOPHYSIOLOGY

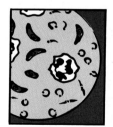

In **gonococcal infections** the gonococcus attaches to and penetrates columnar epithelium, producing a patchy, inflammatory response in the submucosa with a polymorphonuclear exudate. Affected areas in the male are the urethra, Littre's and Cowper's glands, the prostate, seminal vesicles, and the epididymis. Affected areas in the female include the glands of Bartholin and Skene, the urethra, the cervix, and the fallopian tubes. The stratified and transitional squamous epithelia are resistant to the gonococcus; therefore the bladder, upper urinary tract, preputial sac, vulva, vagina, and uterus are infrequently involved. The only exception is prepubescent girls who are susceptible to a gonococcal vulvovaginitis before changes in the vaginal epithelium that accompany puberty. In both sexes primary infections may also affect the pharynx, conjunctivae, and anus.

Direct extension of the infection occurs by way of lymph vessels. In the female, extension most frequently occurs unilaterally or bilaterally to the fallopian tubes, bypassing the uterus. It appears that some cell surfaces of gonococci have greater ability to attach to fallopian tube mucosa. Thus not all gonococcal cervicitis leads to salpingitis. Direct extension in the male most frequently occurs to the epididymis.

Localized infection in any of the above areas may produce cysts and abscesses. The infection may infrequently resolve without treatment if an adequate cellular immune response develops and if there is adequate drainage of the purulent exudate containing the organism. More commonly, the inflammatory exudate is replaced with fibroblasts, and fibrous tissue fills the inflamed tissue. Hardening of the fibrous tissue causes strictures of the lumen of the urethra, epididymis, or fallopian tubes. Complete or partial occlusion of the fallopian tubes results in sterility or increased risk for ectopic pregnancy.

Infection with gonorrhea does result in a short-lived cellular immune response and a longer-lasting humoral immune response, neither of which protects against future infections.

Nongonococcal urethritis and cervicitis are most frequently caused by strains of *Chlamydia trachomatis* that are pathogenic to columnar epithelium in a manner similar to *Neisseria gonorrhoeae*. Symptomatic manifestations are generally less severe than with gonorrhea, with many subclinical infections. Infection with *C. trachomatis* stimulates a cellular and humoral immune response, neither of which is protective against future infections.

COMPLICATIONS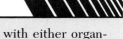

Infection of the fallopian tubes with either organism may result in an acute pelvic inflammatory disease. Exudate may be released into the pelvic cavity, causing a severe peritonitis; or the pelvic inflammatory disease may become chronic, with recurrent inflammatory flare-ups that predispose to pelvic inflammation with normal flora organisms.

Maternal infection during pregnancy can lead to chorioamnionitis and possible disseminated infections in neonates.

Transmission of the pathogens during birth can result in ophthalmia neonatorum and pneumonia in the neonate.

Between 1% and 3% of gonococcal infections become disseminated in the blood, producing septicemia, arthritis, endocarditis, meningitis or skin lesions. Most disseminated infections are asymptomatic before the dissemination. Occasionally an extension of gonococcal or Chlamydial salpingitis in a female leads to perihepatitis.

Both organisms also cause postpartum endometritis in infected women.

Table 9-2

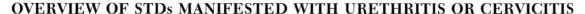

OVERVIEW OF STDs MANIFESTED WITH URETHRITIS OR CERVICITIS

	Gonorrhea	Nongonococcal urethritis (NGU), cervicitis *(Chlamydia)*
Occurrence	Worldwide; highest in 15-30 year olds and among male homosexuals with multiple partners	Worldwide; 3 times more common than gonorrhea
Etiologic agent	*N. gonorrhoeae*, the gonococcus	*C. trachomatis*, less commonly *U. urealyticum*, *T. vaginalis*, *C. albicans*
Reservoir	Humans	Humans
Transmission	Contact with exudates from mucous membranes of infected persons, usually by direct contact	Direct contact with exudates either sexually or during birth
Incubation period	2-7 days	Range 5-10 days for *C. trachomatis*
Period of communicability	Months if untreated	Unknown
Susceptibility and resistance	Universal	Universal; no acquired immunity
Report to local health authority	Mandatory case report	Case report in most states

Reference: Benenson[3]

MEDICAL MANAGEMENT

DRUG THERAPY

Antiinfective agents: **Uncomplicated gonococcal infections in adults and presumption of coexisting Chlamydia infection:**
> Ceftriaxone, 250 mg IM single dose *plus*
> Doxycycline hyclate (Vibramycin), 100 mg PO bid for 7 days, *or*
> Tetracycline (Achromycin; others), 500 mg PO qid for 7 days, *or*
> Erythromycin base or stearate, 500 mg PO qid for 7 days, *or*
> Erythromycin ethylsuccinate, 800 mg PO qid for 7 days.

Alternate regimen for uncomplicated infection:
> Spectinomycin, 2 mg IM once *plus*
> Doxycycline, 100 mg PO bid for 7 days.

If infection was acquired from source proven to not have penicillin-resistant gonorrhea:
> Amoxicillin (Amoxil; others), 3 g PO, single dose with 1 g probenecid PO, *or*
> Ampicillin (Amcill; others), 3.5 g PO, single dose with 1 g probenecid PO, *or*
> Aqueous procaine penicillin G, 4.8 million U IM at two sites with 1 g of probenecid PO *plus* Doxycycline 100 mg PO bid for 7 days.

Pharyngeal gonococcal infection:
> Ceftriaxone, 250 mg IM single dose *or*
> Diprofloxacin, 500 mg po once.

During pregnancy:
> Ceftriaxone, 250 mg IM single dose *plus*
> Erythromycin base or stearate, 500 mg PO qid for 7 days.

Disseminated gonococcal infection (DGI):
> Ceftriaxone, 1 g IM or IV, q 24 h, *or*
> Ceftizoxime, 1 g IV, q 8 h, *or*
> Cefotaxime, 1 g IV, q 8 h.

Adult gonococcal ophthalmia:
> Ceftriaxone, 1 g IM single dose

Infants born to mothers with gonococcal infection:
> Ceftriaxone (50 mg/kg IV or IM, not to exceed 125 mg) single dose.

Infants with gonococcal infection at any site (treat 7 days for ophthalmia or DGI; 10-14 days for meningitis):
> Ceftriaxone, 25-50 mg/kg/day IV or IM q day *or*
> Cefotaxime, 25 mg/kg IV or IM q 12 h.

Gonococcal infections in children who weigh <45 kg (treat children who weigh more with adult regimens):
> Ceftriaxone, 125 mg IM single dose or
> Spectinomycin, 40 mg/kg IM single dose.

Uncomplicated Chlamydia infection only:
> Doxycycline, 100 mg PO bid for 7 days, *or*
> Tetracycline, 500 mg PO qid for 7 days, *or*
> Erythromycin base, 500 mg PO qid for 7 days, *or*
> Erythromycin ethylsuccinate, 800 mg PO qid for 7 days, *or*
> Sulfisoxazole, 500 mg PO qid for 10 days.

The above therapy, recommended by the Centers for Disease Control, 1989 (CDC), is not all inclusive. The recommendations are based on the increase in infections with antibiotic-resistant *N. gonorrhoeae,* such as penicillinase-producing *N. gonorrhoeae* (PPNG), tetracycline-resistant *N. gonorrhoeae* (TRNG), and strains with chromosomally mediated resistance to multiple antibiotics. They also consider the high frequency of concurrent *Chlamydia* infections with gonorrhea. All sexual partners of patients with gonorrhea or *Chlamydia* infection should be examined and treated.

Reference: 37.

DIAGNOSTIC STUDIES AND FINDINGS

Diagnostic Test	Findings
Culture of exudate from urethra, vagina, fallopian tubes, pharynx, or anus	Positive for *N. gonorrhoeae* or *C. trachomatis*
Microscopic examination of gram-stained exudate from urethra or cervix	Positive for gram-negative intracellular diplococci of gonorrhea
Fluorescent antibody (FA) stain and fluorescent microscopic examination	Positive for *C. trachomatis*
ELISA	Detects *C. trachomatis* antibody reaction in specimen
Complement fixation test, immunofluorescent test	For systemic gonococcal infections, fourfold rise in antibody titer between onset of infection and later disease for gonorrhea; Slow-rising titer in sera obtained at 2-wk intervals

All patients with gonorrhea or *Chlamydia* also should be tested for syphilis.

NURSING CARE

See pages 202 to 210.

Syphilis

Syphilis (lues) is a chronic systemic disease characterized by a primary lesion, a secondary eruption involving skin and mucous membranes, long periods of latency, and late seriously disabling lesions of skin, bone, viscera, CNS, and cardiovascular system.

Syphilis is one of several sexually transmitted diseases that have both ulcerative lesions and systemic dissemination. Others are herpesvirus infections and lymphogranuloma venereum (Table 9-3).

PATHOPHYSIOLOGY

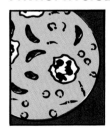

Syphilis is a systemic infection of the vascular system characterized by five distinct stages: incubation, primary and secondary stages, latency, and late syphilis. Incubation begins with the penetration of *Treponema pallidum* into intact mucous membranes or abraded skin. Some of the pathogens remain at the site of invasion while others migrate, within hours, to regional lymph nodes, where some remain while others are disseminated throughout the body. *Treponema* can invade and multiply in any organ system, producing lesions wherever the concentration of the microorganism is the greatest. During this incubation period, blood containing the *Treponema* organisms is infectious.

Vascular pathologic manifestations are the consequence of treponemal tissue invasion at all stages. The inflammatory response in the endothelial tissue produces perivascular infiltration of lymphocytes and plasma cells, resulting in

> For closeups of syphilis infection, see color plates 14 through 18, page xii.

endothelial swelling and an obliterative endarteritis of terminal arterioles and small arteries. Concentric fibroblastic proliferative thickening occurs in the vessels, resulting in eventual foci of tissue necrosis.

The primary stage is characterized by a single lesion at the site of initial invasion containing the *Treponema* and appearing 10 to 90 days after infection. The lesion is firm and hard as a result of intense cellular infiltration accompanied by serum accumulation in connective tissue. The lesion heals spontaneously within 1 to 5 weeks (average of 2 to 3 weeks). A satellite lesion, or bubo, may develop in an inguinal lymph node.

The secondary stage begins as the primary lesion is resolving, lasts 2 to 6 weeks, and is manifested with parenchymal, systemic, and mucocutaneous symptoms that indicate treponemal pathologic manifestations throughout the body. *Treponema* can be recovered from all skin and mucous membrane lesions.

A period of latency, ranging from 1 to 40 or more years, follows the secondary stage. During the first year

Table 9-3

OVERVIEW OF STDs WITH ULCERATIVE LESIONS AND SYSTEMIC DISSEMINATION

	Syphilis	Genital herpes	Herpes type I	Lymphogranuloma venereum
Occurrence	Worldwide; increasing in incidence; highest in 15-30 yr olds and in males, increasing rapidly in females and neonates	Worldwide; increasing rapidly; highest in 15-30 yr olds; most common STD in United States	Worldwide; 70%-90% of adults have antibodies against herpes type 1; primary infection probably occurs by age 5	Worldwide; higher in tropical and subtropical climates
Etiologic agent	*Treponema pallidum*, a spirochete	Herpes simplex virus 2; possibly herpes simplex virus 1	Herpes simplex virus type 1	Several strains of *C. trachomatis*
Reservoir	Humans	Humans	Humans	Humans
Transmission	Direct contact with exudates from lesions on skin and mucous membranes; blood transfusion; congenital	Direct contact with saliva or secretions from mucous membranes and lesions; congenital	Contact with saliva of carriers and active lesions; may be transmitted sexually	Direct contact with open lesions
Incubation period	10 days to 10 wks; usually 3 wks	2-12 days; average of 6 days	2-12 days	4-21 days usually 7-12 days
Period of communicability	Variable; during primary and secondary stages and in mucocutaneous recurrences; 2-4 yrs if untreated	Transient shedding of virus in absence of lesions probably occurs; 7-12 days with lesion	During lesions; virus in saliva found as long as 7 wks after recovery of lesions; transient shedding of virus is common	Variable; weeks to years as long as lesions are present
Susceptibility and resistance	Universal, although only 10% of exposures result in infection; no natural immunity; infection leads to gradually developing resistance to new infections	Universal; immune response does not prevent recurrence	Universal susceptibility	General
Report to local health authority	Mandatory case report	No	No	In some states

References: 3, 37.

of latency there may be recurrence of secondary stage manifestations. Subclinical infection with progressive arterial damage continues for some number of infected persons.

About one third of infected, untreated persons manifest symptoms of late syphilis with clinical evidence of degenerative lesions of the cardiovascular and central nervous systems, the skin, and the viscera. These lesions, called gummas, may be the result of a hypersensitive cellular immune response to the *Treponema* in the tissue. Gummas are granulomatous lesions consisting of a necrotic, coagulated center with obliterative endarteritis of small vessels in the tissue. Lesions of late syphilis, including open gummas on the skin, do not contain *Treponema*. They are therefore not infectious.

Disease manifestations of late syphilis depend on the area of arterial lesions and the extent of circulatory insufficiency. Central nervous system disease may be asymptomatic, meningovascular, or parenchymatous. Parenchymatous neurosyphilis can be seen clinically as paresis (resulting from progressive cortical neuron degeneration) or tabes dorsalis (resulting from posterior column degeneration).

Cardiovascular symptoms frequently result from aortic necrosis with resultant aortic insufficiency.

The immune response in syphilis is not completely understood. Humoral antibodies develop early and persist in untreated persons, but they do not seem to alter the course of the disease. The cell-mediated immune response increases during latency. This may account for the lack of progression to late syphilis for a large portion of untreated persons. Antibody levels will gradually decrease in persons treated in primary and secondary stages.

Congenital transmission of *Treponema* may occur at any time during pregnancy, but the fetus does not develop an inflammatory response to the pathogen until around the fifteenth week of gestation. Treatment of infected pregnant women before the fifteenth week may prevent damage to the fetus. Evidence of congenital syphilitic damage includes early malformations, observed at birth or during the first 2 years of life, and later evidence of developmental deformities (see boxes at right and below.) Infants with congenital syphilis born to untreated or inadequately treated mothers will have active infection and must be treated.

COMPLICATIONS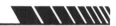

Secondary and tertiary syphilis
Congenital syphilis

NURSING CARE

See pages 202 to 210.

EARLY SYMPTOMS OF CONGENITAL SYPHILIS

Abdomen

Hepatosplenomegaly

Skeletal

Osteochondritis, particularly of the femur and humerus, seen on x-ray examination
Periostitis

Nasopharyngeal

Rhinitis and coryza within first week of life
Frequently bloody mucus

Skin and nails

Dark red, copper-colored maculopapular rash: appears slowly over 3-wks and is followed by a branny desquamation; coppery pigmentation may persist
Suppuration and exfoliation of nails
Loss of hair and eyebrows

Mucous membranes

Fissures on lips, nares, and anus, which bleed easily
Mucous patches on any mucous membrane
Raised moist lesions (condylomata) on areas of skin where there is moisture or friction

Lymph nodes

Generalized lymphadenitis

LATER DEVELOPMENTAL DISABILITIES OF CONGENITAL SYPHILIS

Hutchinson's teeth and mulberry molars
Saddle nose
Interstitial keratitis
Enlarged frontal bossae
Saber shins
Scaphoid scapulae
Short maxilla, high palatine arch, protuberant mandible, and perforation of the hard palate
Deafness
Taboparesis
Mental deficiency

DIAGNOSTIC STUDIES AND FINDINGS

Diagnostic Test	Findings
Darkfield or phase-contrast microscopic examination of exudate or cells from lesions or regional lymph nodes	Positive for *T. pallidum* in primary and secondary stages; not useful for latent or tertiary stages
Nontreponemal serologic tests:	
Venereal disease research laboratory (VDRL)	Useful for screening; many false positive results.
Rapid plasma reagin (RPR)	Increase in nonspecific antibodies 1-3 wks after appearance
Automated reagin test (ART)	of the chancre or 4-6 wks after infection. Become negative
Reagin screen test (RST)	in 6-12 months after treatment of primary syphilis; 12-18 months after treatment of secondary syphilis. Serologic tests may not revert to negative if treatment is delayed beyond 2 yrs; results should be reported quantitatively (i.e., >1:512)
Treponemal serologic tests:	
Fluorescent treponema antibody absorption (FTA-ABS)	Useful for confirmation of positive screening tests. Reported
microhemagglutination assay (MHA-TP)	as nonreactive, borderline, or reactive. These tests become
T. Pallidum hemagglutination assay (TPHA-TP)	reactive earlier in the primary stage and remain reactive longer in latent and late syphilis; remain reactive, even after treatment; results do not vary with disease activity.
Neurosyphilis: Test CSF	
WBC	>5 WBC/mm^3
VDRL	Positive is diagnostic of neurosyphilis (Negative doesn't indicate absence of disease)
Protein	Increased above reference values.

Persons with early syphilis should be tested for other STDs and counseled to be tested for HIV.

MEDICAL MANAGEMENT

DRUG THERAPY

Antiinfective agents: **Primary, secondary, or early syphilis of <1 yr duration:** benzathine penicillin G, 2.4 million U IM single dose.
Of more than 1 yr duration: benzathine penicillin G (Bicillin), 7.2 million U total; 2.4 million U IM/wk for 3 successive wks.
Patients allergic to penicillin: tetracycline (Achromycin; others), 500 mg PO qid for 15 days for infections of <1 yr and for 30 days for infections of longer duration *or*
Doxycycline, 100 mg PO bid for 2 wks for infections of longer duration (pregnant women should not receive tetracycline or doxycycline).
Penicillin-allergic pregnant women should be skin tested and desensitized and then treated with penicillin in a hospital setting (No alternative drug therapies to penicillin are currently effective for treating syphilis in pregnancy, congenital syphilis or neurosyphilis).
Neurosyphilis:
Aqueous crystalline penicillin G, 12-24 million U/day administered 2-4 million U q 4 h IV for 10-14 days *or*
Procaine penicillin, 2-4 million U IM/day plus Probenecid, 500 mg PO qid, both for 10-14 days.
Congenital syphilis:
Aqueous crystalline penicillin G, 100,000-150,000 U/kg/day, administered as 50,000 U/kg IV q 8-12 h *or*
Procaine penicillin, 50,000 U/kg IM, administered once/day for 10-14 days.
If more than 1 day of therapy is missed, restart the entire course.

Reference: 37.

Herpesvirus Infections

Herpes simplex is a systemic viral infection characterized by a localized primary lesion, latency, and a tendency to localized recurrence. Two serologically distinct herpes viral agents, 1 and 2, generally produce distinct clinical syndromes. Herpes simplex virus type 2 (HSV-2) is most often implicated in genital herpes.

For pictures of herpes infections, see color plates 19, 20, and 21, pages xii and xiii.

PATHOPHYSIOLOGY

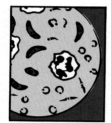

Two antigenically distinct herpes simplex viruses (HSV), types 1 and 2, are responsible for herpes infections. Both are capable of producing infection in epithelial tissue anywhere in the body, but HSV-1 is most often associated with oral, labial, ocular, or skin herpes above the waist, whereas HSV-2 is implicated in 90% of genital, anal, and perianal herpes or oral herpes associated with genital, oral, or sexual transmission. Infections caused by both types of HSV are discussed in this section because of the potential for sexual transmission of both agents and because both produce essentially the same pathologic findings.

All HSV infections have two characteristics in common:

For overview of herpesvirus infection see Table 9-3, page 190.

- Once present in tissue, HSV produces a chronic infection initiated with active self-limiting tissue destruction. The lesions heal, but the organism continues to be viable in the body in the presence of circulating antibodies and in the absence of symptomatic disease.
- There is a latent period during which the genome of the virus is present in tissue in a nondestructive form. Infectious virions cannot be recovered until the virus becomes reactivated and produces recurrent infectious disease. Active infection, either initial or recurrent, need not be symptomatic.

Initial infection refers to the first infection with the HSV type. Initial infection with HSV-1 usually occurs by 4 years and is manifest as a clinical or subclinical gingivostomatitis. Initial infection with HSV-2 usually occurs during the ages of sexual activity and is usually manifested by clinical or subclinical genital herpes.

The organism is transmitted by close contact with saliva or genital secretions of persons with active clinical or subclinical infections either directly or by hand.

The transmitted virus invades and replicates in the parabasal and intermediate epithelial cells of mucous membranes or traumatized skin. Intracellular and extracellular edema and cell lysis cause the cells to lose their intercellular bridges and to undergo a ballooning degeneration. Polymorphonuclear cells infiltrate, forming a thin-walled intradermal vesicle on an erythematous base. Multiple grouped vesicles can be visualized at the sites of tissue inoculation. The superficial epithelium collapses and sloughs, leaving single shallow ulcers, or the vesicles may coalesce into large painful ulcers. Crusting may occur on nonmucous membrane ulcers. All ulcers spontaneously granulate without scarring in about 12 days in initial infections.

The virus may enter the lymphatic system, producing localized lesions there. Rarely, the virus is disseminated to visceral organs, particularly the liver, adrenal glands, lungs, or central nervous system, producing discrete focal areas of necrosis in epithelial tissues in those organs. The virus may also be spread to other external body sites by autoinoculation.

Cellular immune response and nonspecific host defenses appear to inhibit dissemination. Circulating humoral antibodies develop but do not appear to be protective against reinfection or recurrent infection.

Following the primary infections the HSV travels along sensory nerve pathways to a sensory nerve ganglion where it remains in a latent stage. The viral DNA is stored in ganglion neurons in the absence of other viral products. The virus is not pathogenic in this form. It appears that the transient viral shedding may occur during this stage.

The exact mechanism for reactivation of the virus to produce recurrence of lesions is not known; but there are two predominant hypotheses. The **ganglion trigger theory** suggests that a stimulus to latently infected ganglion neurons stimulates the replication of the virus in the neurons. The virus migrates along peripheral nerves to reinvade epithelial cells, producing focal and cellular destruction as in initial infections. The **skin trigger theory** proposes that virus replication in the ganglion neurons is continuous, with viruses regularly reaching the epidermis by way of peripheral nerves. Cellular immune responses block the development of a cellular infectious process unless an external stimulus, such as trauma, overwhelms the defenses.

Recurrence of HSV lesions is generally in the area

of initial inoculation. Genital recurrence is usually associated with HSV-2 and is usually less severe, lasting 4 or 5 days. Genital recurrence is common in women with asymptomatic cervical lesions. Oral HSV-1 infections frequently recur on the lips. Recurrence of either type may be triggered by another infectious disease, menstruation, emotional stress, and immunosuppression.

NURSING CARE

See pages 202 to 210.

COMPLICATIONS

Neuralgia, meningitis (HSV-1), encephalitis (HSV-2), ascending myelitis, urethral strictures, and lymphatic suppuration. In females there is the possibility of an increased risk for spontaneous abortion and cervical cancer. Neonates may become infected during vaginal delivery. Congenital herpes ranges from subclinical infections to severe infections of the skin, eyes, mucous membranes, visceral organs, or central nervous system. Congenital herpes has a high mortality. Many survivors have ocular or neurologic sequelae.

DIAGNOSTIC STUDIES AND FINDINGS

Diagnostic Test	Findings
Microscopic examination of stained smear from base of vesicles	Direct identification of multinucleated giant cells with intranuclear inclusions
Virus tissue culture of specimen from base of vesicles using fluorescent antibody or neutralization techniques	Identification of type 1 or type 2 viral cytopathogenic effect in tissue culture in 24-48 h
Complement fixation or neutralization tests	Fourfold increase in antibody titer in convalescent serum; difficult to differentiate type 1 from type 2
Indirect immunofluorescence and radioimmunoassay	IgM antibodies detected in primary and recurrent infections

Persons with a new infection with herpes should also be examined for syphilis, gonorrhea, and **Chlamydia.**

MEDICAL MANAGEMENT

DRUG THERAPY

Antiinfective agents: **For first clinical episode of genital herpes:** acyclovir 200 mg PO, 5 times/day for 7-10 days, initiated within 6 days of onset of lesions.
For severe infections: acyclovir 5 mg/kg q 8 h IV for 5-7 days or until clinical resolution.
For proctitis: acyclovir 400 mg PO 5 times/day for 10 days.
Recurrent episodes: acyclovir 200 mg PO 5 times/day for 5 days or acyclovir 800 mg PO bid for 5 days.
Suppressive therapy: acyclovir 200 mg PO 2-5 times/day or acyclovir 400 mg PO bid; discontinue after 1 yr.

Reference: 37.

Lymphogranuloma Venereum

Lymphogranuloma venereum is a systemic infection produced by mucosal invasion of a number of closely related strains of *Chlamydia*. The disease has three stages: a primary lesion, regional and disseminated lymphadenitis, and late complications resulting from progression of the regional lymphadenitis.

PATHOPHYSIOLOGY

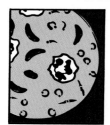 A primary transient nodular or vesicular lesion forms at the site of inoculation. Dissemination of the organism to regional lymph nodes (primarily inguinal lymph nodes) results in lymph node lesions that are initially similar to the inoculation lesion. The lesions are composed of small masses of epithelioid cells and a necrotic center. Satellite lesions are formed in the lymph node, surrounded by a narrow layer of epithelioid cells. The nodes show hyperplasia with an inflammatory cellular infiltration. Spread of the inflammation throughout the nodes causes the nodes to become matted together and form a large abscess. These abscesses develop in one or more areas along the lymphatic system. Untreated, the abscesses may rupture through the skin or other epithelial surfaces to produce chronic draining sinuses or fistulas. If the condition is not treated, it progresses, producing complications resulting from the impaired lymph and draining sinuses.

> For overview of lymphogranuloma venereum, see Table 9-3, page 190.

COMPLICATIONS

Genital elephantiasis and perianal abscesses and fistulas resulting in eventual rectal stricture. Advanced stages of rectal stricture may be manifest as symptoms of painful ileus, distention, complete obstruction, perforation, and peritonitis.

NURSING CARE

See pages 202 to 210.

DIAGNOSTIC STUDIES AND FINDINGS

Diagnostic Test	Findings
Cell culture of lesion exudate or bubo aspirate	Positive for *C. trachomatis*
Complement fixation	Antibody titer of 1:16 or higher within 1-3 wks of infection; fourfold rise in titer between early infection and convalescence; test is nonspecific, since it detects antibodies against all *C. trachomatis* strains
Microimmunofluorescence (micro IF)	Distinguishes between serotypes; tests may not be routinely available

These patients should be examined for other STDs, as well.

MEDICAL MANAGEMENT

DRUG THERAPY

Antiinfective agents: Doxycycline (Vibramycin), 100 mg PO bid for 21 days, *or*
Tetracycline hydrochloride (Achromycin; others), 500 mg PO qid for 21 days, *or*
Erythromycin (Erythrocin; others), 500 mg PO qid for 21 days, *or*
Sulfisoxazole, 500 mg PO qid for 21 days, *or*
Equivalent sulfonamide course

SURGERY

Aspiration of fluctuant lymph nodes as needed (incision and drainage or excision is contraindicated). Strictures or fistulas may require surgery.

Reference: 37.

Chancroid and Granuloma Inguinale

Chancroid, also called "soft sore" or "soft chancre," is an acute, localized, autoinoculable bacterial infection of the genitalia. Necrotizing ulceration occurs at the site of inoculation, frequently accompanied by suppuration of regional lymph nodes. Systemic dissemination does not occur.

Granuloma inguinale (donovanosis) is a mildly communicable, chronic and progressive, autoinoculable bacterial infection of the skin and mucous membranes, external genitalia, inguinal and anal regions, face, and oral cavity. Lesions first appear as small, painless papules or vesicles that become ulcerated and slowly develop into bleeding granulomatous masses. The disease may be difficult to differentiate from carcinoma (Table 9-4).

PATHOPHYSIOLOGY

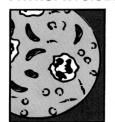

Although both chancroid and granuloma inguinale are manifest as ulcerative lesions, their pathophysiologies differ.

Chancroid

In *chancroid* the transmitted pathogenic bacteria initially invade genital skin or mucous membranes at sites traumatized by sexual contact. A preexisting abrasion facilitates invasion. A small papule is formed, surrounded by a zone of erythema. This erupts to form a shallow and painful ulcer. A purulent exudate results from the extensive necrotic process. The ulcers may enlarge and continue to erode and destroy tissue, or they may become secondarily infected and produce even more rapid destruction of tissue. Fresh lesions may occur from autoinoculation. Extragenital lesions may occur on fingers, tongue, lips, breasts, and eyelids.

> For a picture of a chancroid infection, see color plate 24, page xiii.

Lymphatic dissemination results in a unilateral or bilateral painful inguinal adenitis within 7 to 10 days of the primary lesion. The enlarged lymph gland (bubo) softens, becomes fluctuant, and may rupture spontaneously.

Granuloma Inguinale

The transmission of *granuloma inguinale* is less well understood. The pathogenic bacterium can be found in the rectum of nondiseased patients, suggesting that the organism may be part of the normal GI flora of some persons. Lesions may result from autoinfection, possibly following trauma to the genitalia. The pathogen in the lesions is transmitted sexually, but repeated exposure seems to be necessary for transmission. The dis-

Table 9-4

OVERVIEW OF STDs WITH ULCERATIVE LESIONS WITHOUT SYSTEMIC MANIFESTATIONS

	Chancroid	Granuloma Inguinale (Donovanosis)
Occurrence	Most common in tropical and subtropical climates; increasing in United States	Most common in tropical and subtropical climates and in homosexual males
Etiologic agent	*Haemophilus ducreyi*, a bacterium	*Calymmatobacterium granulomatis*
Reservoir	Humans	Humans
Transmission	Direct sexual contact with exudate from lesions; indirect transmission is rare	Direct sexual contact with lesions or with organism in rectum of nondiseased carriers
Incubation period	3-14 days	8-80 days
Period of communicability	Until lesions heal (can be weeks)	Duration of open lesions
Susceptibility and resistance	General, but highest in uncircumcised males; no evidence of resistance, although women may have more subclinical infections	No evidence of immunity
Report to local health authority	Mandatory case report	Mandatory case report

References: 3, 37, 90, 91.

ease is rare in heterosexual partners of infected persons. Clinical disease is highest in homosexual males.

The organism invades endothelial cells and forms a small, painless papule or nodule at the site of dermal invasion. The epithelium overlapping the lesion softens, erodes, ulcerates, and then produces a gradually enlarging granulomatous ulcerating lesion that bleeds easily. Pronounced marginal epithelial proliferation may simulate early epitheliomatous changes of cancer. The raised mass of granulation tissue looks more like a tumor than an ulcer. Single or multiple lesions may coalesce, or lesions may spread to contiguous tissue. Lesions have variable clinical appearances depending on the area located, mode of spread, tissue resistance, and texture of the skin. The lesions heal by fibrosis at the same time that tissue destruction is occurring in expanding lesions. Resultant scarring may produce urethral occlusion. The inguinal swelling that is sometimes seen with this disease is not a lymphadenopathy, but rather a subcutaneous granuloma.

COMPLICATIONS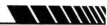

Chancroid
Phimosis and urethral fistulas in males
Females are frequently symptomless
Associated with increased risk for HIV infection
Granuloma inguinale
Hematogenous spread of the pathogen to bones, joints, and liver is rare but has been reported. Lymphatic spread is questionable. Secondary infection and expanding necrosis in untreated lesions may result in complete genital erosion.

NURSING CARE

See pages 202 to 210.

DIAGNOSTIC STUDIES AND FINDINGS

Diagnostic Test	Findings
Chancroid	
Culture or microscopic examination of exudate from bubo or lesions	Positive for *H. ducreyi* bacilli
Tests to rule out other causes of ulcers, particularly syphilis and herpes	
Granuloma inguinale	
Microscopic examination of scrapings from ulcer margin	Donovan bodies can be visualized
Tests to rule out carcinoma; examine for other STDs.	

MEDICAL MANAGEMENT

DRUG THERAPY

Antiinfective agents for chancroid: Erythromycin (Erythrocin), 500 mg PO qid, *or* Trimethoprim/sulfamethoxazole (Septra; Bactrim), tablet containing 160 mg trimethoprim and 800 mg sulfamethoxazole, PO bid for at least 7 days or until ulcers or lymph nodes have healed, *or* Ceftriaxone, 250 mg IM single dose.

Antiinfective agents for granuloma inguinale:
Tetracycline (Achromycin; others), 0.5 g PO qid for 21 days or until lesions heal, *or*
Streptomycin, 0.5 g IM bid for at least 21 days, *or*
Chloramphenicol (Chloromycetin), 0.5 g PO tid for at least 21 days, *or*
Gentamicin (Garamycin), 40 mg IM bid for at least 21 days.

SURGERY

For chancroid: Fluctuant lymph nodes should be aspirated through adjacent normal skin (incision and drainage or excision of nodes is contraindicated).

References: 14, 37, 109.

Molluscum Contagiosum and Condylomata Acuminata

Molluscum contagiosum is a viral disease of the skin that results in pearly pink to white papules with a central exudative pore. Multiple lesions appear on the genitalia and clear spontaneously in 6 to 9 months. Children develop lesions on skin elsewhere on the body.

Condylomata acuminata constitute one of the four major categories of virus-produced warts; this category occurs primarily on the genitalia or perineum. The warts appear as single or multiple, soft pink to brown, elongated lesions, usually in clusters and sometimes as large cauliflower-like masses (Table 9-5).

PATHOPHYSIOLOGY

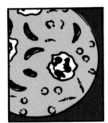

The viruses of both these diseases invade superficial layers of the epidermis, and infect single epithelial cells and stimulate the cells to divide. In the case of condylomata there is excessive proliferation of the cells of the stratum spinosum, constituting the bulk of the wart. Microscopic examination of the infected cells shows aggregates of the virus particles. In the case of molluscum contagiosum, a central pore containing the virus and exudative material develops in the papules.

Both molluscum papules and genital warts appear as multiple lesions on the external genitalia. Genital warts may also be found in the vagina and cervix of females and anterior urethra of males. Perineal and anal warts in females are generally caused by spread, whereas anal warts in males are associated with anal coitus. Genital warts that resemble skin warts suggest hand-to-genital transmission of another category of skin warts.

The papules of molluscum contagiosum clear spontaneously in 6 to 9 months as a result of an immune response. Warts sometimes clear spontaneously, which suggests an immune response. Laryngeal papillomatosis may develop in infants born to mothers with vaginal warts. Also, the enlarged size of some warts may lead to difficulty during a vaginal birth. Secondary infection and bleeding of warts are common. Enlarged or giant condylomata of the penis, although benign, may destroy large areas of the penis. Cancer must be ruled out in this situation. Malignant transformation, both invasive and intraepithelial, has been observed in some warts.

COMPLICATIONS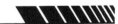

Secondary infection and bleeding of warts
Malignant transformation
Laryngeal warts in neonate

NURSING CARE

See pages 202 to 210.

Table 9-5

OVERVIEW OF STDs WITH NONULCERATIVE LESIONS

	Molluscum contagiosum	Condylomata acuminata (anogenital warts)
Occurrence	Worldwide; 90% of adults have antibodies; four times higher in prepubertal males	Worldwide
Etiologic agent	A member of the poxvirus group	*Papillomavirus*
Reservoir	Humans	Humans
Transmission	Direct sexual contact and indirect contact	Direct sexual contact
Incubation period	2-7 wks	1-20 months (usually 4 months)
Period of communicability	Unknown; probably as long as lesions persist	Unknown; probably as long as lesions persist
Susceptibility and resistance	Usually occurs in small children	General
Report to local health authority	No	No

Reference: 3.

DIAGNOSTIC STUDIES AND FINDINGS

Diagnostic Test	Findings
Molluscum contagiosum	
Microscopic examination of material in core of lesion	Pathognomonic molluscum inclusion bodies can be visualized
Condylomata	
Biopsy	Rule out malignancy
Serology for syphilis	Rule out condylomata of syphilis

> For a picture of genital warts, see color plates 22 and 23, page xiii; for a closeup of molluscum contagiosum, see color plate 25, page xiii.

MEDICAL MANAGEMENT

DRUG THERAPY

No therapy is available to eradicate these infections.

SURGERY

Alternative therapies to remove exophytic warts may include cryotherapy, and electrodesication/electrocautery; carbondioxide laser and conventional surgery for extensive warts.
No treatment should be initiated on cervical warts until results of a Papanicolaou smear are available.
Molluscum lesions may resolve spontaneously or may be removed by curettage after cryoanesthesia or cryotherapy or by the use of caustic chemicals.

Keratolytic agents for removal of condylomata acuminata: Podophyllin, 10%-25% in compound tincture of benzoin to wart only; to be washed off in 1-4 h; four weekly treatments (not to be used during pregnancy or with urethral, oral, cervical, or anorectal warts)

Reference: 37.

Vulvovaginitis

Vulvovaginitis is an inflammation of the superficial mucous membranes of the vulva and vagina caused by a number of microorganisms that are frequently part of the normal vaginal flora in adult women. The inflammation is accompanied by a purulent exudate with characteristics that differ with causative agents. The etiologic agents most frequently associated with vulvovaginitis are *Trichomonas vaginalis* (a protozoan), *Candida albicans* (a yeast form of fungus), and bacteria such as *Gardnerella vaginalis, Corynebacterium vaginale, and Haemophilus vaginalis.* They are responsible for trichomoniasis, candidiasis, and bacterial vaginosis, respectively (Table 9-6). In addition, the inflammation can be caused by mechanical irritants, contact allergens, and ectoparasites (pinworms, lice) (Table 9-7).

PATHOPHYSIOLOGY

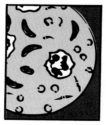

The presence of estrogen in women supports a normal flora of microorganisms in the vagina and anterior urethra. Under certain conditions (alterations in hormonal levels during the menstrual cycle, pregnancy, antibiotic therapy, immunosuppression), imbalance occurs in the normal flora. Certain opportunistic organisms become pathogenic or may be sexually transmitted in large enough numbers to become pathogenic. They colonize on the superficial mucosal layers and produce patches of inflammation and exudate that contain large numbers of the pathogens. The infection rarely extends beyond

Table 9-6

VULVOVAGINITIS CAUSED BY A PATHOGEN

	Trichomoniasis	Candidiasis	Bacterial vaginosis (BV)
Occurrence	Worldwide; highest in females 16-35 yrs; often accompanies other STDs	Worldwide; fungus is part of normal flora in 50% of women 15-45 yrs; most common cause of vaginitis	Worldwide; bacteria are part of normal vaginal flora in many asymptomatic women
Etiologic agent	*Trichomonas vaginalis,* a protozoan	*Candida albicans,* a fungus (yeast)	*Gardnerella vaginalis, Haemophilus vaginalis, Corynebacterium vaginale*
Reservoir Transmission	Humans Direct and indirect contact with vaginal and urethral discharges; transmitted to infant during birth	Humans Direct and indirect contact with excretions from mouth, skin, vagina, and rectum of infected persons and carriers; transmitted to infant during vaginal delivery	Humans Direct contact with vaginal and urethral discharges
Incubation period Period of communicability	4-20 days; average is 7 days Duration of infection	2-5 days in thrush in newborn Duration of lesions	5-7 days Duration of infection
Susceptibility and resistance	General, but clinical disease is mainly in females; exacerbated during menstruation and pregnancy	Many persons have organism but few acquire infection; exacerbated during pregnancy, before menstruation, with oral contraceptives, and antibiotic therapy	General, but clinical disease is only in females; many women have the organism, but not all acquire symptomatic infections; results from change in vaginal pH
Report to local health authority	No	No	No

References: 3, 64, 112.

Table 9-7

VULVOVAGINITIS OF NONPATHOGENIC ORIGIN

Etiology	Epidemiology	Signs and symptoms	Diagnostic studies	Medical plan
Postmenopausal vaginitis (atrophic vaginitis)	Occurs because of decreased estrogen levels	Thin watery discharge; burning and itching	Direct visual examination	Atrophic changes cannot be reversed but can usually be prevented with hormone therapy
Allergic or irritative vaginitis owing to thermal, chemical, and physical causes	Thermal sources: douching with excessively hot water, wearing nylon undergarments Chemical sources: douche solutions, hygiene sprays, soaps, detergents on undergarments, poor personal hygiene Physical sources: retained tampon, diaphragm, toilet paper, condom, or pessary	Redness, burning, and itching of excoriated skin Increase in type and amount of secretions; rash; burning and itching Foul-smelling, serosanguineous, or purulent discharge	Direct visual examination; wet smear; detailed history; bimanual examination	Avoidance of source; secondary infection should be treated according to etiology; oral antihistamines for allergic vaginitis, local cortisone ointment; wearing cotton undergarments

the endocervix. There is a wide range in severity of infections. Many are asymptomatic. The organism may be transmitted to a male sexual partner who may or may not develop symptomatic urethritis. Reinfection of the female from untreated males is common.

The organisms may be transmitted to an infant during birth. Infections in newborns are generally temporary and are limited to the period before maternal estrogens are metabolized by the newborn.

Certain physiologic changes in the host support the pathogenic growth of different organisms. Trichomoniasis is exacerbated during and after menstruation, whereas bacterial infections (bacterial vaginosis), such as *G. vaginalis* vaginitis, are not associated with hormonal changes during the menstrual cycle. *G. vaginalis* vaginitis is associated with an altered vaginal pH; the organism usually does not grow in the normal acid secretions. Yeast infections, such as *candidiasis*, are greatly exacerbated preceding menstruation, during pregnancy, and in women taking oral contraceptives. Candidiasis is also exacerbated by the elimination of normal flora bacteria with antibiotic therapy or with any other condition that compromises skin or mucous membrane defenses.

Whereas *Trichomonas* and *Gardnerella* rarely extend beyond the vulvovaginal or anterior urethral area, *Candida* has the potential for producing infection anywhere in the body where normal defenses are altered. *Candida* is part of the normal GI, oral, and cutaneous flora of many persons, and it may become pathogenic in those areas. Severe infection with invasion and abscess formation, particularly in the GI, tract, may lead to hematogenous dissemination of the yeast to other organs. The organism may also be introduced iatrogenically to internal organs through surgical procedures, catheters, or implanted devices and produce multiple microabscesses in infected tissue. The areas most commonly infected are the central nervous system (particularly the meninges), lungs, peritoneum, heart (myocardium, pericardium, and endocardium), endometrium, eyes, ears, joints, oral cavity, esophagus, skin, and nails. Deep tissue infection is more common in patients with neoplastic disease. Cutaneous infections are more commonly associated with skin injury or continual wetting of the skin. *Candida* infections may involve multiple organs and tissue simultaneously, a particular risk for immunosuppressed individuals.

Vaginal candidiasis may be transmitted to the infant during delivery. A common manifestation of such an infection in the newborn is thrush, an infection in the oral cavity. Creamy white, curdlike patches consisting of desquamated epithelial cells, leukocytes, bacteria, keratin, necrotic tissue, and food debris are formed on the oral mucosa. Scraping of the patches leaves a raw, bleeding, painful surface.

COMPLICATIONS

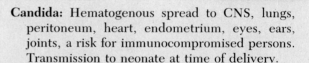

Candida: Hematogenous spread to CNS, lungs, peritoneum, heart, endometrium, eyes, ears, joints, a risk for immunocompromised persons. Transmission to neonate at time of delivery.

Bacterial vaginosis: May cause premature rupture of membranes in pregnant women (not proven).

NURSING CARE

See pages 202 to 210.

DIAGNOSTIC STUDIES AND FINDINGS

Diagnostic Test	Findings
Trichomoniasis	
Culture of vaginal secretions (urethral discharge in AM in males)	Positive for *T. vaginalis*
Microscopic examination of saline wet mount of vaginal secretions	Visualization of motile protozoa
Other STDs should also be ruled out	
Candidiasis	
Microscopic examination of Gram's stain or KOH wet mount preparation of vaginal secretions	Visualization of yeast cells
Culture of vaginal secretions	Positive for *C. vaginale* in symptomatic women; because Candida is part of normal oral flora, culture is not useful in thrush
Bacterial vaginosis	
Culture of vaginal secretions	Positive for *G. vaginalis* or other bacteria in symptomatic women
Microscopic examination of Gram's stain or KOH wet mount preparation of vaginal secretions	Identification of "clue" cells (vaginal epithelial cells with borders obscured by bacteria)

MEDICAL MANAGEMENT

DRUG THERAPY

Antiinfective agents for trichomoniasis: Metronidazole (Flagyl), 2 g PO single dose, *or*
Metronidazole, 500 mg bid for 7 days (contraindicated during the first trimester of pregnancy; asymptomatic women and their sexual partners should be treated to prevent sexual transmission).

Antiinfective agents for vulvovaginal candidiasis: Miconazole nitrate (vaginal suppository 200 mg), intravaginally at HS for 3 days, *or*
Clotrimazole (vaginal tablets 200 mg), intravaginally at HS for 3 days, *or*
Butaconazole (2% cream, 5 g), intravaginally at HS for 3 days, *or*
Teraconazole 80 mg suppository or 0.4% cream, intravaginally at HS for 3 days *or*
Miconazole nitrate (vaginal suppository 100 mg or 2% cream 5 g), intravaginally at HS for 7 days, *or*
Clotrimazole (vaginal tablets 100 mg or 1% cream 5 g) intravaginally at HS for 7 days.
Nystatin and single-dose therapies are not recommended; not necessary to treat male sexual partners unless *Candida balanitis* is present; treatment of candidiasis during third trimester of pregnancy is necessary to prevent oral thrush in newborn.

Antiinfective agents for bacterial vaginosis: Metronidazole (Flagyl), 500 mg PO bid for 7 days (contraindicated during pregnancy), *or*
Clindamycin, 300 mg PO, bid for 7 days.
(Not necessary to treat male sexual partners or asymptomatic women.)

Reference: 37.

---

1 ASSESS (Gonorrhea and Nongonococcal Urethritis and Cervicitis [Chlamydia])

ASSESSMENT	OBSERVATIONS
History	Unprotected sexual contact (vaginal, anal, or oral) with an infected person; multiple sexual partners or unknown partner; history of previous STD
Subjective symptoms	**Male:** May be asymptomatic; dysuria; severe pain of epididymitis; urinary retention with prostatitis **Female:** Usually asymptomatic; dysuria or urinary frequency; pelvic inflammatory disease (pelvic pain, low back pain, dyspareunia, menstrual irregularity, constipation, malaise) **Male and female:** Rectal infection (anal pruritis, burning or tenesmus); pain with defection; pharyngeal infection, sore throat
Genitalia	**Male:** Purulent yellow-white discharge from urethra (clearer discharge with *Chlamydia*); inflammation around meatus; swelling and severe pain in scrotum with epididymitis **Female:** Leukorrhea, usually goes unnoticed
Pelvis (with PID)	**Female:** Rebound tenderness; normal bowel sounds progressing to ileus in untreated persons; nausea and vomiting

ASSESSMENT	OBSERVATIONS
Pharyngeal infection	Usually asymptomatic or inflamed with visible exudate; red, dry tongue
Rectal infection	Bloody and/or mucous diarrhea; purulent discharge
Eyes	Purulent discharge from conjunctiva
Systemic manifestations of disseminated disease	Painful vesicular pustular skin lesions on an erythematous base; petechial skin lesions; symptoms of septicemia, endocarditis, meningitis, arthritis
Body temperature	Low-grade fever, higher with systemic manifestations, PID, or epididymitis

SEE DIAGNOSE, PAGE 207.

1 ASSESS (Syphilis)

ASSESSMENT	OBSERVATIONS
History	Unprotected sexual contact (vaginal, anal, or oral) with an infected person; multiple sexual partners or unknown partner; previous STD

Primary stage: within 10-90 days after exposure (average of 21 days); lasts 1-5 wks

Genitalia	Single painless papule erodes to become a hard, painless indurated chancre without an exudate; located at site of innoculation, usually on glans penis of male and on cervix or external genitalia of female; may be seen on scrotum, anus, rectum, lips, tongue, tonsils, nipple, and fingers; abraded ulcer exudes serous fluid teeming with *T. pallida* organisms
Inguinal lymph nodes	Hard, nonfluctuant, painless, enlarged inguinal lymph nodes

Secondary stage: within 6-12 weeks after infection, lasting a few days to 1 year

Subjective symptoms	Malaise, headache, anorexia, nausea, aching in bones, fatigue, neck stiffness; fever; anemia; jaundice
Skin	Lesions, recurring local or generalized, papulosquamous, macular, papular, or pustular rash; bilateral and symmetric, beginning on trunk and proximal extremities, frequently on soles of feet and palms of hands; lesions are 3-10 mm, nonpruritic, and contain *T. pallida* organisms Condylomata lata: lesions on moist areas coalesce and erode to produce painless, moist, pink to grayish-white, raised plaques Alopecia: nonscarring, temporary hair loss in patches on head and eyebrows
Mucous membranes	Mucous patches: silver-gray superficial erosion surrounded by red periphery on mucous membranes
GI	Epigastric pain or vomiting associated with ulceration

ASSESSMENT	OBSERVATIONS
Latent stage: Lasts a few years to the remainder of person's life.	May have relapses of mucocutaneous symptoms of secondary stage early in latency; otherwise, no symptoms
Late stages (tertiary syphilis): Benign tertiary syphilis of the skin, bone, and viscera (3-10 years after infection)	Gumma lesions (a chronic granulomatous reaction, causing lesions, ulcers, or tumors); lesions are of varying sizes, appear anywhere on the body, and do not contain *T. pallida;* they may occur in palate, nasal septum, and other submucosal tissue, causing disfigurement; gumma lesions in bones cause pain
Cardiovascular syphilis (10-25 years after initial infection)	Aortic valvular insufficiency, thoracic aneurysm, narrowing of coronary ostia
Neurosyphilis (may be asymptomatic or symptomatic)	Meningovascular symptoms: focal neurologic signs depending on area of lesions; seizures Parenchymatous symptoms: paresis—personality changes, ranging from minor to severe psychosis; alteration in intellect and judgment; hyperactive reflexes; tabes dorsalis—ataxia, areflexia, paresthesias, bladder disturbance, impotence; sharp, tearing pain; trophic joint changes; optic atrophy with small, irregular pupils that are not reactive to light but respond normally to accommodation

SEE DIAGNOSE, PAGE 207.

1 ASSESS (Herpes I, Herpes II, and Lymphogranuloma Venereum [LV])

ASSESSMENT	OBSERVATIONS
History	**Herpes II and LV:** unprotected sexual contact (vaginal, anal, or oral) with an infected person; multiple or unknown sexual partners; previous herpes lesions (herpes II)
Subjective symptoms	**Herpes I and II:** burning or pruritis in areas of lesions; fever in initial infection; malaise **LV:** fever, chills, headache, joint pains, anorexia, abdominal pain, urinary retention
Oral cavity	**Herpes I and II:** multiple vesicular and ulcerative lesions on labial and buccal mucosa, tongue, and larynx; erythema of gums; excessive salivation; infection heals in 7-10 days; recurrent infections rare in mouth **LV:** may have lesions in mouth as described under GU/rectal
Lips	**Herpes I:** recurrent "cold sore" or "fever blister" preceded by 1 or 2 days of paresthesia; lesions crust and heal within 3-10 days

ASSESSMENT	OBSERVATIONS
GU/rectal	**Herpes II:** asymptomatic or extensive vesicular lesions with deep ulceration and marked hyperplasia and erythema of cervix, labia, fourchette, and clitoris (sometimes vagina); may extend to anal area, buttocks, and thighs; dysuria, leukorrhea, and marked genital tenderness; scattered vesicles over glans, prepuce, and shaft of the penis (lesions heal in 10 days); urinary retention; urethritis may occur without genital lesions; anal lesions possible **LV:** 2-3 mm painless, discrete, superficial vesicle or nonindurated ulcer at site of inoculation (frequently unnoticed); usually on glans or shaft of penis in males and on labia, vagina, or cervix in females; may be in rectum; rectal inoculation initially produces bloody discharge and tenesmus, and mucopurulent discharge, cramps, and diarrhea later; complications may include elephantiasis of prepuce, penis, scrotum, or vulva; perianal abscess; rectovaginal, rectovesical, and ischiorectal fistulas; rectal stricture 1-10 yrs after infection
Regional lymph nodes	**Herpes I:** enlarged and palpable cervical lymph nodes **Herpes II:** bilateral lymphadenopathy of inguinal lymph nodes in 50% of initial genital infections **LV:** 7-30 days after primary lesion: Initially a firm, tender, discrete, movable inguinal lymph node, which later becomes indolent, fixed, and matted; may be unilateral or bilateral; may subside spontaneously or proceed to form an abscess that may rupture to produce a draining sinus or fistula; female lymph node involvement may be mainly in the pelvic nodes with extension to rectum and rectovaginal septum
Skin	**Herpes I and II:** Clustered vesicular lesions anywhere on body; deep burning; skin edema
Eyes	**Herpes I and II:** Keratitis and conjunctivitis (unilateral or bilateral); periauricular lymphadenopathy

SEE DIAGNOSE, PAGE 207.

1 ASSESS (Chancroid and Granuloma Inguinale)

ASSESSMENT	OBSERVATIONS
History	Unprotected sexual contact (vaginal, anal, or oral) with an infected person; multiple or unknown sexual partners; history of previous STD
Subjective symptoms	**Chancroid:** pain
Genitalia	**Chancroid:** one to 10 primary lesions: inflamed macule/papule/pustule; irregularly shaped and of variable size (1 mm-2 cm); surrounded by a zone of inflammation; erupts to produce a sharply circumscribed, nonindurated ulcer with a granulating base and ragged edges; abundant, purulent exudate; location: frenulum, prepuce, coronal sulcus, glans and shaft of penis, and urinary meatus in males; cervix, vagina, fourchette, labia, and perianal area in females

>>>

ASSESSMENT	OBSERVATIONS
Genitalia—cont'd	Variations in clinical appearance of lesions • Follicular pustules rupture and form ulcers • Dwarf chancroid lesions look similar to herpes lesions • Transient chancroid lesion resolves quickly but is followed by an inguinal bubo • Papular chancroid starts as an ulcer but becomes raised • Giant chancroid frequently follows rupture of inguinal abscess and grows rapidly • Phagedenic chancroid, a small lesion, rapidly extends and becomes necrotic and destructive **Granuloma inguinale:** single or multiple, indurated, sharply defined but irregular papules/nodules; erode to form a beefy, exuberant granulomatous, heaped, clean ulcer, progressing slowly and coalescing with adjacent lesions; serous exudate; location: glans, prepuce, urethra, shaft of penis, and perianal area in males; labia and fourchette in females; lesions bleed easily; if secondarily infected, may have odorous necrotic exudate Variations in clinical appearance • Oral lesions are painful and resemble malignancies • Vaginal and cervical ulcers produce profuse, purulent discharge and irregular bleeding • Cervical ulcers are soft, friable, irregular, and not well-fixed to tissue; resemble cancer • Male genital ulcers may be hypertrophic and verrucose, destructive and necrotic, discoid (buttonlike), or chronic and indolent • Inguinal ulcers and ulcers on female genitalia are generally fleshy and exuberant • Anal ulcers are hypertrophic and verrucose or chronic and indolent
Inguinal area	**Chancroid:** single, unilateral (can be bilateral), tender, and unilocular lymphadenopathy with overlying erythema; suppuration and rupture of fluctuant nodes in 5-10 days may occur, leaving a single, large ulcer **Granuloma Inguinale:** rarely any inguinal involvement; may have a subcutaneous granuloma that suppurates and mimics a lymphadenopathy

SEE DIAGNOSE, PAGE 207.

1 ASSESS (Molluscum and Condylomata)

ASSESSMENT	OBSERVATIONS
History	Sexual contact with infected person; multiple or unknown sexual partner; previous STD
Anogenital area	**Molluscum contagiosum:** multiple, distinct, dome-shaped papules, 1-10 mm, pearly pink to white, with a central pore containing a cheese-like white exudate; may be surrounded by red or scaling skin **Condylomata (warts):** multiple or single, soft pink to brown, elongated lesions, usually in cluster, may be in large masses; painless

SEE DIAGNOSE, PAGE 207.

1 ASSESS (Vulvovaginitis)

ASSESSMENT	OBSERVATIONS
History	Pregnancy or oral contraceptive use
Vulva and vagina	**Trichomoniasis:** inflammation of vaginal walls and endocervix; punctate hemorrhagic lesions; painful coitus; copious loose "frothy" discharge with an odor; ⅓ of patients have yellow-green discharge with bubbles **Candidiasis:** severe perivaginal pruritis; pale or erythematous labia; labial excoriations; erythema extending into vagina and toward anus; tiny papulopustules beyond main area of erythema; discharge thick and adherent (containing curds) or thin and loose; no odor **Bacterial vaginosis:** milder symptoms; less erythema; mild or moderate discharge; thin white grayish white discharge; uniformly adheres to vaginal wall; 25% have gas bubbles in discharge; fishy or aminelike odor to discharge
Lymph nodes	**Trichomoniasis:** May be inguinal lymphadenopathy
Urinary concerns	**Trichomoniasis:** Dysuria or frequency **Candidiasis:** Dysuria

2 DIAGNOSE

NURSING DIAGNOSIS	SUPPORTIVE ASSESSMENT FINDINGS
Potential for infection (patient contacts) related to presence of pathogens in lesions or secretions/exudates from cervix, urethra, eyes, pharynx, or anus	History of unprotected sexual activity or previous STD; laboratory examination of secretions or exudate is positive for pathogen; serologic test is positive for antibodies (for syphilis, herpes, *Chlamydia,* HIV, lymphogranuloma venereum); purulent exudate (for gonorrhea, chlamydia, vulvovaginitis); draining lesions (for syphilis, herpes, lymphogranuloma venereum, chancroid, granuloma inguinale); nonulcerative lesions (for molluscum, condylomata [warts])
Potential for infection (patient complications) related to extension or dissemination of disease if untreated or inadequately treated	The natural history of gonorrhea, *Chlamydia,* syphilis, LV, condylomata, chancroid, and granuloma inguinale is dissemination or extension and tissue destruction unless adequately treated
Knowledge deficit related to transmission, prevention, complications, and medical regimen	Acquiring these STDs suggests lack of understanding of transmission and methods for prevention; STDs are frequently misunderstood and their seriousness underestimated

Other related nursing diagnoses: Those diagnoses related to complications or congenital/perinatal transmission

3 PLAN

Patient goals

1. Patient's infection will not be transmitted to others or back to patient after treatment.
2. Patient's infection will be resolved before extension or dissemination.
3. Patient has knowledge to self-administer antiinfective agents, as prescribed.
4. Patient has information to prevent further episodes of an STD manifestation to prevent transmission of these STDs.

→ › ›

4 IMPLEMENT

NURSING DIAGNOSIS	NURSING INTERVENTIONS	RATIONALE
Potential for infection (patient contacts) related to presence of pathogens in lesions or secretions/exudates from cervix, urethra, eyes, pharynx, or anus	Collect specimen for laboratory examination; collect blood for serology for syphilis, herpes, or *Chlamydia* (see Chapter 3).	For definite diagnosis and treatment.
	Use universal precautions when handling specimens and examining patient.	Lesions and mucous membrane exudates are infectious.
	Examine and treat patient contacts.	To prevent reinfection of patient.
	Serologically screen all pregnant women for syphilis at least once during pregnancy. Rescreen high-risk women during third trimester and again at delivery (testing the mother's blood). Administer antiinfectives as prescribed.	Syphilis is transmitted to the fetus. Adequate treatment of the mother before the 15th wk will prevent damage to fetus. High-risk women are at risk for reinfection during the pregnancy. Infants born of infected mothers are at risk for active infection and severe anomalies.
	Reexamine and treat pregnant women with history of STDs before delivery. Examine newborn for symptoms and administer prophylactics for eyes.	A neonate may become infected on any mucous membrane during a vaginal delivery if mother has a cervical infection.
	Ensure that pregnant women with *Candida* organism are treated during last trimester.	To prevent transmission to neonate during vaginal delivery.
	Report to local health authority if not previously reported by physician or laboratory.	Required by law.
Potential for infection (patient complications) related to extension or dissemination of disease if untreated or inadequately treated	Administer antiinfectives or teach patient to take as prescribed.	Early treatment can prevent complications and transmission of STDs.
	Counsel patient to return for follow-up.	To ensure cure.
	Monitor immunocompromised persons for signs of disseminated infection with herpes and *Candida*.	Immunocompromised are at greater risk for serious systemic disease.
	Monitor body temperature and symptoms of PID and dissemination of gonorrhea and *Chlamydia*.	Early detection of infection and treatment with antiinfective agents may prevent dissemination of the pathogen, severe disease, and fertility problems.
	Monitor for symptoms of complications of tertiary syphilis if patient has been infected over 1 yr.	To initiate supportive care, as needed.
Knowledge deficit regarding transmission, prevention, complications, and medical regimen	See Patient Teaching and Patient Teaching Guides, pages 291-292 and 295.	

5 EVALUATE

PATIENT OUTCOME	DATA INDICATING THAT OUTCOME IS REACHED
Infection is not transmitted to others or back to patient after treatment	Patient contacts are examined and treated.
	Newborn is free of signs of infection (no lesions; nonreactive serology and absence of other symptoms).
	Health care workers have used adequate precautions.
Infection is resolved before extension or dissemination	Absence of signs of secondary or tertiary syphilis; CSF is normal.
	Follow-up serologic tests for syphilis indicate decreasing antibody titers.
	For gonorrhea or *Chlamydia*: Body temperature, urination, and bowel movements are normal. Patient reports absence of nausea and vomiting, dysuria, pain, dysmenorrhea, abnormal menstrual bleeding, or other signs of complications. There is no exudate. Cultures are negative for gonococcus or *Chlamydia*. Patient has been tested for other STDs.
	For LV: Lymph nodes are not swollen, hot, or tender. Mucopurulent exudate no longer drains from lesions or sinuses. Body temperature is normal. Rectum and anal opening are patent. There is no abdominal distention or cramping. Defecation is normal.
	For chancroid: Lesions are healed without scarring. Patient verbalizes intent to return for follow-up.
	For herpes: No signs of CNS disease or infection of visual organs.
Patient has knowledge to self-administer antiinfectives as prescribed	Patient describes medication regimen and intent to take antiinfectives for length of time prescribed.
Patient has information to prevent further episodes of an STD and to prevent transmission of this STD	Patient verbalizes intent to avoid sexual contact until lesions are healed, describes correct use of condom, and verbalizes intent to return for follow-up.

PATIENT TEACHING

GENERAL INSTRUCTIONS:

1. Sexual activity should be avoided until treatment is completed and follow-up examination of secretion/exudates is negative for pathogens (or when herpes lesions are present).
2. Sexual contacts must be examined and treated, even if asymptomatic.
3. Antiinfective agents must be taken for full prescribed course to avoid treatment failure, chronic infection, and complications.
4. If tetracycline is administered, it must be taken for the full prescribed course. It should be taken 1 hour before or 2 hours after meals. The patient should avoid dairy products, antacids, iron, other mineral-containing preparations, and sunlight should be avoided.
5. Condoms may provide protection from future infections (see Patient Teaching Guide on Preventing Sexually Transmitted Diseases, page 292).
6. Counsel patients and their partners to be tested for HIV.

SPECIFIC INSTRUCTIONS:

7. **For gonorrhea or *Chlamydia:*** Patients should return for reexamination 4-7 days after completion of treatment. Care should be taken with vaginal or urethral discharges to avoid contamination of eyes.
8. **For syphilis:** All sexual partners should be referred for examination and treatment (sexual contacts up to 3 months preceding primary infection, up to 6 months preceding secondary stage, and up to 1 year preceding latent stage). Treated patients should return for follow-up serologic tests 3 and 6 months after therapy (1, 2, 3, 6, 9, and 12 months if HIV positive). A systemic reaction (e.g., fever, chills, headache, or tachycardia) 1-2 hours after onset of antibiotic treatment is attributable to endotoxin release from dying spirochetes. The condition is benign and self-limited. Bed rest and aspirin help.
9. **For herpes:** Pregnant women should inform physician of history of genital herpes. Annual Pap smears are recommended. Recurrent episodes of lesions are less painful and less extensive than initial episode. The virus probably cannot be transmitted when there are no lesions present, but this is still being investigated. Proper handwashing following toileting is important to prevent autoinoculation.
10. **For lymphogranuloma venereum:** The sequelae of untreated lymphogranuloma venereum are serious.

Patient must complete the prescribed antibiotic regimen and return for evaluation 3 to 5 days after treatment is begun and weekly or biweekly until the infection is entirely healed.

11. **For chancroid:** Sexual partners should be examined and treated as soon as possible. Sexual contacts 2 weeks before or after onset of chancroid lesions must be treated. Females may be asymptomatic but should be treated. In chancroid the prepuce should remain retracted during therapy and the lesions should be cleaned three times daily. Retraction is contraindicated if there is preputial edema.
12. **For granuloma inguinale:** The patient should return for evaluation within 3 to 5 days of beginning therapy and weekly or biweekly thereafter until all lesions are healed. Total healing of granuloma inguinale takes 3 to 5 weeks. If treatment is stopped prematurely, lesions may become reactivated.
13. **For molluscum and condylomata (warts):** Follow-up examination should take place 1 month after treatment for molluscum so new lesions can be removed.

    Follow-up examinations should be done weekly until all warts have been resolved.

    All women with anogenital warts should have a Pap smear.

    Patients should be informed of the recurrent nature of these conditions.
14. **For vulvovaginitis:** Recurrent infections are common. Patient should return for treatment if symptoms recur.

    Alcohol should be avoided until after 3 days following metronidazole therapy. See instruction number 4 regarding tetracycline.

    Vaginal suppositories for candidiasis should be stored in a refrigerator. Treatment should continue during menstruation. Sanitary pads can be worn to protect clothing.

    Teach the patient to wipe from front to back when toileting.

    Instruct the patient not to douche routinely to avoid removal of normal vaginal flora.

    Instruct the patient to avoid using sprays, soaps, powders, and deodorants; to wear cotton undergarments to permit free airflow to the perineum and to avoid trapping moisture; to wash undergarments in mild detergent and to rinse them twice; to avoid sharing towels and washcloths with others; and to use water-soluble lubricants if necessary before intercourse.

CHAPTER 10

Vector-transmitted Fevers

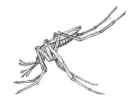

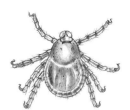

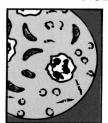

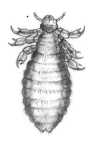

The diseases presented in this section are severe systemic infections of the blood caused by pathogens transmitted to humans by infected vectors, such as ticks and mosquitos. Although there are many such diseases, the four most common are presented in this chapter. These include tick-borne Rocky Mountain spotted fever, Lyme disease, mosquito-borne malaria, and dengue fever (Table 10-1).

Rocky Mountain Spotted Fever

Rocky Mountain spotted fever (RMSF) is an acute rickettsial infectious disease transmitted to humans by infected ticks and manifested by severe systemic symptoms and a macular or maculopapular rash. The disease is severe, with a 10% to 20% fatality rate in the untreated. The rate increases with age.

PATHOPHYSIOLOGY

Rickettsiae, similar to viruses, are intracellular parasites that replicate and metabolize only within host cells. The pathogens are carried in the feces of their respective arthropods and are deposited on the skin while the arthropod feeds on humans. Rickettsiae are subsequently rubbed or scratched into the open skin lesion produced by the arthropod bite.

Initially, a local neutrophilic inflammatory response occurs at the site of skin inoculation. Later, mononuclear cells infiltrate and phagocytose the rickettsiae. This local tissue reaction may result in an eschar. The rickettsiae then replicate and are disseminated within mononuclear cells throughout the vascular system.

See Table 10-1, page 213, for an overview of Rocky Mountain spotted fever.

Once in the blood, rickettsiae invade the cytoplasm of vascular endothelial cells, replicate there, and cause the cells to burst. A rapidly progressive systemic angiitis with severe systemic manifestations develops, heralding the acute onset of this disease. Vascular endothelial edema, fibrin and platelet deposition, and microthrombi development lead to obstruction and occlusion of small blood vessels with resultant hemorrhage, tissue infarction, and necrosis.

Other vascular changes include increased permeability with perivascular accumulation of neutrophils, macrophages, and lymphocytes, and plasma loss into tissues. The mechanism for this process is unknown. It is hypothesized that the vascular permeability results from an allergic response of the host to the toxin produced by the pathogen.

Vascular lesions are widely disseminated and most frequently affect the skin, myocardium, skeletal muscles, kidneys, and central nervous system. Disease symptoms, following the initial systemic manifestations, result from the localization of the vascular lesions and tissue infarctions and the loss of circulating plasma. A petechial skin rash that becomes purpuric, clouded sensorium, edema, hypotension, and peripheral vascular circulatory collapse are characteristic. Myocardial involvement with symptoms of myocarditis results from the focal vascular lesions plus a diffuse mononuclear cell infiltration. A shift in intracellular water and electrolytes in terminal stages of the disease may result in increases in circulating volume and tissue edema.

For picture of rash from Rocky Mountain spotted fever, see color plates 29 through 31, page xiv.

Both antibiotic therapy and the development of circulating antibodies during the second week of acute disease arrest the progression of rickettsiae but do not completely eradicate them. The pathogen remains latent in cells, and relapses, although uncommon, do occur.

COMPLICATIONS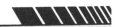

Shock
Disseminated intravascular coagulation
Thrombosis and gangrene
Renal failure
Coma
Death (associated with delay in diagnosis)
Neurologic sequelae (deafness, visual and speech
   disturbances, mental confusion)
Cardiac sequelae (dysrhythmias)

DIAGNOSTIC STUDIES AND FINDINGS

Diagnostic Test	Findings
Immunofluorescence of skin tissue	Identification of rickettsiae during third or fourth day of disease (not very sensitive)
Serology	Increase in antibody titers can be detected after 7-10 days of illness in the untreated but may be delayed for 4 wks if antibiotic therapy is begun early; titers decrease rapidly during late convalescence
Confirmatory: Indirect fluorescent antibody	IFA titer ≥1:64
Complement fixation	Fourfold rise in titer during second wk or single titer ≥1:16.
Probable: Indirect hemagglutination, latex agglutination, or microagglutination	Fourfold rise in titer during second wk or single titer ≥1:128
Blood components	WBC normal; prolonged prothrombin time and partial prothrombin time; decreased platelets; normocytic anemia; hyponatremia; hypochloremia; hypoalbuminemia; thrombocytopenia; hypofibrinogenemia

Table 10-1

OVERVIEW OF VECTOR-TRANSMITTED FEVERS

	Tick-borne fevers		Mosquito-borne fevers	
	Rocky Mountain spotted fever	**Lyme disease**	**Malaria**	**Dengue**
Occurrence	United States: spring and summer; in western United States incidence is highest in adult males; in eastern United States, highest in children; ⅔ of cases are from NC, SC, Va, Md, Mo, Ga, Tenn, Okla, and Mont	Increasing in United States, possibly because of better diagnosis; seen in summer; endemic along coast from Mass to Va, in Wis, Minn, Calif, Ga, and Ore	Endemic in tropics and subtropics; acquired by travelers to those areas; over 1,000 cases/yr in the United States; increasing possibly due to spread of chloroquine resistance	Endemic in tropical areas; recent epidemics in Central America, Mexico, the Caribbean, and the Rio Grande valley; mosquitoes carrying the virus have been migrating north to the United States, although most cases seen in the United States are in travelers to endemic areas
Etiologic agent	*Rickettsia rickettsii*	*Borrelia burgdorferi*, a spirochete (identified in 1982)	*Plasmodium vivax, P. malariae, P. falciparum, P. ovale*	Flavivirus, four immunologically distinct serotypes (types 1, 2, 3, and 4)
Reservoir	Ticks	Ticks that feed on deer, wild rodents	Humans	Mosquitoes and humans as one reservoir
Transmission	Bite from tick; contamination with tick's feces	Tick bite or contact with tick feces	Bite from infected female *Anopheles* mosquito, blood transfusion, or congenital	Bite from infected mosquito; *Aedes* species, particularly *A. albopictus* and *A. aegypti*
Incubation period	3-14 days	3-32 days	Dependent on strain of *Plasmodium* agent; average is 12-30 days; may be as long as 8-10 months	3-15 days, average is 5-6 days
Period of communicability	Not communicable person to person	Not communicable person-to-person	Untreated cases may be a source of mosquito infection for 1-3 yrs; stored blood is infected for 16 days	Infected persons are a source of infection for mosquitoes 1 day before and 5 days after disease onset; mosquitoes are infective for the remainder of their lives (1-4 months)
Susceptibility and resistance	General; infection confers lifetime immunity	General population; reinfection occurs	General; tolerance present in adults in endemic areas; black Africans show a natural resistance	General; children have less severe cases; immunity to one subtype of virus follows infection with that type
Report to local health authority	In some states where disease is endemic	In 31 states	Mandatory case report	Report during epidemics

Data from Benenson.[3]

MEDICAL MANAGEMENT[57]

DRUG THERAPY

Antiinfective agents: Tetracycline (Achromycin; others), 25-50 mg/kg/day PO in 4 divided doses until patient is afebrile for 48 h, or for 5-7 days, *or*
Chloramphenicol (Chloromycetin), 50-100 mg/kg/day PO in four divided doses until patient is afebrile for 48 h, or for 5-7 days.
Either of above may be given IV in appropriate doses during initial toxic stage.

Cardiac glycosides: Digitalis for cardiac decompensation.

Narcotic analgesics: Codeine or meperidine (Demerol) for severe headache.

GENERAL MANAGEMENT*

IV fluids and electrolytes (to be administered cautiously).
Sedation of delirious patients with paraldehyde or chloral hydrate.
High-protein, high-calorie diet.
Transfusion of serum albumin.
Packed red cells for anemia.
Oxygen for pulmonary complications.
Refrigerated blanket for fever control.

*Depends on severity of disease and complications.

1 ASSESS

ASSESSMENT	OBSERVATIONS
History	Recent exposure to ticks or tick-infested area
Subjective symptoms	Sudden onset of symptoms: fever, chills, severe headache, extreme myalgias and arthritic type of pain, prostration
Body temperature	39°-40°C (102°-104°F); AM remissions; fever lysis in 2-3 wks if untreated
Eyes	Injected and suffused conjunctiva; photophobia
Skin	Eschar at site of tick bite Macular rash (3-5 mm) on mucous membranes, face, palms, and soles, beginning on third to fifth day; red to purple colored; blanches on pressure; begins on face and extremities; spreads in a centripetal fashion, involving the trunk last; if untreated, rash becomes maculopapular to petechial to purpuric; areas coalesce with possible necrosis and gangrene Jaundice
Respiratory	Nonproductive cough may be present; rapid respiration
Lymph nodes	Unilateral postauricular adenopathy if bite was on the head
Abdomen	Hepatosplenomegaly, GI distress, anorexia; constipation

ASSESSMENT	OBSERVATIONS
Central nervous system	Mental dullness and lethargy, progressing to delirium, stupor, convulsions, coma, and death; may have focal neurologic signs, such as deafness, tinnitus, nuchal rigidity, tremor, vertigo; hallucinations, paranoid behavior, and extreme irritability
Cardiovascular	Early: bradycardia Later: tachycardia, gallop rhythm; hypotension and tractable shock, possibly leading to death
Urinary	Oliguria or anuria in the event of circulatory collapse; incontinence in severely ill
Complications	Pneumonia; hemorrhage; iritis; nephritis; hemiplegia; deafness; impaired vision; persistent tachycardia

2 DIAGNOSE

NURSING DIAGNOSIS	SUPPORTIVE ASSESSMENT FINDINGS
Hyperthermia related to infection	Chills; body temperature 39°-40°C (102°-104°F), AM remissions; fever lysis in 2-3 wks if untreated
Pain related to systemic angitis (vascular rupture, and hemorrhage)	Severe headache, arthralgia
Altered tissue perfusion (generalized) related to vascular endothelial damage and reaction to pathogen toxin	Hypotension and other symptoms of shock and hemmorhage; oliguria or anuria
Sensory/perceptual alterations (visual) related to disease process	Injected and suffused conjunctiva; photophobia
Impaired skin integrity related to rash and altered peripheral circulation	Eschar at site of tick bite; macular, maculopapular, petechial, or purpuric rash; necrosis or gangrene
Activity intolerance related to disease severity	Extreme myalgias and arthritis type of pain; prostration
Altered nutrition: less than body requirements related to increased metabolism caused by infection and fever	Liver involvement, jaundice; prolonged high fever
Potential for injury related to CNS changes	Mental dullness and lethargy, progressing to delirium, stupor, convulsions, and coma; focal neurologic signs (e.g., tremor, vertigo, hallucinations, and paranoid behavior)
Potential for infection related to environmental risk factors	History of exposure to tick-infested areas

Other related nursing diagnoses: Constipation

➤ ➤ ➤

3 PLAN

Patient goals

1. Patient's body temperature will be maintained within the normal range; comfort and safety will be maintained for patients experiencing fever.
2. Patient will obtain relief from pain.
3. Patient will demonstrate improved generalized tissue perfusion and cellular oxygenation.
4. Patient will not be confused or frightened by environmental stimuli during time of alteration in vision; visual function will return to normal.
5. Skin will return to prepathogenic state.
6. Patient will achieve adequate rest to conserve energy during active disease and will return to preillness level of activity during convalescence.
7. Nutrition will be adequate for body requirements.
8. Patient will not experience injury.
9. Patient will have information to prevent further episodes of vector-borne infections.

4 IMPLEMENT

NURSING DIAGNOSIS	NURSING INTERVENTIONS	RATIONALE
Hyperthermia related to infection	See inside back cover, interventions 1-15.	
Pain related to systemic angitis, vascular rupture, and hemorrhage	Administer analgesics regularly as prescribed.	To relieve severe headache.
	Do not administer aspirin.	Aspirin affects coagulability, increasing risk of bleeding complications of disease.
Altered tissue perfusion (generalized) related to vascular endothelial damage and reaction to pathogen toxin	Administer antibiotics as soon as ordered.	To prevent vascular damage.
	Regularly check vital signs and intake and output. Monitor for signs of shock (hypotension, cyanosis, tachycardia, absent peripheral pulses, urinary output <30 ml/h).	To detect signs of shock and hemorrhage for immediate intervention.
	Administer oxygen.	To maintain adequate circulating oxygen.
	Maintain unconscious patient in a supine position and give nothing by mouth.	To prevent aspiration in unconscious patient.
	Measure intake and output. (Maintain indwelling catheter in unconscious patient.) Output should equal intake.	Accurate measurement is essential because patients are at risk for shock and renal failure.
	Administer IV fluids slowly in enough quantity to maintain 1,500 ml/day urine output.	To ensure proper hydration without overload.
	Monitor IV infusion rate hourly. Monitor for edema. Stop IV line if anuria occurs.	To prevent and detect overhydration.
Sensory-perceptual alterations (visual) related to vascular damage to retina	Minimize unnecessary environmental stimuli; continuously interpret environment for patient; supervise patient closely and restrain if necessary; administer sedatives as prescribed.	To prevent hallucinations, confusion, and injury.

NURSING DIAGNOSIS	NURSING INTERVENTIONS	RATIONALE
Impaired skin integrity related to rash and altered peripheral circulation	Turn and reposition frequently.	To prevent pressure over bony prominences or purpuric or necrotic areas.
	Observe distal extremities, nose, and genitalia.	To detect and report signs of impaired circulation.
	Observe entire body for petechiae.	To detect and report signs of hemorrhage.
Activity intolerance related to disease severity	Provide opportunity for adequate rest until patient's energy returns.	To prevent excess demands on patient's metabolic and circulatory processes.
	Reassure patient that the loss of energy is temporary.	To relieve patient's anxiety.
Altered nutrition: less than body requirements related to increased metabolism caused by infection and fever	Offer frequent, small, high-protein, high-calorie feedings.	To compensate for increased metabolic needs.
	Administer nasogastric feedings to unconscious patient.	To supply nutrition.
Potential for injury related to CNS changes	Constantly supervise delirious or convulsing patient; use padded headboard and side rails; administer sedatives as prescribed.	To prevent injury and decrease uncontrolled muscle activity.
Potential for infection related to environmental risk factors	See Patient Teaching Guide.	

5   EVALUATE

PATIENT OUTCOME	DATA INDICATING THAT OUTCOME IS REACHED
Body temperature is maintained within the normal range. Comfort and safety are maintained	Body temperature is between 37°-38°C (96.8°-100°F) oral. Vital signs are normal. Skin is cool to touch and free of excess perspiration; patient's clothing and bedding are dry. Patient is free of headache and malaise. Patient experiences no injury from seizures. Body fluids are adequate.
Patient obtains relief from pain.	Patient expresses relief from headache and moves without signs of pain.
Patient demonstrates improved generalized tissue perfusion and cellular oxygenation.	Peripheral pulses are palpable. Blood pressure, pulse, and respirations are normal. Patient is awake and oriented and communicates coherently; sensory and visual perceptions are normal. Urinary output is between 1,500 and 3,000 ml/day or equal to intake. There is no edema. Serum albumin, sodium, and chloride levels are normal. Prothrombin time, partial thromboplastin time, platelets, fibrinogen, and RBC count are normal. Pneumonia, renal failure, gangrene, mental or neurosensory sequelae, or cardiac dysrhythmias are not present.

PATIENT OUTCOME	DATA INDICATING THAT OUTCOME IS REACHED
Patient is not confused or frightened by environmental stimuli; visual function returns to normal.	Patient does not experience injury or express fear of the environment. Patient reads or engages in diversional activity without impairment of vision.
Skin returns to pre-pathogenic state.	Skin and mucous membranes are warm, moist, and normal colored. There are no purpuric or necrotic skin lesions.
Patient will achieve adequate rest during active disease and return to preillness level of activity during convalescence.	Patient rests comfortably during acute illness; sleeps for uninterrupted periods of time; gradually increases self-care activities and diversional activities.
Nutrition is adequate for body requirements.	Patient has not lost weight during course of the illness. Energy level is adequate after convalescence, allowing patient to perform all ADLs. There are no signs of anemia or hypoalbuminemia.
Patient does not experience injury.	Patient is protected from falls or any trauma.
Patient has information to prevent further episodes of vector-borne infections.	Patient describes practices that decrease exposure to pathogens or vectors in the environment.

PATIENT TEACHING

1. Patient understands that relapses may occur and recurrence of symptoms should be reported to physician immediately so antibiotic therapy can be resumed rapidly.
2. Patient knows to avoid tick-infested areas and to check body surfaces every 3 to 4 hours for attached ticks if working or playing in infested areas.
3. Instruct patient to remove ticks as follows:

   - Wear gloves and do not touch ticks with hand (to prevent contaminations with tick feces).

   - Remove tick with tweezers or forceps, using a firm, steady traction (to avoid leaving mouthparts in skin).

4. Inform patient that deticking dogs minimizes the tick population near residences.
5. Instruct patient on use of insect repellants applied to clothing and uncovered skin as useful for repelling ticks. The most effective repellant is *N-N-Diethyl-m*-toluamide (Deet).

Lyme Disease

Lyme disease is a multisystem illness caused by a tick-borne spirochete. The illness closely mimics other rheumatic diseases. It usually occurs in stages characterized by different clinical manifestations and by exacerbations and remissions. The best clinical marker is erythema migrans, an annular skin lesion that appears at the site of a tick bite. Flu-like symptoms may be present initially. Neurologic, cardiac, or arthritic abnormalities emerge weeks or months later.

PATHOPHYSIOLOGY

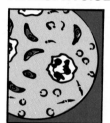

The spirochete, *Borrelia burgdorferi*, is introduced into the skin by the bite of ixodid ticks. These ticks, which vary by geographic areas, are very small. The spirochete produces an endotoxin, which causes initial vascular and cellular inflammation. Later pathologic changes appear to result from the immune response to the pathogen. In some cases the spirochete remains localized in the initial skin lesion and regional lymph nodes. At other times, the spirochete spreads hematogeneously and develops secondary lesions similar to the first. In either

See Table 10-1, page 213, for an overview of Lyme disease.

For picture of rash of Lyme disease see color plates 26 through 28, page xiv.

case, the pathogen can invade and replicate in any tissue. The spirochete has been cultured from blood, skin, cerebrospinal fluid, and joint fluid and has been observed in specimens of skin and myocardial, retinal, and synovial lesions. It appears that the spirochete is active during all stages of the disease in untreated persons.

The immune response is suppressed initially. After the first weeks of infection, mononuclear cells produce active immune responses to spirochetal antigens. There is often evidence of B cell hyperactivity. Antigen-reactive mononuclear cells concentrate in joint fluid when arthritis is present. Synovia show pathologic changes similar to other chronic inflammatory arthritis.

IgM antibodies peak during the third to sixth weeks after disease onset. IgG antibodies rise slowly, peaking months later when arthritis is present.

COMPLICATIONS

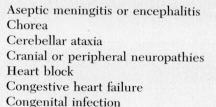

Aseptic meningitis or encephalitis
Chorea
Cerebellar ataxia
Cranial or peripheral neuropathies
Heart block
Congestive heart failure
Congenital infection

NURSING CARE

Nursing care will vary depending on the stage in the disease that the infected person is experiencing when presenting to the health care providers. Providing support during the diagnosis is important. Patient teaching is the same as that for RMSF.

SYMPTOMS OF LYME DISEASE

Erythema migrans, an annular skin lesion that expands over a period of days to weeks and develops central clearing. The lesion is warm to touch but is not painful.

Plus some combination of the following:

- Flu-like symptoms (e.g., malaise, fatigue, fever, headache, stiff neck, myalgia, migratory arthralgias, and lymphadenopathy)
- Inflamed, painful arthritis in large joints
- Limb weakness, sensory loss
- Confusion, memory loss
- Bell's palsy

DIAGNOSTIC STUDIES AND FINDINGS

Diagnostic Test	Findings
Serology*	
Indirect immunofluorescent antibody	≥1:128
Enzyme-linked immunosorbent assay optical density	≥.40
Erythrocyte sedimentation	Sometimes elevated
Rheumatoid factor	Negative

*Serologic tests are not very sensitive in early stages of the disease (many false negatives occur). Diagnosis is based on serologic findings plus history of tick bite, presence of erythema migrans, and involvement of at least two of three organ systems usually affected by Lyme disease (e.g., the joints, nervous system, and cardiovascular system).

MEDICAL MANAGEMENT[130]

DRUG THERAPY

Early disease: Tetracycline, 250 mg qid PO for adults for 10 days,* or
Phenoxymethyl penicillin, 500 mg qid PO for 10 days,* or
Erythromycin, 250 mg, qid, PO for 10 days.*

For meningitis: Penicillin G, IV, 20 million U/day, in divided doses for 10 days.

For heart block: Penicillin G, IV, 10-20 million U/day for 10 days.
Corticosteroids.

For established arthritis: Benzathine penicillin, IM, 2.4 million U/wk for 3 wks (total dose 7.2 million U) or
Penicillin G, IV, 20 million U/day in divided doses, for 10-20 days.

*Continue for 20 days if symptoms persist.

Malaria

Malaria is a severe systemic infection caused by one of four protozoan parasites of the *Plasmodium* genus. The parasite is transmitted to humans through mosquito bites. Disease severity varies with the type of plasmodium causing the infection, with some plasmodia killing more than 10% of untreated individuals. The duration of acute malarial disease is long, sometimes lasting months, with recurrent fever in treated individuals. Relapses occur irregularly for years in untreated persons.

PATHOPHYSIOLOGY

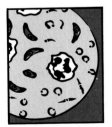

Four species of plasmodia produce malaria in humans, and more than one species may be present in any given malarial infection. The life cycle of the plasmodium is important to the pathophysiology of the disease. The sexual stage of the cycle occurs only in the intestines of the *Anopheles* mosquito, producing sporozoites that are discharged in mosquito saliva. The asexual development of the pathogen occurs in humans. There are two phases to the asexual cycle within humans, the exoerythrocytic and the erythrocytic. The exoerythrocytic phase begins when plasmodium sporozoites from mosquito saliva are inoculated into human blood and are carried to the liver, where they invade hepatocytes. There they form cystlike structures that rupture and release hundreds of merozoites into the blood when they mature. Once in the blood parasites never reinvade the liver. Two of the species, *P. vivax* and *P. ovale*, may retain some merozoites in the liver in a dormant form. Release of these at a later time causes relapsing malaria. Infection induced by transfusion of blood containing the life cycle form of merozoites does not progress through the exoerythrocytic phase but begins directly with the erythrocytic phase.

See Table 10-1, page 213, for an overview of malaria.

The erythrocytic phase of the plasmodium life cycle is responsible for pathologic findings in the human host. Plasmodium merozoites invade select erythrocytes that contain surface receptors that attract the plasmodia. The absence of these RBC receptors in black Africans protects them from symptomatic malaria. Once in erythrocytes the merozoites feed and grow into trophozoites. Trophozoites feed on hemoglobin, metabolizing the globin fraction and depositing the heme fraction as hematin granules into the cytoplasm. Trophozoites sexually segment into numerous merozoites. This causes the erythrocytes to rupture and release merozoites into the circulation, enabling them to reinvade additional erythrocytes within seconds.

The process of erythrocytic invasion, asexual multiplication of the plasmodia, and erythrocytic rupture continues until antibodies develop within the host to control the parasite or until the host is treated with sufficient antimicrobial agents. An antibody response is adequate to limit all malarial plasmodia except *P. falciparum*, which, in the absence of treatment, may overwhelm the host with severe fulminating disease, resulting in death.

Symptomatic attacks of chills, fever, and diaphoresis coincide with completion of the erythrocytic life cycle of the plasmodium in humans. The length of time between attacks varies with the *Plasmodium* species: every 42 to 48 hours in *P. vivax*, 48 hours in *P. falciparum*, 50 hours in *P. ovale*, and 72 hours in *P. malariae*.

The erythrocytic activity of the parasite produces the following pathophysiologic changes: fever and its physiologic consequences, hemolytic anemia, tissue hypoxia resulting from anemia and alterations in the microcirculation, and coagulation defects resulting from immunopathologic events.

Fever with marked vasodilation leads to a decrease in effective plasma volume with a resultant orthostatic hypotension and an increased secretion of ADH and aldosterone. Diaphoresis and vomiting that accompany the toxic fever result in fluid and electrolyte loss and possible hyponatremia.

Anemia triggers the spleen to store erythrocytes, resulting in splenomegaly. Anemia also results in tissue hypoxia, particularly in the kidneys, lungs, liver, and central nervous system, with resultant dysfunction to those systems. Erythrocyte invasion also causes erythrocytes to adhere to vascular endothelium, slowing the blood flow and accentuating tissue hypoxia, edema, and vascular pathologic findings and hemorrhage.

The immune response is pathologic, as well as protective. Excess immunoglobulin production triggers hypersplenism and plays a role in the further development of anemia and in the development of neutropenia and thrombocytopenia. Laboratory evidence of coagulation defects in some patients can be observed.

COMPLICATIONS

Renal failure
Hepatic failure
Pulmonary edema
Perivascular edema and hemorrhage in cerebral cortex

DIAGNOSTIC STUDIES AND FINDINGS

Diagnostic Test	Findings
Microscopic examination of stained peripheral blood smear (taken at least twice daily, within 6-12 hours after chills)	Identification of plasmodia in blood Detection of granular, brownish pigment within monocytes or neutrophils, or identification of parasitized RBC If more than 5% of RBCs are affected, *P. falciparum* should be suspected
Indirect fluorescent antibody	Increase in antibody titer after 1 wk of illness Useful for screening blood donors but should not be relied on for diagnosis
In uncomplicated malaria: Blood	Leukopenia, monocytosis, hemolytic anemia (normocytic, normochromic), decreased platelets
VDRL	False positive
With complications: Blood	Decreased fibrinogen; platelets <50,000/mm³; decrease in factors V, VII, VIII and X; prolonged prothrombin and partial thromboplastin times
Urine	Proteinuria; increased serum creatinine
Liver enzymes	Increased serum transaminase and indirect serum bilirubin

Table 10-2

DRUGS USED IN THE PROPHYLAXIS OF MALARIA[3,43,53]

Drug	Adult dose	Pediatric dose
Chloroquine phosphate (Aralen)	300 mg base (500 mg salt) orally, once/wk*	5 mg/kg base (8.3 mg/kg salt) orally once/wk, up to maximum adult dose of 300 mg base*
Hydroxychloroquine sulfate (Plaquenil)	310 mg base (400 mg salt) orally, once/wk*	5 mg/kg base (6.5 mg/kg salt) orally, once/week, up to maximum adult dose*
For travelers to areas with chloroquine-resistant *P. falciparum*		
Mefloquine (Lariam)	228 mg base (250 mg salt) orally, once/wk*	15-19 kg: ¼ tab/wk* 20-30 kg: ½ tab/wk* 31-45 kg: ¾ tab/wk* >45 kg: 1 tab/wk*
Doxycycline	100 mg orally, once/day beginning 2 days before travel	>8 years of age: 2 mg/kg of body weight orally/day up to adult dose of 100 mg/day
Proguanil	200 mg orally, once/day in combination with weekly chloroquine	<2 years: 50 mg/day 2-6 years: 100 mg/day 7-10 years: 150 mg/day >10 years: 200 mg/day
Primaquine	15 mg base (26.3 mg salt) orally, once/day for 14 days	0.3 mg/kg base (0.5 mg/kg salt) orally once/day for 14 days
Pyrimethamine-sulfadoxine (Fansidar)	3 tablets (75 mg pyrimethamine and 1,500 mg sulfadoxine), orally as a single dose	5-10:1/2 11-20:1 21-30:1 1/2 31-45:2 >45:3

*Drug should be taken once each week for 4 weeks after leaving an area with malaria.

MEDICAL MANAGEMENT

Uncomplicated infections with *P. ovale*, *P. vivax*, and *P. malariae* can be treated in an outpatient setting. Patients infected with *P. falciparum* should be hospitalized.

DRUG THERAPY[3]

For uncomplicated infection with all species except chloroquine-resistant *P. falciparum;* chloroquine phosphate (Aralen), PO, 25 mg/kg (base) administered over 3 days: 15 mg/kg the first day (10 mg initially and 5 mg 6 h later), 5 mg/kg the second day, and 5 mg/kg the third day.

For emergency treatment of severe infections or for persons unable to retain orally administered medications:
  Chloroquine hydrochloride (Aralen hydrochloride), IM, 200 mg base q 6 h for 3 days.
  Quinine dihydrochloride, 20 mg base per kg, diluted in 500 ml of normal saline, glucose, or plasma, administered slowly IV (never push and never give IM); repeat in 8 h at 10 mg base per kg (no more than three doses/per 24 h)

For infection caused by chloroquine-resistant *P. falciparum:*
  Quinine sulfate, PO, 25-30 mg/kg/24 h in 3 divided doses for 7-10 days, plus
  Tetracycline, 15 mg/kg in 4 doses daily for 7 days.

For prevention of relapses from *P. vivax* and *P. ovale*

Primaquine phosphate, PO, 0.25 mg base/kg/day for 14 days (26.3 mg/day for average adult) following treatment with chloroquine phosphate.

Chemoprophylaxis for people traveling to areas where malaria is endemic, prophylaxis to begin once weekly for 2 wks before entering and 4 wks after leaving an endemic area. Available drugs and dosage in Table 10-2.

Those traveling to areas with high risk for acquiring *P. falciparum* malaria, and who are not sensitive to sulfonamides or pyrimethamine and who are not pregnant, can be given one dose of sulfadoxine-pyrimethamine (Fansidar) to have in their possession while traveling to take if symptoms develop.

GENERAL MANAGEMENT

IV fluids and electrolytes; restrict fluids in cerebral edema; monitor body weight and fluid intake and output.
Assisted ventilation and intubation in pulmonary edema.
Transfusion of packed RBCs in anemia.
Transfusion of whole blood in shock.
Corticosteroids in cerebral edema.
Heparin, low-molecular weight dextran, or fresh frozen plasma in coagulopathy.
Peritoneal or hemodialysis in renal failure.

1 ASSESS

ASSESSMENT	OBSERVATIONS
History	Recent travel to an area where malaria is endemic
Subjective symptoms	Myalgia; fatigue, malaise; slight chills; paroxysms of chills, fever, and diaphoresis
Chill phase **Skin**	Cold, pale skin; cyanotic nail beds; severe shaking chills lasting 1-2 h
Fever phase **Body temperature**	Fever of 39°-41°C (103°-106°F) lasting 3-6 h, decreasing suddenly by lysis
Vital signs	Tachycardia, tachypnea, hypotension
Systemic manifestations	Severe headache, nausea and vomiting, cough
Diaphoresis phase	Profuse sweating; weakness leading to sleep
Between attacks **Abdomen**	Hepatomegaly in *P. vivax* and *P. falciparum;* splenomegaly in *P. vivax;* abdominal pain
Lungs	Scattered rales
Systemic	Energy returns to normal between attacks in all but *P. falciparum* infections
Vital signs	Tachycardia persisting between fever episodes
Additional symptoms in *P. falciparum* infections **GI**	Severe prolonged vomiting and diarrhea leading to dehydration and electrolyte imbalance
Skin	Jaundice resulting from hepatic dysfunction
Neurologic	Delirium, convulsions, coma; altered intellectual function, behavior changes, focal neurologic signs, positive Babinski's sign, tremors, and hemiparesis
Respiratory	Pulmonary congestion and respiratory distress

2 DIAGNOSE

NURSING DIAGNOSIS	SUPPORTIVE ASSESSMENT FINDINGS
Potential for infection related to environmental exposure to malaria-carrying mosquitos	Plans to travel to areas where malaria is endemic or has history of travel to such areas without following prophylactic measures
Hyperthermia related to erythrocytic life cycle of plasmodia	Fever of 39°-41°C (103°-106°F) lasting 3-6 h, which decreases suddenly by lysis and is followed by profuse sweating and weakness, leading to sleep

NURSING DIAGNOSIS	SUPPORTIVE ASSESSMENT FINDINGS
Hypothermia related to diaphoresis and hypotension	Severe shaking chills lasting 1-2 h
Altered cerebral, cardiopulmonary, and renal tissue perfusion related to anemia and hemorrhagic complications	Tachycardia; tachypnea; hypotension; cold, pale skin; cyanotic nail beds; delirium, convulsions, coma; altered intellectual function, behavior changes, focal neurologic signs, positive Babinski's sign, tremors, hemiparesis
Potential for injury related to disease complications and chemotherapeutic agents	Potential complications, particularly when *P. falciparum* is involved, including renal, hepatic, and pulmonary failure and CNS damage. Antimalarial drugs have many toxic side effects.

Other related nursing diagnoses: Depends on extent of complications (e.g., fluid volume excess in renal failure)

3 PLAN

Patient goals

1. Infection will be prevented in persons experiencing risk factors.
2. Patient will be free of infection and complications of malaria.
3. Patient's body temperature will be maintained within the normal range; comfort and safety are maintained for patients experiencing fever and chills.
4. Patient will demonstrate improved cerebral, renal, and cardiopulmonary tissue perfusion and cellular oxygenation.
5. Patient will not experience injury.
6. Patient will self-administer antiinfective agents as prescribed.

4 IMPLEMENT

NURSING DIAGNOSIS	NURSING INTERVENTIONS	RATIONALE
Potential for infection related to environmental exposure to malaria-carrying mosquitos	Employ blood and body fluid precautions for duration of illness (see Chapter 13, Patient Teaching, and Patient Teaching Guide).	To prevent transmission of pathogen.
	Administer antiinfective agents as soon as prescribed.	To prevent complications of untreated disease.
Hyperthermia related to erythrocytic life cycle of plasmodia	See inside back cover, Interventions 1-15.	
Hypothermia related to diaphoresis and hypotension	Provide hot drinks and application of external heat.	To provide comfort during chills.
Altered cerebral tissue perfusion related to anemia and/or hemorrhagic complications	Monitor and report changes in level of consciousness, behavior, or neurologic signs.	For immediate medical intervention for cerebral edema or cerebral hemorrhage.
	Monitor delirious patient on one-to-one basis.	To ensure patient safety.

NURSING DIAGNOSIS	NURSING INTERVENTIONS	RATIONALE
Altered cardiopul-monary tissue per-fusion related to anemia and/or hem-orrhagic complica-tions	Monitor for signs of pulmonary congestion. Limit fluid intake if necessary. Prepare to assist ventilation if needed.	Pulmonary edema is a common complica-tion of malaria.
Altered renal tissue perfusion related to anemia and/or hem-orrhagic complica-tions	Monitor intake and output and body weight to report edema or urinary output <intake.	Renal failure is a common complication of malaria.
	Monitor patient receiving IV drugs. Limit intake if necessary.	To prevent overhydration.
Potential for injury related to disease complications and chemotherapeutic agents	Monitor for potentially fatal skin reactions to Pyrimethamine-sulfadoxine (Fansidar).	To discontinue drug immediately.
	Monitor for signs of toxic reactions to qui-nine (tinnitus, headache, nausea, altered vision) and hypersensitivity (bronchos-pasm, hemolytic anemia, thrombocytope-nia).	To detect cardiotoxicity, hypotension, and widening of QRS complex.
	Use caution when palpating abdomen.	To prevent splenic rupture.
	Caution patient against lifting heavy ob-jects.	To prevent splenic rupture, which is a com-mon complication of malaria.

5 EVALUATE

PATIENT OUTCOME	DATA INDICATING THAT OUTCOME IS REACHED
Infection is pre-vented in persons experiencing risk factors	Persons traveling to areas where malaria is endemic describe plans to self-administer pro-phylactic antiinfective agents and behaviors to reduce exposure to mosquito.
Patient is free of in-fections and com-plications of malaria	No parasites are detected in peripheral blood smears 4 or 5 days after treatment. Adult oral body temperature is consistently around 37°C (98.6°F) for 4 to 5 days after treat-ment. Paroxysms of chills and diaphoresis that accompany fever are absent. Leukocyte, monocyte, erythrocyte, and platelet counts are normal. Coagulation factors V, VII, VIII, and X are normal. Prothrombin time and partial thromboplastin time are normal. Serum transaminase, indirect bilirubin, and creatinine levels are normal. Serum sodium level is normal. Urine protein is normal.
Body temperature is maintained within normal range; com-fort and safety are maintained	Body temperature is between 36°-38°C (96.8°-100°F), oral. Vital signs are normal. Skin is cool to touch and free of excess perspiration; patient's clothing and bedding are dry. Pa-tient is free of headache and malaise. Patient experiences no injury from seizures. Body fluids, serum electrolyte, urine output, and specific gravity are normal.
Patient demon-strates improved tissue perfusion and cellular oxy-genation	Patient is alert and oriented to surroundings, speaks coherently, and has memory for re-cent and past events; behavior and affect are appropriate to the situation. All neurologic signs are normal. Breath sounds are clear. There is no dyspnea or cyanosis. Urine output is 1,500 to 3,000 ml or equal to input. There is no evidence of edema. Blood pressure, pulse, and respirations are normal.

PATIENT OUTCOME	DATA INDICATING THAT OUTCOME IS REACHED
Patient does not experience injury	Same data as above plus no signs of hemorrhage.
Patient self-administers antiinfective agents as prescribed	Patient completes full course of antiinfective therapy. No preventable drug interactions or allergic reactions are experienced. If untoward reactions are experienced, the patient discontinues the drug and contacts the physician immediately.

PATIENT TEACHING

1. Patients infected with *P. vivax* or *P. ovale* may still have plasmodia in the liver after treatment; remissions are possible. They should continue with prescribed medication for 14 days following initial treatment and should report recurrence of symptoms immediately.
2. All patients should return for blood examination 4 or 5 days after completion of treatment.
3. Patients should discontinue medications and seek medical help if they experience any reactions.
4. Persons taking doxycycline prophylactically during travel to areas where *P. falciparum* is endemic should be reminded that photosensitivity is possible when taking tetracyclines.
5. Overdose of antimalarial drugs can be fatal. These drugs should be stored in child-proof containers out of the reach of children.
6. Chemoprophylaxis is not completely protective. Travelers who develop symptoms should seek medical assistance immediately. Early treatment is most effective and safe.
7. Travelers to malaria-endemic countries should follow recommendations for prophylaxis.
   - Comply with pharmacologic prophylaxis (see Medical Management).
   - Wear clothing that covers as much skin as possible, particularly during the evening and night.
   - Frequently apply insect repellent on uncovered skin or clothing. Products containing *N,N*-Diethyl-*m*-toluamide (Deet) are the most effective.
   - Sleep only in screened areas and use mosquito netting if necessary.
   - Stay indoors during the evening and night when the *Anopheles* mosquito is likely to bite.
   - Use pyrethrum-containing flying insect spray in living and sleeping areas during the evening and night.
   - Permethrin (Permanone) may be sprayed on clothing.
8. Some persons exposed to Deet have experienced toxic encephalopathy. This risk can be minimized by applying the repellant sparingly on exposed skin; avoid inhaling, ingesting, or getting in the eyes. Do not apply to children's hands or to wounds or irritated skin. If reaction occurs, wash treated skin and seek medical care.

Dengue (Breakbone Fever)

Dengue (breakbone fever) is an acute viral febrile illness of short duration that is transmitted to humans through mosquito bites. The risk for dengue is increasing in the southern United States because of movement of infected mosquitos northward from Mexico. Two forms of the disease, a benign and a hemorrhagic form, occur.

PATHOPHYSIOLOGY

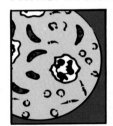

The pathologic agents producing dengue are four immunologically distinct viruses that require both *Aedes* mosquitos and humans for their viability. An *Aedes* mosquito that feeds on an infected person during the symptomatic viremic stage of dengue becomes infective after an incubation period of 8 to 10 days. Infective mosquitos transmit the virus to every person they bite. In tropical and subtropical areas where *Aedes* organisms survive year-round, dengue is an endemic, and sometimes epidemic, disease in the population. Epidemics or disease outbreaks may occur anywhere that *Aedes* mosquitos are present by the introduction of either infective mosquitos or persons into the area.

See Table 10-1, page 213, for an overview of dengue.

Dengue occurs in two clinical disease forms: classic (benign) dengue and the more severe dengue hemorrhagic fever. Either form may be produced by any of the four viral serotypes. The mechanism for the development of two different dengue diseases is unknown. One hypothesis is that the form of the disease varies with differences in virulence within viral strains. A second hypothesis is that a primary infection with one viral serotype may result in the benign form of the disease but predispose one to an immunopathologic response to a subsequent infection with another serotype, resulting in dengue hemorrhagic fever.

The pathologic process is similar in both disease forms, although more extensive and life-threatening in dengue hemorrhagic fever. Once injected, the virus replicates at the site of inoculation and in local lymphatic tissue. Viruses invade the blood within days, producing a viremia that lasts 4 to 5 days after symptomatic disease onset. The viremia results in endothelial swelling, mononuclear cell infiltration, increased vascular permeability, and perivascular edema. Extravasation of blood from dermal vessels produces a maculopapular or petechial rash. Leukopenia and lymphadenopathy are common. Symptom severity varies in the benign form.

In the hemorrhagic form of the disease, the increased vascular permeability is more severe, with extensive extravasation of blood and fluid into serous cavities and hemorrhage and congestion within many organs, particularly the spleen, liver, kidneys, pleura, and peritoneum. Blood changes include a thrombocytopenia, increase in platelet agglutinability, mild or moderate disseminated intravascular coagulation, and hemoconcentration. A rising hematocrit concentration on the third day of illness is a sign of impending life-threatening hypovolemic shock, the dengue shock syndrome. Vascular and blood component pathologic findings coincide with the development of an immune response and may result from the action of circulating antigen-antibody complexes, the activation of complement, or the release of vasoactive amines.

Virus serotype-specific IgM antibodies develop early during the febrile period of both forms of the disease and persist for 8 weeks. This initial antibody response is followed within 1 or 2 days by a rise in IgG antibodies that persists for more than 40 years and confers lifetime immunity against the specific dengue serotype. Secondary infections with another dengue serotype initiate an early and extremely high IgG antibody response that cross reacts against the infecting serotype, the initial serotype, and other flaviviruses. This immune response is thought to play a role in the pathogenesis of dengue hemorrhagic fever.

Patients may spontaneously recover from dengue hemorrhagic fever or progress to hypovolemic shock.

SYMPTOMS OF DENGUE

Benign dengue

Prodome: 12 hours; malaise, anorexia

Abrupt onset: chills, severe frontal headache, ocular pain, severe and incapacitating myalgia, arthralgia, and backache

Mild pharyngitis

Nausea and vomiting

Epigastric pain

Fever of 40°C (104°F), unremitting and persisting for 3 to 7 days

Diphasic course with "saddle back" temperature curve

Tachycardia for first few days of fever

Bradycardia during last days of fever

Injected conjunctivae

Generalized tender lymphadenopathy

First 1 or 2 days: transient erythematous flush over face, neck, and upper trunk, disappearing within 1 day

Third to fifth day: distinct macular or maculopapular rash on trunk, spreading centrifugally to face and extremities; petechiae on palate, in the axillae, and on the lower extremities at the end of the febrile period

Subjective symptoms during convalescence

Prolonged fatigue and depression

Hemorrhagic dengue

Same symptoms as benign dengue with the following additions:

Hemorrhagic symptoms during the febrile period: positive tourniquet test, purpura, epistaxis, gingival bleeding, hematemesis, melena, and hematuria

Jaundice

Hepatomegaly

Severe epigastric or generalized abdominal pain

Shock phase

Rapid, weak pulse

Hypotension; narrow pulse pressure

Rapid drop in body temperature

Cool, clammy, edematous skin

Circumoral cyanosis

Untreated shock leads to tissue anoxia, coma, metabolic acidosis, hyperkalemia, and death within 12 to 24 hours.

Laboratory findings in dengue hemorrhagic fever include decreased serum albumin and sodium; decreased platelets, fibrinogen, and coagulation factors V, VII, IX, and X; decreased C3 serum complement; a 20% or greater increase in hematocrit; the presence of fibrin split products in plasma and an increase in prothrombin time; and an increase in BUN and serum transaminase proportional to kidney and liver dysfunction, respectively.

NURSING CARE

Nursing care for persons with dengue is primarily supportive. It is essential to prevent this infection by preventing contact with infected mosquitos. See Patient Teaching for prophylaxis for malaria in addition to the following:

1. During illness, the person with dengue must protect self from mosquito vectors to prevent transmission to others.
2. Patient can prevent future infections by protecting self from mosquito vectors with screened living quarters, protective clothing, and insect repellents on exposed skin and clothing when in the proximity of mosquitoes. *Aedes* mosquitoes enter homes and usually bite during the day.
3. Mosquitos can be controlled around living quarters by eliminating potential breeding places, particularly any water-filled containers.
4. Persons living close to the patient may have been exposed to mosquito vectors infected with dengue. They should be monitored for early diagnosis of dengue.
5. Prolonged weakness and depression are characteristic of the convalescent period.

CHAPTER 11

Childhood and Vaccine-Preventable Diseases

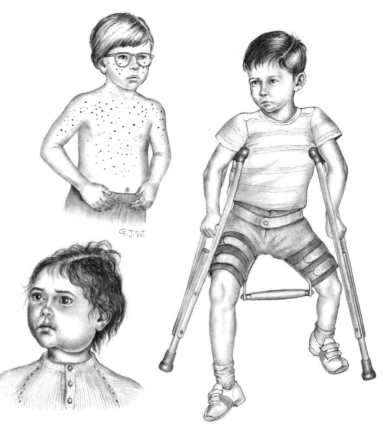

G.J.W.

The infectious diseases presented in this chapter, with the exception of chickenpox, are preventable with routine immunization. Each is presented separately. An overview of all of the diseases is presented in Table 11-1.

Chickenpox

Chickenpox (varicella) is an acute, highly communicable viral disease common in childhood and young adulthood. It is characterized by a sudden-onset fever, mild malaise, and a skin eruption that is maculopapular for a few hours and vesicular for 3 to 4 days, leaving a granular scab.

PATHOPHYSIOLOGY

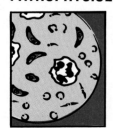

The varicella-zoster (V-Z virus, a herpesvirus, enters the body by way of the respiratory mucous membranes and produces systemic disease and skin lesions. The lesions are generally superficial unilocular vesicles, with the fluid containing more polymorphonuclear cells than mononuclear cells. Lesions generally occur in successive crops with several stages of maturity present at one time. They are generally more abundant on covered areas of the body, but they may appear everywhere including the scalp, conjunctivae, and upper respiratory tract.

Lesions have been found in the lungs, liver, spleen, adrenal glands, and pancreas. Complications include conjunctival involvement, secondary bacterial infections, viral pneumonia, encephalitis, aseptic meningitis, myelitis, Guillain-Barré syndrome, and Reye's syndrome. Disease is severe in those with deficiencies in

For overview of chickenpox, see Table 11-1, page 232.

For picture of lesions of chickenpox, see color plates 35 through 37, page xv.

cell-mediated immunity. After recovery the virus is believed to remain in the body in an asymptomatic latent stage, possibly localized in the dorsal root ganglia.

Reactivation of the infection with the V-Z virus can occur later in life or during times of altered immune status. It leads to the disease manifestation of herpes zoster, in which there is a localized eruption of vesicles with an erythematous base. The vesicles are restricted to the skin areas supplied by sensory nerves of a single or associated group of dorsal root ganglia.

COMPLICATIONS

Conjunctival ulcers
Secondary bacterial infections
Viral pneumonia
Encephalitis and meningitis
Myelitis
Guillain-Barré syndrome
Reye's syndrome

Table 11-1

OVERVIEW OF CHILDHOOD AND VACCINE-PREVENTABLE DISEASES

	Chickenpox	Diphtheria	Mumps (infectious parotitis)	Pertussis (Whooping Cough)
Occurrence	Worldwide; in metropolitan areas 75% of the population has had chickenpox by age 15 yrs, and 90% by young adulthood	Formerly a prevalent disease; rare in United States with immunization; affects unimmunized children under 15 yrs and adults	Occurs commonly in winter and spring; ⅓ of those exposed have subclinical infections; incidence decreasing with immunization	Common in children; worldwide; decline in incidence in areas with active immunization programs
Etiologic agent	Varicella-zoster (V-Z) virus, a member of the *Herpesvirus* group	*Corynebacterium diphtheriae*, with many toxigenic strains	A type of paramyxovirus; antigenically related to parainfluenza viruses	*Bordetella pertussis*, the pertussis bacillus
Reservoir	Humans	Humans	Humans	Humans
Transmission	Direct and indirect contact with droplets from respiratory passages; an extremely contagious disease	Direct or indirect contact with exudate from mucous membranes of infected person or carrier; raw milk may also be a vehicle	Direct contact with saliva droplets from infected person	Direct contact with droplets from respiratory passages
Incubation period	2-3 wks; commonly 13-17 days	2-5 days	2-3 wks; commonly 18 days	7-14 days; commonly 7-10 days
Period of communicability	1-2 days before onset of rash and until lesions have crusted over (not more than 6 days after first appearance of vesicles)	Variable; until bacilli have disappeared from discharges and lesions (usually in 2 wks); a carrier may shed bacilli for 6 months	6 days before parotid symptoms to 9 days after; most communicable 48 h before parotid swelling	7 days after exposure to 3 wks after onset; highly communicable in early catarrhal stage before cough; not communicable after 3 wks even though cough may persist
Susceptibility and resistance	General; one attack confers long-term immunity; second attacks are rare	Unimmunized children most susceptible; infants born of immune mothers have passive immunity for 6 months; recovery from clinical disease confers temporary immunity	General; immunity is lifelong and develops after clinical and subclinical disease; placental transfer of antibodies occurs	General; children under 7 yrs most susceptible; no passive immunity from mother; attack confers prolonged, but not lifetime immunity
Report to local health authority	In some areas	Case report required	Case report required in some areas	Case report required

Data from Benenson.[3]

Diagnostic Test	Findings
Electron microscopy or tissue culture of vesicular fluid from lesions	Visualization of V-Z virus during first 3 days after eruption
Giemsa-stained scrapings from lesions	Multinucleated giant cells
Serology:	
Immunofluorescence	Increase in long-lasting antibodies 2 wks after rash
Complement fixation	Increase in antibodies up to 2 months after infection, with subsequent decrease in antibodies

Poliomyelitis	Rubella (German measles)	Measles (rubeola)	Tetanus
Worldwide; commonly in summer and early autumn; highest in children and adolescents but does affect nonimmune adults; United States incidence decreasing with immunization	Worldwide and endemic; most common in winter and spring; primarily a disease of children but does occur in unimmunized adolescents and adults	Worldwide; endemic and epidemic occurrences; seen more in adolescents and adults since routine immunization of children	Worldwide; occurs sporadically and affects all ages; rare in United States with immunization; common among agricultural workers, parenteral drug abusers, and the elderly
Polio virus, types 1, 2, and 3; all are paralytogenic	Rubella virus	Measles virus, a type of paramyxovirus	*Clostridium tetani*, the tetanus bacillus (an anaerobic pathogen)
Humans, particularly children with subclinical infections	Humans	Humans	Intestines of humans and animals
Direct and indirect contact with respiratory discharges and feces; fecal-oral route more common than respiratory transmission	Direct or indirect contact with nasopharyngeal secretions of infected persons; transplacental transmission leads to congenital rubella syndrome	Direct or indirect contact with nasal secretions from infected persons; highly communicable	Tetanus spores enter body through a wound contaminated with soil and feces; necrotic tissue favors the growth of the bacillus
3-35 days; commonly 7-14 days	14-23 days; commonly 16-18 days	Commonly 10 days; 8-13 days until fever; 14 days until rash	3-21 days; commonly 10 days
Highly communicable during first days after onset of symptoms; virus is in throat secretions in 36 h and in feces in 72 h after infection and remains 1 wk in throat and 6 wks in feces	From 1 wk before and 4 days after appearance of rash; highly communicable; infants with congenital rubella syndrome may shed virus for months after birth	A few days before fever to 4 days after appearance of rash	Not directly transmitted
General; paralytic infections are rare and risk increase with age; infection confers long-term immunity; second attacks are result of another virus type	General; infants born with passive immunity from mother lasting 6-9 months; one attack confers lifetime immunity for most, but reinfections (mostly asymptomatic) have been documented	General; acquired immunity from infection is permanent; artificial active immunity may not be permanent	General; recovery from tetanus does not confer permanent immunity; temporary active immunity provided by tetanus toxoid
Case report required	Case report required	Case report required	Case report required

MEDICAL MANAGEMENT[3,10]

DRUG THERAPY

Acyclovir (Zovirax) or Vidarabine (Ara-A, Vira-A) may be helpful for immunocompromised persons if administered early in the disease.

Zoster immune globulin (ZIG) (for high-risk persons only), 125 U/10 kg body weight up to maximum of 625 U IM within 96 h of exposure.

GENERAL MANAGEMENT

Relief of pruritus.
Management of fever.
Treatment of complications: encephalitis (Chapter 4).
Viral pneumonia.
Strict isolation of hospitalized patients until all lesions have crusted (Chapter 13).

1 ASSESS

ASSESSMENT	OBSERVATIONS
History	Exposure within past 2-3 wks to person with chickenpox
Subjective symptoms	Headache, anorexia, malaise, chills
Body temperature	Fever: 38°-39° C (101°-103° F) during prodrome
Upper respiratory concerns	Coryza during prodrome
Skin and mucous membranes	Lesions in various stages of development; may have lesions on buccal mucosa, palate, or conjunctivae

2 DIAGNOSE

NURSING DIAGNOSIS	SUPPORTIVE ASSESSMENT FINDINGS
Potential for infection (patient contacts) related to virus in respiratory secretions	Open skin lesions; diagnostic tests positive for virus in lesion exudate
Impaired skin integrity related to lesions	Lesions in various stages of development
Hyperthermia related to infection	Fever: 38°-39° C (101°-104° F); headache, anorexia, malaise

3 PLAN

Patient goals

1. Infection will not be transmitted to patient contacts.
2. Patient will be free of secondary bacterial infection of skin and mucous membranes. Skin will be free of lesions and scars.
3. Body temperature will be maintained within normal range. Comfort and safety will be maintained for patient experiencing fever.

4 IMPLEMENT

NURSING DIAGNOSIS	NURSING INTERVENTIONS	RATIONALE
Potential for infection (patient contacts) related to virus in respiratory secretions	Observe strict isolation of hospitalized patients until all lesions have crusted (see Chapter 13).	To prevent transmission to others.
	Refer high-risk patient to physician for prophylactic treatment with zoster immune globulin.	To lessen risk for infection.
Impaired skin integrity related to lesions	Bathe or encourage patient to bathe regularly.	To remove exudate.
	Apply calamine lotion or cornstarch.	To relieve itching.
	Caution patient against scratching lesions.	To prevent spread of exudate and potential scarring and introduction of bacteria into lesions.
Hyperthermia related to infection	See inside back cover.	

5 EVALUATE

PATIENT OUTCOME	DATA INDICATING THAT OUTCOME IS REACHED
Infection has not been transmitted	Patient contacts and health personnel have not acquired chickenpox. Immunocompromised patient contacts have received zoster immune globulin.
Patient is free of secondary bacterial infection of skin and mucous membranes; skin is free of lesions and scars	Crusts are shed. Warm, moist, natural color returns to skin and mucous membranes. Patient is not observed scratching lesions.
Body temperature is maintained within normal limits; comfort and safety are maintained	Body temperature is between 36° and 38° C (96.8° and 100° F) oral. Pulse and respirations are between normal limits. Skin is cool to touch and free of excess perspiration; patient's clothing and bedding are dry. Patient is free of headache and malaise associated with fever. Reye's syndrome is prevented.

➔ ❯ ❯

PATIENT TEACHING ■■■■■■■■■■■■■■■■■■■■■■■■■■■■■■■■■■■■■■■

1. Chickenpox is usually a benign condition with complete recovery. However, complications do occur. Report to physician any symptoms appearing during convalescence, such as a secondary rise in fever, headache, or respiratory or neurologic symptoms.
2. Chickenpox is communicable 1 to 2 days before onset of the rash until lesions have crusted over. The disease is transmitted by droplets of respiratory secretions. The incubation period is 2 to 3 weeks.
3. Avoid trauma or scratching of lesions to prevent secondary infection and scars. Daily bathing without irritating soaps is encouraged.
4. Manage fever by taking antipyretic agents and tepid sponge baths, wearing minimal clothing and maintaining a cool environment. Avoid giving children aspirin because it has been implicated in Reye's syndrome. (See Patient Teaching Guide on Fever, page 302.)
5. Manage itching with applications of calamine lotion or cornstarch. Avoid greasy lotions and creams. Maintain a cool environment to relieve itching associated with perspiration.
6. Encourage intake of foods and fluids as tolerated. Popsicles and soft drinks may appeal to young children.
7. Immunocompromised patient contacts should be referred to a physician for prophylactic treatment with zoster immune globulin.

Diphtheria

For overview of diphtheria, see Table 11-1, page 232.

Diphtheria is an acute communicable disease in which a bacterial toxin affects the mucous membranes of the respiratory tract. The disease is manifest as fibropurulent exudative membranes, commonly on the tonsils and pharynx but also on the larynx, nasal passages, skin, conjunctivae, and genitalia, and as systemic symptoms resulting from toxin dissemination.

PATHOPHYSIOLOGY

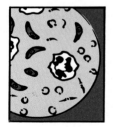 *Corynebacterium diphtheriae*, widely available in the nasopharynx of carriers and persons with inapparent infection, invades and multiplies in the nasopharynx of susceptible persons. The pathogen produces a toxin that is disseminated by the blood and lymph throughout the body. The toxin first causes necrosis of the local tissue, resulting in a fibrinopurulent exudative membrane characteristic of this disease. The membrane appears as grayish membrane patches surrounded by a red zone of inflammation on the tonsils, pharynx, larynx, nasal mucosa, or skin. Edema is present in adjacent and underlying tissue and in the cervical lymph nodes. Laryngeal edema and the extension of the membrane into the trachea, bronchial tree, and alveoli may result in suffocation. Nasopharyngeal diphtheria and laryngeal diphtheria are the most severe types. Nasal diphtheria is mild and marked by one-sided nasal excoriations and discharge. Cutaneous diphtheria lesions are variable and may resemble impetigo.

Disseminated toxin inhibits protein synthesis primarily in the heart, peripheral nerves, and muscle tissue. Effects of toxin absorption appear early and include fatty degeneration, edema, and interstitial fibrosis in the myocardium and in the myelin sheath of peripheral nerves. Damage to peripheral nerves results in peripheral motor and sensory palsies. The spleen and kidneys also may be affected. Otitis media, peritonsillar abscess, and albuminuria are less severe complications. Severe toxemia may result in a life-threatening myocarditis, motor or sensory paralysis, pharyngeal and respiratory paralysis, and pneumonia. ECG changes and an increase in SGOT levels may be present.

COMPLICATIONS \\\\\\\\\\\

Peripheral motor or sensory paralysis
Toxemia
Myocarditis
Pharyngeal or respiratory paralysis
Pneumonia

DIAGNOSTIC STUDIES AND FINDINGS

Diagnostic Test	Findings
Bacteriologic examination of lesions using Loeffler's methylene blue stain	Positive for *C. diphtheriae*
Test for toxigenicity by inoculation of an animal with serum from patient	Necrosis at site of inoculation; animal will become ill if toxin is present in patient's serum
Hemagglutination and RIA	Positive for agglutinating antibodies
Schick skin test	0.1 ml of active diphtheria toxin and 0.1 ml of an inactive toxin (for a control) are injected at two different sites on person; read at 24 and 48 hrs; increased redness, edema, and flaking of skin at test site between two readings indicate no circulating antitoxin; this is a test for susceptibility
Differential diagnosis	Rule out acute tonsillitis, septic sore throat, infectious mononucleosis, scarlet fever, Vincent's angina, syphilis, and candidiasis

MEDICAL MANAGEMENT[3,146]

DRUG THERAPY

Immunologic agents: Diphtheria antitoxin administered IM in mild infections and IM and IV (diluted) in severe infections; dosages vary with severity of infection and number of days since disease onset:
Tonsillar: 20,000 U
Pharyngeal: 20,000-40,000 U
Tonsillar and uvular: 40,000 U
Nasopharyngeal: 60,000-100,000 U
Laryngeal: 20,000 U
Laryngeal with other: 20,000-100,000 U.

Corticosteroids: May be used to prevent or ameliorate myocarditis.

Antiinfective agents: Local application of penicillin solution plus IM antitoxin for cutaneous diphtheria.
Aqueous procaine penicillin, 600,000 to 2 million units IM daily for 10 days.
Erythromycin (Robimycin), 50 mg/kg body weight/day for 1 wk for carrier state.
Active or passive immunization for prevention and prophylaxis for case contacts (Chapter 13, inside front cover).

GENERAL MANAGEMENT

Laryngeal and tracheal suction.
Intubation.
Nasogastric feedings if pharyngeal paralysis occurs.
Positive-pressure ventilation if respiratory paralysis occurs.
Bed rest with minimal exertion for 4 to 6 wks.
IV administration of glucose and amino acids if oral feeding is impossible; otherwise, soft diet.
Strict isolation until two nasopharyngeal cultures 24 h apart are negative; for cutaneous diphtheria, contact isolation (see Chapter 13).

SURGERY

Tracheostomy.

1 ASSESS

ASSESSMENT	OBSERVATIONS
History	Inadequately immunized; exposure during past 2-5 days to diphtheria
Body temperature	Moderately elevated: 38°-39° C (100°-102° F)
Head and neck	Edema of neck and lymph nodes
Nasopharynx	Presence of edema and gray membranous patches on tonsils, pharynx, larynx, or nasal passages; difficulty in swallowing
Breathing pattern	Noisy, labored; may be sudden obstruction; neck muscle retraction; suprasternal and substernal retraction
Activity patterns	Restlessness as a sign of impaired oxygenation
Cardiovascular	Sudden slowing of pulse and beginning irregularity; pallor
Neurologic: peripheral nerves	Palatal paralysis: nasal tone to voice (tenth day) Oculomotor paralysis: strabismus (third wk) Ciliary paralysis: dilation of pupils and blurring of vision (third wk) Facial paralysis: loss of tone of cheek muscles; flattening of one side of face; inability to blow out cheeks equally (third wk) Pharyngeal paralysis: difficulty in swallowing; regurgitation of food through nose (third or fourth wk) Laryngeal paralysis: hoarseness or aphonia (third to fifth wk) Paralysis or paresis in extremities: weakness, numbness, and tingling in extremities Paralysis of diaphragm: difficulty in breathing; cyanosis (fifth or sixth wk)

2 DIAGNOSE

NURSING DIAGNOSIS	SUPPORTIVE ASSESSMENT FINDINGS
Potential for infection (patient contacts) related to presence of pathogen in mucous membrane exudate	Patient and family history of inadequate immunization Throat culture positive for *C. diphtheriae;* serology positive for agglutinating antibodies indicating infection; positive Schick skin test, indicating susceptibility
Ineffective airway clearance related to edema of membrane on pharynx and larynx	Edema of neck and lymph nodes; presence of edema and gray membranous patches on pharynx and larynx; difficulty in swallowing; hoarseness, aphonia
Ineffective breathing pattern related to respiratory muscle paralysis	Sudden noisy labored breathing; restlessness as sign of impaired oxygenation; cyanosis
Decreased cardiac output related to myocardial inflammation	Sudden slowing of pulse and beginning irregularity; pallor
Hyperthermia related to action of toxin	Chills, feels hot; fever
Impaired swallowing related to pharyngeal edema and muscle paralysis	Pain; regurgitation of food through nose; refusal to take oral fluids or food; facial paralysis

NURSING DIAGNOSIS	SUPPORTIVE ASSESSMENT FINDINGS
Impaired verbal communication related to palatal nerve paralysis	Nasal tone to voice
Sensory-perceptual alterations (visual) related to oculomotor and ciliary paralysis	Strabismus; dilation of pupils and blurring of vision
Impaired physical mobility and activity intolerance related to paralysis or paresis in extremities	Weakness, numbness, and tingling in extremities

3 PLAN

Patient goals

1. Patient will be free of infection and complications of diphtheria. Infection will not be transmitted to patient's contacts.
2. Airway will be patent, and aspiration of secretions will be avoided.
3. Patient will demonstrate a normal respiratory pattern, oxygen intake, and blood gas levels.
4. Circulation will be maintained.
5. Body temperature will be maintained within the normal range. Comfort and safety will be maintained for patient experiencing fever.
6. Adequate fluid and nutrition intake will be maintained while swallowing is impaired. Oral intake will improve during convalescence.
7. Patient will be able to communicate needs. Speech will return to normal.
8. Patient will not be confused or frightened by environmental stimuli during time of alteration in vision. Visual function will return to normal.
9. Patient will maintain function, comfort, and skin integrity while immobile. Patient will demonstrate increasing strength and movement during convalescence.

4 IMPLEMENT

NURSING DIAGNOSIS	NURSING INTERVENTIONS	RATIONALE
Potential for infection (patient contacts) related to presence of pathogen in mucous membrane exudate	Collect specimen (as described in Chapter 3).	Incorrect collection and handling of specimens may destroy the pathogen or contaminate the specimen with environmental organisms, interfering with accurate diagnosis and treatment. Improper handling can also contaminate health care workers.
	Administer antiinfective agents as prescribed. Initiate universal blood and body secretion precautions and other isolation procedures as indicated. Dispose of contaminated equipment, body fluids, and dressings as required.	Antiinfective therapy and isolation procedures should be initiated as soon as possible to prevent transmission to health care workers, other patients, and patient contacts.
	Employ strict isolation precautions until two nasopharyngeal cultures 24 h apart are negative. Utilize protective isolation procedures as indicated. Prevent patient exposure to infected visitors/staff. Limits visitors if necessary.	To limit exposure of susceptible patients to additional pathogens.

→ → →

NURSING DIAGNOSIS	NURSING INTERVENTIONS	RATIONALE
	Participate in follow-up of patient contacts.	To ensure that they are examined and treated.
	Report to local health authority.	Reporting is required by law to facilitate public health monitoring and control of outbreaks.
	Participate in community immunization programs to provide immunizations to high-risk populations.	Even distribution of immunized persons in the community decreases risk for outbreaks and epidemics of vaccine-preventable diseases.
Ineffective airway clearance related to edema of membrane on pharynx and larynx	Assess for symptoms of obstruction (e.g., neck muscle retraction, suprasternal retraction, dyspnea, and restlessness).	To intervene immediately.
	Have tracheostomy tray available; administer tracheostomy care.	To maintain patent airway.
	Elevate head of bed and change position every 2 h and prn.	To prevent pooling of secretions and to relieve pressure on diaphragm.
Ineffective breathing pattern related to respiratory muscle paralysis	Monitor respiratory rate, depth and use of accessory muscles; monitor skin color for cyanosis; monitor restlessness and breath sounds.	Airway obstruction and diaphragmatic paralysis may lead to inadequate O_2 intake.
	Administer O_2 as prescribed.	To maintain adequate circulating O_2.
	Elevate head of bed.	To reduce pressure on diaphragm.
Decreased cardiac output related to myocardial inflammation	Assess for changes in pulse (rate, rhythm, quality) and in BP. Look for sudden decrease in pulse rate and onset of irregularity and pallor.	To intervene immediately.
	Employ complete bed rest; minimize anxiety.	To decrease stress on cardiovascular system.
	Prepare to provide cardiopulmonary assistance; administer O_2 as needed.	To maintain circulating oxygen.
	Administer sedatives and analgesics, as ordered, with caution.	To avoid further depression of circulatory system.
Hyperthermia related to action of toxin	See inside back cover.	
Impaired swallowing related to pharyngeal edema and muscle paralysis	Assess intake and output and ability to swallow.	To prevent aspiration.
	Provide frequent, small feedings of soft foods and liquids as can be swallowed, administer IV fluids, as prescribed, **for patient who cannot swallow.**	To provide adequate fluids and nutrients to compensate for increased metabolic needs.

NURSING DIAGNOSIS	NURSING INTERVENTIONS	RATIONALE
	Suction oral cavity prn.	To prevent aspiration.
Impaired verbal communication related to palatal nerve paralysis	Anticipate needs of patient who is unable to communicate. Provide communication board or other communication assistance device.	To minimize anxiety and meet basic needs.
Sensory-perceptual alterations (visual) related to oculomotor and ciliary paralysis	Assess for blurring of vision or crossing of eyes (strabismus); interpret environment for patient. Protect patient as necessary.	To determine functional ability of patient; to ensure patient safety.
	Reassure patient that vision changes are temporary.	To relieve anxiety.
Impaired physical mobility and activity intolerance related to paralysis or paresis in extremities	Assess for onset of peripheral nerve paralysis.	To determine functional ability of patient.
	Maintain bed rest; turn every 2 h; position in correct body alignment.	To prevent contractures, foot drop, or decubiti.
	Employ complete bed rest for up to 6 wks; provide total hygiene and feeding.	To reduce neurologic and cardiovascular stress; to conserve patient's energy.

5　EVALUATE

PATIENT OUTCOME	DATA INDICATING THAT OUTCOME IS REACHED
Patient is free of infection and complications of diphtheria; infection is not transmitted	There is no secondary infection in nasopharynx. There is no edema, erythema, or membranous patches. Two nasopharyngeal cultures are negative. Infection has not been transmitted to others in the environment. All patient contacts are adequately immunized for diphtheria.
Airway is patent and aspiration of secretions is avoided	The patient can swallow secretions. Patient has not aspirated. Breathing is quiet.
Patient demonstrates normal respiratory pattern, oxygen intake, and blood gas levels	Breathing is unlabored, with normal rhythm. Skin, nails, lips, earlobes, and mucous membranes are warm and moist, with natural color. Patient is not restless.
Circulation is maintained	Vital signs are normal. Peripheral pulses can be felt. Skin is warm and normal colored.
Body temperature is maintained within normal range; comfort and safety are maintained	See inside back cover.

➤ ➤ ➤

PATIENT OUTCOME	DATA INDICATING THAT OUTCOME IS REACHED
Adequate fluid and nutrition intake are maintained; oral intake improves	Skin turgor is good. Secretions are thin. Urine output equals intake. Weight loss is avoided. Energy improves. Patient eats regular diet during convalescence.
Patient communicates needs and speech returns to normal	Health care workers respond to patient's nonverbal cues. During convalescence there are no signs of facial paralysis. Patient is able to speak coherently, without nasal tone to voice.
Patient is not confused or frightened by environmental stimuli; visual function returns to normal	Facial expression is calm and serene; breathing is regular; there are periods of motionlessness. There is no startle response to stimuli. During convalescence, the patient correctly identifies letters on Snellen eye chart from distance of 20 ft. Pupils are normal and reactive.
Patient maintains function, comfort, and skin integrity while immobile; patient demonstrates increasing strength and movement	Patient moves extremities and changes body position in bed. Patient is able to sit, stand, or walk during convalescence without signs of contractures, foot drop, or pain.

PATIENT TEACHING

1. Diphtheria is transmitted by direct or indirect contact with exudates from mucous membranes of infected persons. It is communicable from 2 weeks to 6 months, until organism is no longer in lesions or exudates. Onset for patient contacts is between 2 to 5 days from exposure to the infection.
2. Transmission of the infection to others can be prevented by careful handwashing and avoidance of contact with secretions and disinfection of articles with exudates.
3. Diphtheria can be prevented by active immunization (see Patient Teaching Guide on Immunizations, page 304).
4. Manage fever by taking antipyretic agents and tepid sponge baths, wearing minimal clothing, and maintaining a cool environment. Avoid chilling. Avoid giving children aspirin. Encourage intake of fluids and food as tolerated (popsicles and soft drinks may appeal to young children). (See Patient Teaching Guide on Fever, page 302).
5. Report the recurrence of any symptom to physician. Convalescence may be prolonged; this is a severe disease.
6. Contacts should be referred to a physician for early diagnosis, treatment, and prophylaxis with passive immunization.

Mumps (Parotitis)

Mumps (**parotitis**) is an acute, communicable systemic viral disease characterized by localized unilateral or bilateral edema of one or more of the salivary glands, with occasional involvement of other glands.

PATHOPHYSIOLOGY

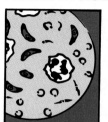

The paramyxovirus invades and multiplies in the parotid gland or the superficial epithelium of the upper respiratory passages, enters the blood, and subsequently localizes in glandular or nervous tissue. Interstitial tissue edema and infiltration with lymphocytes occur in the affected gland. Cells of the glandular ducts degenerate, producing an accumulation of necrotic debris and polymorphonuclear leukocytes in the lumina, resulting in plugging of the ducts or tubules. The parotid and testes are the glands most frequently involved, but mumps may also affect the pancreas, other salivary glands, ovaries, breast, and thyroid. Testicular atrophy follows mumps orchitis, but sterility is rare. The intensity of symptoms in mumps is variable; at least 30% of infections are asymptomatic. Elevated cerebrospinal fluid protein concentrations are common even in the absence of clinical symptoms of meningoencephalitis. Glucose levels may be depressed.

For overview of mumps, see Table 11-1, page 232.

For closeup of mumps infection, see color plate 38, page xvi.

COMPLICATIONS

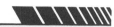

Meningoencephalitis
Pericarditis
Deafness
Male sterility (rare)
Nephritis
Arthritis

DIAGNOSTIC STUDIES AND FINDINGS

Diagnostic Test	Findings
Cell cultures from saliva, urine, CSF specimens (not ordinary procedures)	Positive for virus up to 7 days after onset of infection; in urine up to 2 wks after infection onset
Serology: complement fixation, hemagglutination, neutralization	Fourfold increase in antibody titer between acute and convalescent stages; neutralization is a more time-consuming and expensive procedure
Serum amylase determination	Elevated early in acute illness
CSF analysis	Protein: elevated; glucose: depressed

MEDICAL MANAGEMENT

DRUG THERAPY

Steroids for treatment of orchitis.
Analgesics for pain.
Active immunization for prevention (see Chapter 13, inside front cover).

GENERAL MANAGEMENT

Relief of pain with heat or cold applications.
Fluid diet until patient tolerates solid food.
Support of scrotum (small pillow or Alexander bandage).
Respiratory isolation of hospitalized patients for 9 days after onset of swelling (see Chapter 13).

1 ASSESS

ASSESSMENT	OBSERVATIONS
History	Inadequate immunization for mumps; exposure within 2-3 wks to person with mumps
Subjective symptoms	Feeling hot or chilled; headache; pain in parotid glands, testes, or other glands (tender to touch); parotid pain is aggravated by eating
Body temperature	38°-39° C (100°-103° F) for 3-4 days; higher if orchitis is present
Head and neck	Variable parotid swelling lasting up to 1 wk; severe parotid pain aggravated by eating, particularly sour substances; parotid gland (or other glands) tender to touch; hooked lobe of parotid gland (extending under earlobe) can be palpated
Testes	Swollen and tender to touch; patient has severe pain
Breasts	Inflammation and pain associated with mastitis
Abdomen	Pain from pancreatitis or oophoritis

2 DIAGNOSE

NURSING DIAGNOSIS	SUPPORTIVE ASSESSMENT FINDINGS
Potential for infection (patient) related to risk for secondary infections	Laboratory evidence of mumps
Potential for infection (patient contacts) related to virus in saliva	Inadequate immunization; exposure to mumps
Pain related to glandular edema	Severe pain in parotid glands and testes (less commonly in breasts, ovaries, and pancreas)
Hyperthermia related to infection	Feeling hot and/or chilled; headache; elevated temperature; flushed, hot skin
Impaired swallowing related to infection in parotid gland	Pain on eating and swallowing; swollen parotid gland
Anxiety related to fear of sterility	Adult male patient may express fear of sterility associated with mumps

3 PLAN

Patient goals

1. Patient will be free of infection and complications of mumps.
2. Infection will not be transmitted to patient's contacts.
3. Patient will obtain relief from pain.
4. Body temperature will be maintained within the normal range; comfort and safety will be maintained for patient experiencing fever.
5. Adequate fluid and nutrition intake will be maintained while swallowing is impaired. Oral intake will improve during convalescence.
6. Patient will demonstrate reduction in fear of disease condition and residual disability.

4 IMPLEMENT

NURSING DIAGNOSIS	NURSING INTERVENTIONS	RATIONALE
Potential for infection (patient) related to risk for secondary infection	Monitor for signs indicating complications of mumps. Refer to physician.	For early diagnosis and medical management.
Potential for infection (patient contacts) related to virus in saliva	If patient is hospitalized, employ respiratory isolation for 9 days after onset of swelling.	To prevent transmission to others (see Chapter 13).
	Ensure that patient contacts are immunized for mumps.	Adequate immunization is an effective method of prevention.
Pain related to glandular edema	Administer analgesics as prescribed.	To relieve pain.
	Give liquid or soft diet as prescribed.	To minimize pain with swallowing.
	Apply warm or cold compresses, whichever is more comfortable to patient.	To relieve pain.
	Support scrotum with small pillow or an adhesive tape bridge between the thighs (or nest of cotton for infant).	To relieve pressure on testes.
Hypothermia related to infection	See inside back cover.	
Impaired swallowing related to infection in parotid gland	Encourage liquid or soft, bland diet as prescribed. Allow patient to drink from a straw.	To minimize mouth movement, which is painful.
Anxiety related to fear of sterility	Inform patient that testicular atrophy does not result in impotence and that sterility is extremely rare.	To allay anxiety regarding effects of orchitis.

5 EVALUATE

PATIENT OUTCOME	DATA INDICATING THAT OUTCOME IS REACHED
Patient is free of infection and complications of mumps	There are no signs of glandular edema or pain. Body temperature is normal. No signs of complications.
Infection is not transmitted to patient contacts	Appropriate isolation procedures are implemented on hospitalized patients soon after infection is confirmed. Patient demonstrates behavior to prevent transmission of pathogens to others. Patient's contacts are adequately immunized for mumps.
Patient obtains relief from pain	Facial expression is calm and relaxed. Posture is normal. Muscles are relaxed when patient is resting and motionless. There is no pain in any glandular area.
Body temperature is maintained within normal range	See inside back cover.

➡ ➤ ➤

PATIENT OUTCOME	DATA INDICATING THAT OUTCOME IS ACHIEVED
Adequate fluid and nutrition intake is maintained; oral intake improves	Skin turgor is good. Elimination is adequate. Intake is adequate for needs.
Patient demonstrates reduction in fear of residual disability	Patient discusses any concerns about future sexual function.

PATIENT TEACHING

1. Mumps is transmitted by direct contact with saliva of infected persons. It is communicable from 6 days before parotid swelling to 9 days afterward. Disease onset is between 2 to 3 weeks after exposure to infection.
2. Transmission of the infection to others can be prevented by handwashing and avoiding contact with respiratory secretions.
3. Mumps can be prevented by active immunization (see Patient Teaching Guide on Immunizations, page 304).
4. Manage fever by taking antipyretics and tepid sponge baths, wearing minimal clothing, and maintaining a cool environment. Avoid chilling. Avoid giving children aspirin. Encourage intake of fluids and food as tolerated. Popsicles and soft drinks may appeal to young children. (See Patient Teaching Guide on Fever, page 302).
5. Manage other symptoms with analgesics for pain, soft, bland foods and liquid diet, scrotal support for testicular pain, and local application of warm or cold compresses.
6. Report the following complications to physician: headache, photophobia, hearing disturbance, stiff neck, joint pain, kidney pain, convulsions, or disturbance in gait.
7. Contacts should be referred to a physician for active immunization.
8. Convalescence is usually complete with no residual disability.

Pertussis (Whooping cough)

Pertussis (whooping cough) is an acute communicable bacterial infection of the mucous membranes of the tracheobronchial tree, characterized by paroxysms of repeated and violent coughing. Paroxysms are terminated by a prolonged, high-pitched inspiratory whoop and the expulsion of clear, tenacious mucus. This disease is most severe in children under 1 year of age and in persons living in poverty.

PATHOPHYSIOLOGY

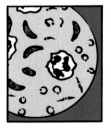

The toxigenic *Bordetella pertussis* bacillus enters the respiratory passages by airborne droplets of respiratory secretions from persons with asymptomatic infections or with clinical disease. The organism reproduces in the mucous membranes of the trachea, bronchi, and bronchioles, producing a toxin that causes necrosis to the ciliated mucosa. There are three stages of the disease: catarrhal, paroxysmal, and convalescent. A serous exudate is produced initially in the catarrhal stage, lasting 1 to 2 weeks. This is followed by a viscid mucopurulent exudate that is irritating to the mucosa. The exudate, which is difficult to expel, initiates severe spasmodic coughing (paroxysms) that may persist for 1 to 2 months. Coughing may also be initiated by toxin stimulation to the central nervous system.

Local necrosis of the tracheal and bronchial epithelium is extensive, with an associated peribronchial and interstitial inflammatory infiltrate. Unexpelled mucous plugs may produce areas of atelectasis and emphysema. Paratracheal and bronchial lymphadenopathy may be present. Edema, congestion, and hemorrhage may occur in lung tissue, and edema and petechial hemorrhages are commonly found in brain tissue. These pathologic findings result from anoxia during the prolonged paroxysms of coughing. Paroxysms may also result in epistaxis, scleral hemorrhage, periorbital edema, vomiting, exhaustion, aspiration, and aspiration pneumonia. Also, umbilical and inguinal hernias and rectal prolapse may result from increased intra-abdominal pressure during paroxysms.

The convalescent stage is characterized by a cessation of whooping and vomiting with a gradual decrease in the number of paroxysms over a 2- to 3-week period. Some patients develop exacerbations of paroxysms of cough, whooping, and vomiting during subsequent respiratory infections.

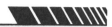

For overview of pertussis, see Table 11-1, page 232.

COMPLICATIONS

Hernia
Rectal prolapse
Scleral hemorrhage
Secondary bacterial infection (otitis media, pneumonia)
Seizures

DIAGNOSTIC STUDIES AND FINDINGS

Diagnostic Test	Findings
Direct fluorescent antibody staining of nasopharyngeal secretions during catarrhal stage	Positive for *B. pertussis*
WBC count	Leukocytes: 15,000 to 40,000/mm^3; may be as high as 175,000 to 200,000/mm^3
Differential WBC count	90% lymphocytes

MEDICAL MANAGEMENT[154]

DRUG THERAPY

Antiinfective agents: Erythromycin (Erythrocin), 35-50 mg/kg/24 h PO in 4 divided doses for 14 days. Betnesol, 0.075 mg/kg/24 h PO.

Corticosteroids: Hydrocortisone sodium succinate (Solu-Cortef), 30 mg/kg/24 h for 2 days IM; to be reduced gradually and discontinued by eighth day.
Active immunization for prevention (Chapter 13 and inside front cover).
Prophylaxis for case contacts (Chapter 13 and inside front cover).

GENERAL MANAGEMENT

Suction of respiratory secretions.
Ventilatory assistance, if needed.
Oxygen administration.
Parenteral fluid and electrolyte therapy.
Small, frequent feedings.
Postural drainage following paroxysms.
Respiratory isolation for 3 wks after onset of paroxysms or 7 days after antimicrobial therapy (Chapter 13).

1 ASSESS

ASSESSMENT	OBSERVATIONS
History	Inadequate immunization for pertussis; exposure to pertussis during past 3 wks
Respiratory	Catarrhal stage: normal respirations; dry, hacking cough Paroxysmal stage (after 1 or 2 wks): paroxysms of cough (40-50/24 hrs in severe cases) followed by high-pitched inspiratory whoop; vomiting frequently follows paroxysm Convalescent stage: paroxysms and vomiting become gradually less frequent and prolonged
Mucous membranes	Catarrhal stage: serous rhinorrhea, sneezing, lacrimation, conjunctivitis Paroxysmal stage: tenacious mucus; epistaxis
Skin	Color may be cyanotic following paroxysms; loss of turgor because of dehydration
Body temperature	Normal or low-grade fever; elevated in secondary infection
Head and neck	Venous engorgement of face and neck during paroxysms; scleral hemorrhages and periorbital edema may be present
Neurologic	Anoxic convulsions
Activity patterns	Exhaustion following paroxysms
Abdomen	Umbilical or inguinal hernia complications

2 DIAGNOSE

NURSING DIAGNOSIS	SUPPORTIVE ASSESSMENT FINDINGS
Potential for infection (patient) related to risk for secondary infection	History of inadequate immunization; examination of nasopharyngeal secretions positive for *B. pertussis;* laboratory evidence of leukocytosis and lymphocytosis; fever; serous rhinorrhea, sneezing, lacrimation, conjunctivitis
Potential for infection (patient contacts) related to pathogen in respiratory secretions	Same as above
Ineffective airway clearance related to tenacity of mucus	Tenacious mucus; vomiting follows paroxysms
Ineffective breathing pattern related to coughing spasms	Extended paroxysms of coughing; cyanosis and exhaustion following paroxysms; anoxic convulsions
Potential fluid volume deficit related to severe vomiting and inability to swallow	Loss of skin turgor; vomiting; exhaustion
Activity intolerance related to coughing spasms and decreased O_2	Exhaustion following paroxysms

NURSING DIAGNOSIS	SUPPORTIVE ASSESSMENT FINDINGS
Potential for injury related to coughing spasms	Umbilical or inguinal herniation; convulsions; venous engorgement of face and neck during paroxysms; scleral hemorrhages and periorbital edema may be present
Hyperthermia related to infection	Normal or low-grade fever; elevated in secondary infection

3 PLAN

Patient goals

1. Patient will be free of infection and complications of pertussis.
2. Infection will not be transmitted to patient's contacts.
3. Airway will be patent and aspiration of secretions will be avoided.
4. Patient will demonstrate normal respiratory pattern, oxygen intake, and blood gas levels.
5. Fluid and electrolyte balance will be maintained.
6. Patient will achieve adequate rest to conserve energy during active disease and will return to preillness level of activity during convalescence.
7. Patient will not experience injury.
8. Body temperature will be maintained within the normal range. Comfort and safety will be maintained for patients experiencing fever.

4 IMPLEMENT

NURSING DIAGNOSIS	NURSING INTERVENTIONS	RATIONALE
Potential for infection (patient) related to risk for secondary infection	Collect nasopharyngeal specimen for examination (see Chapter 3).	Incorrect collection and handling of specimens may destroy the pathogen or contaminate the specimen with environmental organisms, interfering with accurate diagnosis and treatment. Improper handling can also contaminate the health care worker.
	Administer antiinfective agents as soon as prescribed.	Early detection of infection and treatment may prevent severe disease and death.
	Monitor temperature and respiratory status.	To detect signs of secondary infection for early treatment.
Potential for infection (patient contacts) related to pathogen in respiratory secretions	Employ respiratory isolation for 3 wks after onset of paroxysms or for 7 days after onset of antimicrobial therapy (see Chapter 13).	To prevent transmission to health care workers, other patients, and patient contacts.
	Refer patient contacts to physician.	To ensure that patient contacts are examined, treated, and/or immunized.
	Ensure that case of pertussis is reported to local health authority.	Required by law.
Ineffective airway clearance related to tenacity of mucus	Place infant on lap with infant's head down during paroxysms.	To drain secretions.
	Suction pooled secretions if necessary.	To maintain patent airway.
	Provide moist air.	To liquify secretions.

→ > >

NURSING DIAGNOSIS	NURSING INTERVENTIONS	RATIONALE
Ineffective breathing pattern related to coughing spasms	Assess patient's skin color and behavior.	To detect symptoms of anoxia.
	Provide oxygen by mask.	To restore breathing after paroxysms.
	Assist respiration if necessary.	To maintain oxygen.
	Monitor breathing for signs of atelectasis or pneumonia.	To report to physician for intervention.
Potential fluid volume deficit related to severe vomiting and inability to swallow	Assess skin turgor and urinary output	For signs of dehydration.
	Give frequent, small liquid feedings or parenteral fluids if vomiting is excessive.	To maintain adequate fluids.
Activity intolerance related to coughing spasms and decreased O_2	Provide for rest in a nonstimulating environment.	To compensate for exhaustion from paroxysms.
Potential for injury related to coughing spasms	Provide convulsion precautions (padded bed, side rails, and tongue blade).	To protect from trauma during convulsions.
	Monitor for complications from excessive coughing.	To report to physician for early intervention.
Hyperthermia related to infection	See inside back cover.	

5 EVALUATE

PATIENT OUTCOME	DATA INDICATING THAT OUTCOME IS REACHED
Patient is free of infection and complications of pertussis	Blood leukocyte count is normal. Bacterial culture is negative. Breathing patterns are normal. Body temperature is normal.
Infection is not transmitted	Patient contacts are free of infection. Children are immunized for pertussis. Infection is reported to local health department.
Airway is patent and aspiration of secretions is avoided	Patient does not aspirate secretions during paroxysms of coughing and returns to normal coughing and breathing patterns during convalescence.
Patient demonstrates normal respiratory pattern, oxygen intake, and blood gas levels	Skin, nails, lips, and earlobes are warm and moist, with natural color. Breathing pattern, rhythm, rate, and depth are regular. Oxygen saturation, carbon dioxide, P_{O_2}, and P_{CO_2} are normal.

PATIENT OUTCOME	DATA INDICATING THAT OUTCOME IS ACHIEVED
Fluid and electrolyte balance is maintained	Skin turgor is good; secretions are thin. Urine output equals intake. Urine specific gravity is normal.
Patient achieves adequate rest and returns to preillness level of activity	Patient moves and cares for self at level of development. There is no weakness or malaise. Breathing during activity is regular.
Patient does not experience injury	Patient experiences no injury associated with seizures.
Body temperature is maintained within normal range; comfort and safety are maintained	See inside back cover.

PATIENT TEACHING

1. Pertussis is transmitted by direct contact with droplets from respiratory passages. It is communicable from 7 days after exposure to 3 weeks after disease onset (highly communicable during early catarrhal stage). Disease onset is 7 to 12 days from exposure to the infection.
2. Transmission of the infection to others can be prevented by handwashing, avoidance of inhaling respiratory secretions, and disinfection of items contaminated with respiratory secretions.
3. Pertussis can be prevented by active immunization (see Patient Teaching Guide on Immunizations, page 304).
4. Manage fever by taking antipyretic agents and tepid sponge baths, wearing minimal clothing, and maintaining a cool environment. Avoid chilling. Avoid giving children aspirin. Encourage intake of fluids and food as tolerated. Popsicles and soft drinks may appeal to young children (see Patient Teaching Guide on Fever, page 302).
5. Manage other symptoms: moist air in environment, frequent liquids, soft foods, and bed rest.
6. Report the following symptoms of complications to physician: convulsions, rise in fever, or recurrence of respiratory symptoms, whooping, or vomiting.
7. Contacts should be referred to a physician for early diagnosis, treatment, and prophylaxis with a booster dose of pertussis vaccine.
8. Convalescence is slow, with gradual cessation of whooping and vomiting over a 2 to 3 week period. Subsequent respiratory infections predispose to recurrence of symptoms.

Poliomyelitis

Poliomyelitis is an acute communicable systemic viral disease affecting the central nervous system with variable severity ranging from subclinical infection, to a nonfebrile illness, to an aseptic meningitis, to paralytic disease, and possibly to death.

PATHOPHYSIOLOGY

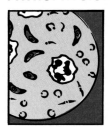

Three immunologically distinct polioviruses produce poliomyelitis, an infection that occurs 100 times more frequently in a subclinical form than in clinical disease. The polioviruses are all enteroviruses; that is, they multiply in the intestinal tract and can be recovered from the feces of cases and subclinical cases. Transmission of the virus is primarily by the fecal-oral route and sometimes by direct contact with respiratory secretions.

Once in a susceptible host, the virus multiplies in the lymphoid tissue of the throat and ileum, producing follicular necrosis. A transient viremia follows with subsequent viral invasion of the central nervous system producing cell damage primarily in the anterior horn cells of the spinal cord, in the medulla and pons, in the midbrain, and in the motor area of the precentral gyrus. Damage to the motor neurons results from destruction within the body of the cells. Damage may be reversible at this point, with complete recovery, or it may progress to necrosis and phagocytosis of the neurons resulting in clinical disease concomitant with the extent and concentration of neuron destruction.

Clinical paralysis results when there is extensive damage to motor neurons associated with any one functional motor group. Skeletal muscle fiber groups atrophy rapidly from absence of innervation from associated destroyed motor neurons. Paralysis is characteristically asymmetric, involving the lower extremities and muscles of respiration and swallowing.

Clinical poliomyelitis may be seen in three phases: a systemic stage, a phase of central nervous system involvement, and the paralytic stage. The onset of the systemic phase is acute, with low-grade fever, headache, nausea, abdominal tenderness, occasional vomiting, and the presence of a mild tonsillitis or pharyngitis. These symptoms subside within 24 to 36 hours, and the infectious process is terminated for about 80% of patients.

> For overview of poliomyelitis, see Table 11-1, page 232.

A small percentage of patients manifest signs of the second phase within 1 to 4 days, with a higher fever, frontal headache, vomiting, strained anxious expression on the face, dermal hypersensitivity, and hyperhidrosis, particularly around the head and neck. The symptoms may end here or progress to the paralytic stage, with nuchal and spinal stiffness from spasm of back and hamstring muscles, positive spinal fluid findings, hypertension, and paralysis.

Paralysis may affect different parts of the body depending on the area of central nervous system damage, giving rise to the differentiation of types of paralysis as spinal, spinobulbar, bulbar, ataxic, encephalitic, or meningitic. Complications are associated with the areas of muscle paralysis or weakness and the effect on body functioning. They include intercostal and respiratory paralysis, pharyngeal, facial, and palatal paralysis, and paralysis of eye muscles and of the urinary bladder.

COMPLICATIONS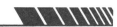

Motor paralysis

DIAGNOSTIC STUDIES AND FINDINGS

Diagnostic Test	Findings
Culture of feces	Positive for poliovirus 2 days after exposure to 5 days after exposure
Culture of nasopharyngeal secretions	Positive for poliovirus 2 days after exposure to 7 days after disease onset
Neutralization and complement fixation tests	Increase in IgA antibody titer 7 days to 4 months after exposure; antibodies persist for a few years
CSF	Protein: 80-200 mg/dl
Differential diagnosis	Rule out aseptic meningitis, suppurative meningitis, toxic neuronitis, brain trauma, encephalitis, diphtheria, leptospirosis, lymphocytic choriomeningitis, infectious mononucleosis

MEDICAL MANAGEMENT

DRUG THERAPY

Active immunization for prevention (see Chapter 13 and inside front cover).

GENERAL MANAGEMENT

Respiratory assistance.
Tracheostomy.
Suction.
Indwelling catheter for urinary bladder paralysis.
Oxygen.
IV fluids; nasogastric feeding.
Complete bed rest.
Hot, moist packs to muscles in spasm.
Passive range of motion exercises for paralytic disease.
Muscle reeducation during convalescence.
Stabilizing prosthesis may be used later in convalescence.
Enteric precautions for 7 days after disease onset (see Chapter 13).

1 ASSESS

ASSESSMENT	OBSERVATIONS
History	Inadequate immunization; contact within the past 4 wks with a person with polio or with the feces of a person who had just received oral polio vaccine
Systemic stage	
Subjective symptoms:	Headache
Body temperature	37°-38° C (99°-101° F)
Abdomen	Abdominal tenderness; nausea
Pharynx	Erythema of throat and tonsils
CNS involvement	
Body temperature	38°-39° C (100°-102° F)
Abdomen	Vomiting
Head	Strained, anxious expression; frontal headache
Skin	Hypersensitive to touch; profuse perspiration, particularly around head and neck
Neuromuscular system	Pain and stiffness in neck, back, and legs

→ > > >

ASSESSMENT	OBSERVATIONS
Paralytic stage includes all of above plus:	
Level of consciousness	Drowsiness, stupor, or restlessness
Neuromuscular concerns	Pain and spasm (neck, back, and legs); hyperactive deep tendon reflexes followed by absence of reflexes; asymmetric paralysis (variable parts of body): legs, arms, abdomen, back, face, urinary bladder, pharyngeal, and respiratory; paralysis of face may be observed by an inability to pull up the corner of the mouth when smiling, flattening on one side, or an inability to close one eye
Oropharynx	Patient may be unable to stick out tongue, or tongue may deviate to one side; palate and uvula may deviate to one side; voice may have nasal tone; liquid may be regurgitated through nose; difficulty in swallowing; aphonia may be present
Breathing patterns	Dyspnea, respiratory stridor; rib cage fixed in inspiration because of spasm of sternocleidomastoid, platysma, and trapezius muscles; movement of diaphragm and intercostal muscles may be absent
Blood pressure	May be elevated
Urinary elimination	Distended bladder; no urinary output

2 DIAGNOSE

NURSING DIAGNOSIS	SUPPORTIVE ASSESSMENT FINDINGS
Potential for infection (patient contacts) related to virus in feces and respiratory secretions	History of inadequate immunization; laboratory evidence of poliovirus infection
Ineffective breathing pattern related to paralysis of muscles of respiration	Dyspnea, respiratory stridor; cyanosis; restlessness
Ineffective airway clearance related to paralysis of facial and pharyngeal muscles	Paralysis of face and pharynx; regurgitation of liquid through nose; difficulty in swallowing; erythema of throat and tonsils; aphonia
Hyperthermia related to infection	Profuse perspiration, particularly around head and neck; body temperature: 37°-38° C (99°-101° F) early; 38°-39° C (100°-102° F) later
Impaired physical mobility and self-care deficit (all ADLs) related to motor neuron damage with paralysis	Pain and spasm (neck, back, and legs); asymmetric paralysis
Potential fluid volume deficit related to difficulty in swallowing	Difficulty swallowing; nausea and vomiting
Altered nutrition: less than body requirements related to difficulty in swallowing	Difficulty swallowing; regurgitation of food through nose; nausea and vomiting

NURSING DIAGNOSIS	SUPPORTIVE ASSESSMENT FINDINGS
Urinary retention related to paralysis	Distended bladder; no urinary output
Potential for injury related to CNS infection	Drowsiness, stupor, or restlessness
Pain related to muscle spasms	Frontal headache; pain and stiffness in neck, back, and legs; skin hypersensitive to touch; abdominal tenderness; strained, anxious expression
Impaired verbal communication related to paralysis	Facial and orpharyngeal paralysis; aphonia

3 PLAN

Patient goals

1. Patient will be free of infection and complications of polio. Infection will not be transmitted to patient's contacts.
2. Patient will demonstrate normal respiratory pattern, oxygen intake, and blood gas levels.
3. Airway will be patent and aspiration of secretions will be avoided.
4. Body temperature will be maintained within the normal range. Comfort and safety will be maintained for patients experiencing fever.
5. Patient will maintain function, comfort, and skin integrity while immobile and will demonstrate increasing strength and movement during convalescence.
6. Patient will have daily living needs met while acutely ill. Patient will return to preillness level of function.
7. Fluid and electrolyte balance will be maintained.
8. Nutrition needs will be met.
9. Urine will be eliminated and patient will resume normal voiding patterns.
10. Patient will not experience injury.
11. Patient will obtain relief from pain.
12. Patient will communicate needs. Speech will return to normal.

4 IMPLEMENT

NURSING DIAGNOSIS	NURSING INTERVENTIONS	RATIONALE
Potential for infection (patient contacts) related to virus in feces and respiratory secretions	Collect fecal and nasopharyngeal specimen for laboratory examination (see Chapter 3).	Incorrect collection and handling of specimen may destroy the pathogen or contaminate the specimen with environmental organisms, interfering with accurate diagnosis and treatment. Improper handling can also contaminate the health care worker.
	Employ enteric precautions for duration of hospitalization (Chapter 13).	To prevent the spread of fecally shed virus to others.
	Participate in follow-up of patient contacts to ensure immunization.	Adequate immunization is an effective method of prevention.
	Report to the local health authority.	Reporting is required by law to facilitate public health monitoring and control of outbreaks.
Ineffective breathing pattern related to paralysis of muscles of respiration	Monitor for dyspnea, avoidance of speech, abnormal chest movement, respiratory stridor, or cyanosis.	To provide assistance early.

> > >

NURSING DIAGNOSIS	NURSING INTERVENTIONS	RATIONALE
	Initiate ventilatory assistance with respirator or positive-pressure breathing and O_2 as prescribed.	To maintain adequate O_2 intake.
	Gradually wean from respirator, as prescribed, during convalescence.	To restore respirations to normal patterns.
Ineffective airway clearance related to paralysis of facial and pharyngeal muscles	Monitor for inability to swallow. Provide suctioning or tracheostomy care as prescribed. Feed with nasogastric tube if swallowing is impaired.	To prevent aspiration of secretions, food, or fluids.
Hyperthermia related to infection	See inside back cover.	
Impaired physical mobility related to motor neuron damage with paralysis	Position (on a firm mattress with a footboard, no pillow) in a dorsal or prone position with extremities extended.	To maintain perfect alignment to prevent muscle contractures and foot drop.
	Turn every 2 h.	To prevent pooling of secretions and pressure on skin.
	Perform range of motion exercises tid.	To prevent contractures.
Self-care deficit (all ADLs) related to paralysis	Feed patient, starting with fluids and increasing toward normal diet as tolerated. Provide frequent oral hygiene for comfort. Bathe patient daily during convalescence; omit bathing during acute stage (to minimize stimuli). Help with bowel and bladder elimination.	To provide all ADLs patient cannot perform for self.
	Refer for home nursing care if needed at time of hospital discharge.	To provide care that patient cannot.
Potential fluid volume deficit and altered nutrition: less than body requirements related to difficulty swallowing	Monitor intake, output, urine specific gravity, skin turgor, patient's weight, and serum electrolytes.	To detect and report signs of deficits.
	Encourage frequent small feedings; administer IV and nasogastric tube feedings for patient who can't swallow.	To provide fluids and nutrients.
Urinary retention related to paralysis	Monitor for distended bladder. Insert indwelling catheter if necessary.	To empty bladder.
	Intermittent catheterization (q 4 h) is preferred.	Less risk for infection.
	Provide bladder retraining during convalescence.	To increase bladder capacity.
Potential for injury related to CNS infection	Monitor mental status.	To detect alteration in consciousness.
	Supervise closely; keep bed rails up.	To protect stuporous or confused patient.

NURSING DIAGNOSIS	NURSING INTERVENTIONS	RATIONALE
Pain related to muscle spasms	Employ complete bed rest in a quiet, non-stimulating environment.	To minimize stress on the already compromised system.
	Handle and move patient as little as possible; support body parts completely when moving patient.	To prevent pain.
	Apply hot, moist packs to muscles.	To relax muscles in spasm.
Impaired verbal communication related to paralysis	Anticipate patient's needs. Observe and encourage nonverbal communication.	To relieve anxiety and attend to patient's needs.

5 EVALUATE

PATIENT OUTCOME	DATA INDICATING THAT OUTCOME IS REACHED
Patient is free of infection and complications of polio	Fecal and nasopharyngeal cultures are negative. Body temperature is normal.
Infection is not transmitted to patient's contacts	Appropriate isolation procedures are implemented on hospitalized patients soon after infection is confirmed.
	Reportable infections are reported to the local health department.
	Patient care staff remain free of signs of infection.
Patient demonstrates normal respiratory pattern, O_2 intake, and blood gas levels	Breathing pattern, rhythm, and depth are regular. Respiratory rate is normal. O_2 saturation and CO_2 levels are normal. Patient breathes without assistance. Skin, nails, lips, earlobes, and mucous membranes are warm, moist, with natural color. Patient is not restless.
Airway is patent and aspiration of secretions is avoided	Patient can swallow and cough secretions. Breathing is quiet.
Body temperature is maintained within normal range	See inside back cover.
Patient maintains function, comfort, and skin integrity and demonstrates increasing strength and movement	Patient participates in muscle-building physical therapy. Mobility is adequate. Patient ambulates independently with mechanical devices if needed. Arms, legs, feet, and spine are in good alignment. There are no contractures. There are no decubiti.
Patient has daily living needs met and returns to preillness function	Patient is fed, bathed, toileted, dressed, turned, and provided oral hygiene while ill. Patient resumes all ADLs after acute illness, or arrangements are made for home help if needed.

→ → →

PATIENT OUTCOME	DATA INDICATING THAT OUTCOME IS REACHED
Fluid and electrolyte balance is maintained	Skin turgor is good; skin and mucous membranes are moist. Urine output and specific gravity are normal. Serum electrolyte levels are normal.
Nutrition needs are met	Weight is maintained at preillness level. Energy levels improve during convalescence.
Urine is eliminated and patient resumes normal voiding patterns	Urine output is normal. Patient empties bladder completely on own during convalescence.
Patient does not experience injury	Patient is monitored completely; does not fall or sustain injury.
Patient obtains relief from pain	Facial expression is calm and relaxed; posture is normal; muscles are relaxed when patient is resting and motionless.
Patient communicates needs; speech returns to normal	Health care providers are able to anticipate patient's needs while ill; patient communicates nonverbally; speaks intelligibly following illness.

PATIENT TEACHING

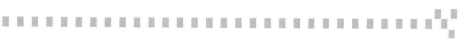

1. Poliomyelitis is transmitted by direct and indirect contact with throat secretions and feces. It is communicable from onset of respiratory symptoms, for 1 week by respiratory contact and for 6 weeks by fecal-oral contact. Disease onset is 3 to 35 days from exposure to the infection.
2. Transmission of the infection to others can be prevented by handwashing and disinfection of articles contaminated with feces and respiratory secretions.
3. Poliomyelitis can be prevented by active immunization (see Patient Teaching Guide on Immunizations, page 304).
4. Manage fever by taking antipyretic agents and tepid sponge baths, wearing minimal clothing, and maintaining a cool environment. Avoid chilling. Avoid giving children aspirin. Encourage intake of fluids and food as tolerated. Popsicles and soft drinks may appeal to young children. (See Patient Teaching Guide on Fever, page 302).
5. Report the following symptoms of complications to the physician: high fever, severe frontal headache, vomiting, muscle spasms, neck and back stiffness, paralysis, or difficulty in swallowing or breathing.
6. Contacts should be referred to a physician for early detection and treatment. Active immunization may be too late if exposure has already occurred.
7. Convalescence may be prolonged and will depend on the amount of physical function that person has. Refer patient and/or family for home care and physical and occupational therapy if necessary.

Rubella (German measles)

Rubella (German measles) is a mild, febrile, highly communicable viral disease characterized by a diffuse punctate macular rash. Symptoms in the prodromal period include low-grade fever, coryza, malaise, headache, lymphadenopathy, and conjunctivitis. Infection during the first trimester of pregnancy may lead to infection in the fetus and may produce a variety of congenital anomalies: the congenital rubella syndrome.

PATHOPHYSIOLOGY

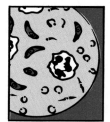

Rubella is a usually mild disease caused by a specific virus that invades and is present in nasopharyngeal secretions, blood, urine, and feces. The virus is transmitted primarily through contact with nasopharyngeal secretions of persons with clinical and subclinical infections 7 days before to 5 days after the appearance of the rash. The virus may also be transmitted transplacentally, producing active infection in the fetus. This may result in death to the fetus or congenital damage (congenital rubella syndrome). Infants born with congenital rubella syndrome generally have the virus in their nasopharyngeal secretions, stools, and urine for up to 1 year after birth, indicating the presence of a chronic infection.

In acquired rubella the virus invades the lymph glands from the nasopharynx, producing a lymphadenopathy. It subsequently enters the blood, stimulating an immune response that is responsible for the development of the rash. Once the rash appears, the virus can no longer be found in the blood, and prodromal symptoms of a viremia subside. There may be a temporary leukopenia during acute infection. The disease is generally mild, particularly in children. Complications are rare. They include a transitory arthritis, an extremely rare encephalitis, and hemorrhagic manifestations that subside in 2 weeks. In the latter case there is a decrease in blood platelets and an increase in clotting time.

Congenital rubella syndrome is a much more serious manifestation, affecting about 25% of infants born to mothers who were infected with rubella virus during their first trimester. Infection later in the pregnancy carries a lesser risk for congenital damage. The syndrome is characterized by a variety of permanent or transitory defects including cataracts, microphthalmia, microcephaly, mental retardation, deafness, patent ductus arteriosus, arterial or ventral septal defects, congenital glaucoma, retinopathy, purpura, hepatosplenomegaly, neonatal jaundice, and bone defects. There is a high risk for death during the first 6 months, generally from congenital heart disease and sepsis.

For closeup of rubella rash, see color plates 39-40, page xvi.

For overview of rubella, see Table 11-1, page 232.

The pathologic mechanisms producing the syndrome are not clear, but they appear to be the direct result of viral invasion and infection of developing tissue of the placenta and embryo. One hypothesis is that persistent infection with the virus may lead to mitotic arrest of cells, causing retardation in organ growth. Maternal infection may also result in placental and fetal vasculitis resulting in retarded growth of the fetus. Also, chromosomal breakage has been found in cultured cells from children with congenital rubella syndrome.

COMPLICATIONS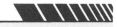

Transitory arthritis
Encephalitis
Hemorrhagic manifestations
Congenital rubella syndrome

DIAGNOSTIC STUDIES AND FINDINGS

Diagnostic Test	Findings
Culture of pharyngeal secretions (also blood, urine, or stool)	Positive for rubella virus in pharyngeal secretions 7 days before rash in post-natal rubella Virus present up to 1 yr following birth in congenital rubella syndrome; decreasing with age
Acquired rubella: serology	
Hemagglutination inhibition (HI)	Fourfold increase in antibody titer between acute and convalescent stages; hemagglutination antibodies develop quickly and are long lasting; used to determine immunity
Complement fixation (CF)	Complement fixation antibodies develop slowly; can be detected within 2 wks of onset Titers of 1:8 to 1:64 indicate recent infection
Solid-phase radioimmunoassay (SPRIA)	Increase in IgG and IgM antibodies; increase in short-lasting IgM indicates recent infection
Congenital rubella: serology	
Hemagglutination inhibition (HI) Complement fixation (CF)	Increase in IgM antibodies from birth to 5 months is diagnostic Passively acquired maternal IgG antibodies will decrease after 1 month in infant's serum Increase in IgG within 6 months-1 year indicates active immune response in infant

MEDICAL MANAGEMENT

DRUG THERAPY—ACQUIRED RUBELLA

Antipyretics for temperature control.
Antibiotic treatment of otitis media, an infrequent complication.
Active and passive immunization for prevention (Chapter 13, inside front cover).

DRUG THERAPY—CONGENITAL RUBELLA SYNDROME

Treatment of sepsis.
Treatment of congestive heart failure.

GENERAL MANAGEMENT—CONGENITAL RUBELLA SYNDROME

Rehabilitation of children who survive infancy.
Strict isolation of neonates with rubella until throat culture is free of virus (Chapter 13).

SURGERY—CONGENITAL RUBELLA SYNDROME

Correction of various anomalies.

1 ASSESS

ASSESSMENT	OBSERVATIONS
Acquired rubella	
History	Inadequate immunization for rubella; exposure to person with symptoms of rubella within the past 2-3 wks
Body temperature	37°-38° C (99°-101° F) during 1- to 5-day prodrome in adult and adolescent; subsiding after rash appears Elevated temperature with rash in children
Upper respiratory	Coryza, sore throat, cough during prodrome
Head and neck	Postauricular, postcervical, and occipital lymphadenopathy (small, shotty, and occasionally tender nodes can be palpated during prodrome and a few days after rash fades) Mild conjunctivitis and headache possible later complication
Skin	Light pink to red, discrete macular rash, rapidly becoming papular; appearing on the first day of the rash on face and trunk and by the second day on the upper and lower extremities; rash fades within 3 days Purpura is a rare complication, appearing several days to several weeks after the rash
Oral cavity	Reddish spots, pinpoint or larger, on soft palate during prodrome or on first day of rash (Forchheimer spots)
Musculoskeletal	Self-limiting polyarthritis possible complication Inflammation and pain in proximal interphalangeal and metacarpophalangeal joints of hand and knee and ankle joints (begins within 5 days of rash and persists for <2 wks)
Neurologic	Symptoms of complicating encephalitis very rare; usually during first few days after rash
Congenital rubella syndrome	A variety of defects may be present. Some are listed here:
CNS	Encephalitis; psychomotor retardation
Head and neck	Microencephaly; large anterior fontanelle
Cardiovascular	Patent ductus arteriosus; septal and aortic arch defects; pulmonary artery and valvular stenosis; myocardial necrosis
Eyes	Cataracts; retinopathy; corneal clouding; glaucoma
Ears	Deafness
Lungs	Interstitial pneumonitis
Hematopoietic	Anemia; hepatitis; thrombocytopenia
Skin	Purpura; jaundice
Abdomen	Inguinal hernia; hepatomegaly; splenomegaly
Lymphatic	Generalized lymphadenopathy
Skeletal	Metaphyseal rarefaction; growth retardation

→ >>>

2 DIAGNOSE

NURSING DIAGNOSIS	SUPPORTIVE ASSESSMENT FINDINGS
Acquired rubella	
Potential for infection (patient contacts) related to virus in pharyngeal secretions	Immunization and exposure history; culture of pharyngeal secretions (also of blood, urine, or stool) positive for rubella virus in pharyngeal secretions 7 days before rash in postnatal rubella; virus present up to 1 yr following birth in congenital rubella syndrome; decreasing with age
Hyperthermia related to infection	Body temperature is 37° to 38° C (99° to 101° F) during 1-5 day prodrome
Congenital rubella syndrome*	
Altered parenting (potential) related to congenital anomalies	Severe anomalies and/or illnesses of infant with congenital rubella syndrome

*Remainder of diagnoses depend on needs of infants and on the type of anomaly present. These will not be dealt with here.

3 PLAN

Patient goals

1. Patient is free of infection and complications of rubella. Infection is not transmitted to patient's contacts.
2. Body temperature is maintained within the normal range. Comfort and safety are maintained for patients experiencing fever.
3. Parents bond with infant with congenital rubella syndrome. They are aware of resources for support and rehabilitation and will use them if needed.

4 IMPLEMENT

NURSING DIAGNOSIS	NURSING INTERVENTIONS	RATIONALE
Potential for infection (patient contacts) related to virus in pharyngeal secretions	**For acquired rubella:** isolate child from pregnant women. Select nursing personnel who are not at risk for rubella infection to care for patient.	To prevent perinatal infections and their congenital sequelae.
	If patient is hospitalized, employ contact isolation for 5 days after rash. For congenital rubella, employ contact isolation until three throat cultures after 3 months are free of virus.	To prevent transmission of infection.
	Ensure adequate immunization of patient contacts.	Adequate immunization is an effective method of preventing rubella.
	Administer immune globulin, as indicated, for unimmunized persons exposed to rubella.	To increase their resistance to these infections.
Hyperthermia related to infection	See inside back cover.	

NURSING DIAGNOSIS	NURSING INTERVENTIONS	RATIONALE
Altered parenting (potential) related to congenital anomalies	Explain and interpret infant's disease to parents. Allow parents to express feelings of anxiety and guilt. Allow parents to have adequate contact with isolated infant and to participate in infant's care as much as possible. Support bonding. Refer parents to support group if needed. Reassure parents that defects are not hereditary.	To help provide support system for parents who are grieving.

5 EVALUATE

PATIENT OUTCOME	DATA INDICATING THAT OUTCOME IS REACHED
Patient is free of infection and complications of rubella	Temperature is 37° C (98.6° F). Joints are not inflamed or tender. There are no signs of encephalitis or purpura. Lymph nodes are not palpable. Skin is free of rash. Infection has not been transmitted. Leukocyte and platelet counts and bleeding time are normal.
Infection is not transmitted	Hospital personnel and patient contacts are free of infection. They are immunized for rubella or have received immune globulin.
Body temperature is maintained within normal range; comfort and safety are maintained	See inside back cover.
Parents bond with infant with congenital rubella syndrome. Parents are aware of resources for support and rehabilitation and will use them if needed	Parents hold and cuddle newborn; talk positively about family's future. Parents discuss their needs and infant's needs and are aware of resources for help and describe how they can use the resources.

PATIENT TEACHING

1. Rubella is transmitted by direct or indirect contact with nasopharyngeal secretions and transplacentally. It is communicable from 1 week before to 4 days after onset of rash; infants with congenital rubella may shed virus for months. Disease onset is between 14 to 23 days from exposure to the infection.
2. Transmission of the infection to others can be prevented by control of contact with respiratory secretions and handwashing.
3. Rubella can be prevented by active immunization (see Patient Teaching Guide on Immunization, page 304).
4. Manage fever by taking antipyretic agents and tepid sponge baths, wearing minimal clothing, and maintaining a cool environment. Avoid chilling. Avoid giving children aspirin. Encourage intake of fluids and food as tolerated. Popsicles and soft drinks may appeal to young children. (see Patient Teaching Guide on Fever, page 302).
5. Report the following symptoms of complications to a physician: inflammation and pain in joints; severe headache, altered consciousness; bleeding or bruising.
6. Contacts should be referred to a physician for active or passive immunization.
7. Inform women patients that pregnant women should not be given rubella vaccine and that women should avoid pregnancy for 3 months after receiving rubella vaccine.
8. Convalescence should be uneventful.

Measles (Rubeola)

Measles (rubeola) is an acute, highly communicable viral disease manifest as a prodromal fever, conjunctivitis, coryza, bronchitis, Koplik's spots on the buccal mucosa, and a characteristic red blotchy rash. The rash appears on the third to seventh day on the face, becomes generalized, lasts 4 to 7 days, and sometimes ends in a branny desquamation.

PATHOPHYSIOLOGY

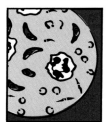

The virus of measles (rubeola) is a paramyxovirus that can be found in the blood, urine, and pharyngeal secretions of infected persons. It is transmitted directly and indirectly through contact with respiratory secretions of infected persons during the catarrhal phase of the illness (from 4 days before to 5 days after the onset of the rash). The virus invades the respiratory epithelium and multiplies there. It spreads by way of the lymph system, producing hyperplasia of lymphoid tissue. A primary viremia results and spreads the virus in leukocytes to the reticuloendothelial system. The infected reticuloendothelial cells necrose, an increased amount of virus is released, and a reinvasion of leukocytes with a secondary viremia results. With the secondary viremia the entire respiratory mucosa becomes infected, producing upper respiratory symptoms. Edema of the mucosa may predispose to secondary bacterial invasion and complications such as otitis media and pneumonia.

Within a few days after the occurrence of generalized involvement of the respiratory tract, Koplik's spots appear on the buccal mucosa and a dermal rash develops. The virus appears to invade the cells of the epidermis and oral epithelium, producing histologic changes and stimulating a cell mediated immune response manifested by the rash. The onset of the rash, following respiratory prodrome, coincides with the production of serum antibodies. Uncomplicated disease lasts 7 to 10 days. There are frequently leukopenia and lymphocytosis. Leukocytosis later in the disease occurs if there is a secondary bacterial infection.

Complications of measles involve the respiratory tract and central nervous system. Pneumonia may result from direct invasion of the virus or by secondary bacterial infection. Encephalitis resulting from direct viral invasion of the brain affects many persons subclinically. Gross evidence of edema, congestion, and petechial hemorrhages can be seen in the brain and spinal cord. Symptoms range from mild to severe. Many patients are left with neurologic sequelae. Rarely, a subacute sclerosing panencephalitis develops several years after infection.

> For an overview of measles (rubeola), see Table 11-1, page 232.

> For closeup of rash of koplik spots of measles, see color plates 41-43, page xvi.

COMPLICATIONS

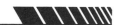

Secondary bacterial infections (otitis, pneumonia)
Viral pneumonia
Encephalitis
Delayed subacute sclerosing panencephalitis

DIAGNOSTIC STUDIES AND FINDINGS

Diagnostic Test	Findings
Tissue culture of secretions from nasopharynx, conjunctiva, and culture of blood or urine	Positive for measles virus
Hemagglutination inhibition	Detects long-lasting antibodies; therefore useful for determining immune status; fourfold increase in antibodies between acute and convalescent stages is diagnostic
Complement fixation tests	Detect short-lasting antibodies during and shortly after rash; titer as high as 1:512
Neutralization tests	Lack of antibodies indicates susceptibility

MEDICAL MANAGEMENT

DRUG THERAPY

Antiinfection therapy for secondary infections only.
Antipyretics for temperature control.
Active immunization for prevention (Chapter 13, inside front cover).
Passive immunization for high-risk contacts: immune globulin, 0.25 ml/kg to maximum of 15 ml within 6 days of exposure.

1 ASSESS

ASSESSMENT	OBSERVATIONS
History	Inadequate immunization status (see inside front cover for update on assessing immunization status of those previously immunized for measles); exposure to person with measles (rubeola) during past 8-14 days.
Subjective	Headache; feels hot or chilled.
Body temperature	Up to 40° C (104° F) during prodrome; decrease in 3-5 days (when rash appears)
Upper respiratory	Hacking cough; coryza within 24 h of fever, increasing in intensity until rash appears, gradually subsiding within 5-10 days
Eyes	Periorbital edema; conjunctivitis, subsiding with appearance of rash; photophobia
Head and neck	Lymphadenopathy
Oral cavity	Koplik's spots on buccal mucosa, most often opposite second molars; appear 2-4 days after onset of prodrome; resemble tiny grains of bluish white sand surrounded by inflammatory areola
Skin	Irregular macules appear on face and neck and in front of and behind the ears 3-4 days after onset of prodrome; rash rapidly becomes maculopapular, spreading to trunk and extremities within 24-48 hrs; at this time it begins to fade from the face; rash is brownish-pink in color and irregularly confluent; petechiae or ecchymoses may be present in severe cases; rash fades in 4-7 days, leaving a brownish desquamation; acute thrombocytopenic purpura with hemorrhage may be a complication
Neurologic	Symptoms of encephalitis, a rare complication, within 2 days-1 wk of onset of rash; secondary elevation of temperature; headaches; seizures; altered state of consciousness
Ears	Otitis media may result as a secondary infection
Abdomen	Symptoms of secondary acute appendicitis
Activity level	Severe lethargy or prostration after onset of rash may indicate a secondary bacterial infection
Breathing patterns	Dyspnea may indicate secondary bacterial infection

→ > >

2 DIAGNOSE

NURSING DIAGNOSIS	SUPPORTIVE ASSESSMENT FINDINGS
Potential for infection (patient) related to risk for secondary infection	History of inadequate immunization or of exposure to measles; laboratory evidence of infection
Potential for infection (patient contacts) related to virus in nasal secretions	Laboratory evidence of infection
Hyperthermia related to infection	Feels hot or chilled; headache; lethargy; body temperature up to 40° C (104° F) during prodrome
Sensory-perceptual alterations (visual) related to viremia	Photophobia; periorbital edema, conjunctivitis

3 PLAN

Patient goals

1. Patient will be free of infection and complications of measles. Infection will not be transmitted to patient's contacts.
2. Body temperature will be maintained within the normal range. Comfort and safety will be maintained for patients experiencing fever.
3. Patient will not be confused or frightened by environmental stimuli during time of alteration in vision. Visual function will return to normal.

4 IMPLEMENT

NURSING DIAGNOSIS	NURSING INTERVENTIONS	RATIONALE
Potential for infection (patient) related to risk for secondary infection	Collect specimen (as described in Chapter 3).	Incorrect collection and handling of specimens may destroy the pathogen or contaminate the specimen with environmental organisms, interfering with accurate diagnosis and treatment. Improper handling can also contaminate health care workers.
	Monitor systemic and local responses suggesting bacterial infection with a pathogen (elevated body temperature, localized inflammatory response, pain); report findings.	Early detection of bacterial infection and treatment with antiinfective agents may prevent dissemination of the pathogen, severe disease, and death.
	Utilize protective isolation procedures as indicated. Prevent patient exposure to infected visitors/staff. Limit visitors, if necessary.	To limit the exposure of patients to additional pathogens.

NURSING DIAGNOSIS	NURSING INTERVENTIONS	RATIONALE
Potential for infection (patient contacts) related to virus in nasal secretions	Initiate universal blood and body secretion precautions and other isolation procedures as indicated. Dispose of contaminated equipment, body fluids, and dressings as required. If patient is hospitalized, employ respiratory isolation for 4 days after onset of rash.	Isolation procedures should be initiated as soon as possible to prevent transmission to health care workers, other patients, and patient's contacts.
	Participate in follow-up of patient contacts.	To ensure that patient contacts are examined, treated, and immunized.
	Report to the local health authority.	Reporting is required by law to facilitate public health monitoring and control of outbreaks.
Hyperthermia related to infection	See inside back cover.	
Sensory-perceptual alterations (visual) related to viremia	Assess patient for photophobia. Dim lights if photophobia is present.	To prevent pain.
	Cleanse eyelids with warm water.	To remove crusts or secretions.

5 EVALUATE

PATIENT OUTCOME	DATA INDICATING THAT OUTCOME IS REACHED
Patient is free of infection and complications of measles	Vital signs are within normal limits. Cultures of body secretions, excretions, and exudates are negative for colonized pathogens. WBC count is within normal limits. There are no signs of injury associated with complications.
Infection is not transmitted to patient's contacts	Patient care staff members wash hands after providing care to each patient and follow universal blood and body secretions procedures with all patients.
	Appropriate isolation procedures are implemented on hospitalized patients soon after infection is confirmed.
	Patient or family describes transmission of pathogen, demonstrates proper procedures for handling infective materials, and demonstrates proper handwashing and other behaviors necessary to prevent transmission.
	All patient contacts are adequately immunized or examined and treated for infection.
Body temperature is maintained within normal range; comfort and safety are maintained	See inside back cover.
Patient is not confused or frightened by environmental stimuli. Visual function returns to normal	Pupils are normal and reactive. Patient is calm and rests comfortably during acute illness. There is no startle response to environmental stimuli. During convalescence the patient correctly identifies letters on a Snellen eye chart at a distance of 20 ft.

→ › ›

PATIENT TEACHING

1. Measles (rubeola) is transmitted by direct or indirect contact with nasal secretions. Virus remains viable in air for over 2 hours. It is communicable from a few days before fever to 4 days after appearance of rash.
2. Transmission of the infection to others can be prevented by avoidance of contact with respiratory secretions of infected persons.
3. Measles can be prevented by active immunization (see Patient Teaching Guide Immunizations, page 304).
4. Manage fever by taking antipyretic agents and tepid sponge baths, wearing minimal clothing, and maintaining a cool environment. Avoid chilling. Avoid giving children aspirin. Encourage intake of fluids and food as tolerated. Popsicles and soft drinks may appeal to young children. (See Patient Teaching Guide on Fever, page 302).
5. Manage other symptoms: dim lights if photophobia is present; employ bed rest.
6. Report the following symptoms of complications to physician: secondary rise in fever, ear pain, abdominal pain, nose bleeds or bruising, shortness of breath, coughing, headache, seizures, or alterations in alertness.
7. Contacts should be referred to a physician for active immunization within 72 hours of exposure or immune globulin up to 6 days after exposure.
8. Convalescence in uncomplicated disease lasts 7 to 10 days. Recovery is usually complete.
9. Note instructions for revaccination of adolescents and young adults on inside front cover.

Tetanus

Tentanus (lockjaw) is an acute neurointoxication induced by the tetanus bacillus growing anaerobically at the site of an injury. It is manifested as tonic rigidity and painful, intermittent tonic spasms of the masseter and cervical muscles and muscles of the trunk and extremities. Abdominal rigidity, a position of opisthotonus, generalized spasms induced by sensory stimuli, and a facial expression known as risus sardonicus are characteristic. Fatality is high.

PATHOPHYSIOLOGY

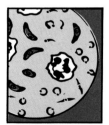

Tetanus spores enter through a trivial or extensive injury to the skin. The anaerobic organism multiplies in the wound, even after the injury has healed, producing a lethal toxin. The toxin (tetanospasmin) reaches the central nervous system by the bloodstream or by centripetal passages along peripheral motor nerves. The toxin binds with central nervous system tissue and spinal motor ganglia. There it interferes with the release of an inhibitory transmitter and induces a hyperexcitability of motor neurons, resulting in tonic rigidity and spasms of facial, cervical, masseter, respiratory, abdominal, and extremity muscles. The bound toxin cannot be neutralized by an antitoxin.

The permanency of pathologic changes in the central and peripheral nervous system in patients who recover has not been determined. Neonatal tetanus generally leaves no permanent neurologic sequelae. Central nervous system findings in fatal cases range from mild congestion to definite hemorrhage, areas of demyelination, gliosis and tissue necrosis in the cerebral hemispheres.

For overview of tetanus, see Table 11-1, page 232.

COMPLICATIONS

Pathologic changes in other parts of the body result from anoxia caused by respiratory impairment, asphyxial convulsions, toxic degeneration, and inanition. Pulmonary complications are frequent in tracheotomized patients. In striated muscles changes such as hemorrhage and rupture also occur throughout the body. The risk for further pathologic change increases with duration of the disease. Cardiac, pulmonary, and musculoskeletal complications are common.

There are no definitive diagnostic studies. The organism is rarely recovered from the site of the lesion, and there is no detectable antibody response. Clinical findings are important for differential diagnosis.

Tetanus must be differentiated from meningitis, poliomyelitis, encephalitis, rabies, strychnine poisoning, reactions to phenothiazides, tetany, peritonsillar abscess, and peritonitis.

MEDICAL MANAGEMENT[3,137]

DRUG THERAPY

Antitoxin serum therapy (two types).
Hyperimmune human tetanus immune globulin, 500-6000 UIM (1 dose), or hyperimmune equine or bovine serum, 10,000-20,000 IU IV or IM (1 dose).
Sensitivity test dose of 0.01-0.05 ml undiluted antitoxin should be administered IM and patient observed for 15-30 min for anaphylactic-type reaction before administering full dose.

Sedative-relaxant therapy: Thiopental sodium (Pentothal sodium), 0.4% IV drip; Phenobarbital (Luminal), 3-5 mg/kg body weight IM, IV, or PO q 3-6 h; Paraldehyde (Panal), 0.15 mg/kg IM q 4-6 h.

Psychotherapeutic agents: Chlorpromazine (Thorazine), 0.5 mg/kg IM or IV q 4-8 h; 100 mg IV (up to 300 mg/24 h) used for relaxant effect and emergency control of seizures in adults; 25-50 mg PO q 6 h for mild cases.

Antianxiety agents: Meprobamate (Miltown Injectable), 200-400 mg for patients >5 yr IM q 3 h.
Diazepam (Valium), 0.2 mg/kg IM or IV q 3-4 h; dosage may be increased with severity of seizures up to 9.5 mg/kg/24 h for adults.

Muscle relaxants: Methocarbamol (Robaxin), IM or IV; initial dose of 15 mg/kg; maximal dose of 50 mg/kg/24 h divided into 4-6 doses to be infused at rate of 3 mg/min.
Neuromuscular block is indicated only in severe cases when above agents are ineffective; agents used include tubocurarine chloride, demethyl tubocurarine chloride, gallamine triethiodide, and succinylcholine chloride; assistive or controlled respiration must be available.

Beta-adrenergic blockers: Propranolol (Inderal), 0.2 mg aliquots, to total of 2 mg IV for adults or 10 mg q 8 h intragastric; used for treatment of cardiovascular sympathetic overactivity syndrome.
Active or passive immunization (Chapter 13).

GENERAL MANAGEMENT

Intermittent positive-pressure breathing (IPPB).
Suction of respiratory secretions.
Control of environment to reduce stimulation.
Hyperalimentation, nasogastric feedings, or IV fluids, plus liquid feedings as patient's condition warrants.
Indwelling catheter to control urinary retention.
Physical therapy to prevent contractures and to facilitate return of muscle function and ambulation during convalescence.
Care of vertebral compression fractures.
Control of delayed allergic anaphylactic reactions to antitoxin.
Treatment of local lesions and tetanus prophylaxis in wound management to prevent tetanus.
Aseptic care of umbilical stump and circumcision wound to prevent tetanus.

SURGERY

Tracheostomy or laryngotracheal intubation as needed to aid respiration.
Surgical care of local lesion by removal of foreign bodies only (debridement or amputation of locus of infection is not indicated).

DIAGNOSTIC STUDIES AND FINDINGS

Diagnostic Test	Findings
CSF Examination	Increased spinal pressure
Hematology	Moderately elevated WBC count; slight decrease in blood platelets and prothrombin time; low prothrombin levels, impaired thrombin generation, and increased fibrinolytic activity; decreased serum iron and iron-binding capacity
Serum enzymes	Increased serum enzymes: SGOT (serum glutamic oxaloacetic transaminase), SGPT (serum glutamic pyruvate transaminase), CPK (creatinine phosphokinase), serum aldolase, alkaline phosphatase
Blood gas levels	Metabolic acidoses; hypoxemia
ECG	Sinus tachycardia and transient electrocardiograph changes
EEG	Abnormal

1 ASSESS

ASSESSMENT	OBSERVATION
History	May be history of slight to severe wound or burn to skin; inadequate immunization
Body temperature	Early: 38°-40° C (101°-104° F) or afebrile Terminal: 43°-44° C (110°-112° F)
Musculoskeletal	Early: stiff neck, tight jaw, incipient stiffness of arms and legs Later: locked jaw (trismus); spasms of facial muscles with raising of eyebrows, wrinkling of forehead, and drawing out of mouth corners (risus sardonicus) Difficulty in swallowing, rigid muscles
Neurologic	Early: restlessness, irritability Later: convulsions; paralysis of one or more cranial nerves in cephalic tetanus
Respiratory	Dyspnea; asphyxia and cyanosis result from viselike constriction of chest muscles
Cardiovascular	Dysrhythmias; tachycardia; hypertension; easy bruising or bleeding
Skin	Pain, tingling at site of injury; profuse perspiration
Urinary elimination	Urinary retention (bladder distension and absence of urine output)
Bowel elimination	Constipation (absence of bowel movement)

2 DIAGNOSE

NURSING DIAGNOSIS	SUPPORTIVE ASSESSMENT FINDINGS
Ineffective breathing pattern related to spasm of chest muscles	Hypoxemia and metabolic acidosis; dypsnea; asphyxia and cyanosis; restlessness

NURSING DIAGNOSIS	SUPPORTIVE ASSESSMENT FINDINGS
Ineffective airway clearance and impaired swallowing related to spasms of neck and facial muscles	Locked jaw (trismus); spasms of facial muscles
Decreased cardiac output related to effects of toxin and anoxia on heart muscle	Abnormal ECG, dysrhythmias, tachycardia, hypertension, cyanosis
Hyperthermia related to effect of toxin	Body temperature 101°-104° F (early) to 110°-112° F (terminal); profuse perspiration; convulsions
Potential for injury related to effects of toxin on multiple organ systems	Convulsions; abnormal clotting factors; bleeding; altered mobility (rigid muscles); tissue hypoxia (cyanosis)
Urinary retention related to motor neuron changes	Bladder distention and absence of urine output
Constipation related to motor neuron changes	Absence of bowel movement; abdominal distention
Impaired physical mobility related to muscle spasm	Stiff neck, rigid muscles; sedation used to control seizures
Potential for infection (patient) related to impaired functional state	Patient is at risk for nosocomial infections because of severity of present illness

3 PLAN

Patient goals

1. Patient will demonstrate normal respiratory pattern, oxygen intake, and blood gas levels.
2. Airway will be patent and aspiration of secretions will be avoided.
3. Adequate fluid and nutrition intake will be maintained while swallowing is impaired. Oral intake will improve during convalescence.
4. Circulation will be maintained.
5. Body temperature will be maintained within the normal range. Comfort and safety will be maintained for patients experiencing fever.
6. Patient will not be injured.
7. Urine will be eliminated and patient will resume normal voiding patterns.
8. Patient will return to normal pattern of bowel elimination.
9. Patient will maintain function, comfort, and skin integrity while immobile. Patient will demonstrate increasing strength and movement during convalescence.
10. Patient will be free of secondary infection. Patient's family will be adequately immunized for tetanus.

4 IMPLEMENT

NURSING DIAGNOSIS	NURSING INTERVENTIONS	RATIONALE
Ineffective breathing pattern related to spasm of chest muscles	Observe for signs of respiratory failure in sedated patients; provide respiratory assistance as needed.	To intervene rapidly.
	Administer O_2 as prescribed.	To maintain adequate oxygen intake when breathing is compromised.

→ › ›

NURSING DIAGNOSIS	NURSING INTERVENTIONS	RATIONALE
Ineffective airway clearance related to spasm of neck muscles	Assess for airway patency. Provide frequent aspiration of secretions and care of tracheostomy or endotracheal tube.	To maintain patent airway.
Impaired swallowing related to spasm of neck and facial muscles	Administer IV therapy as prescribed. Monitor intake and output.	To detect and provide fluids not provided orally; to replace fluids lost with fever and to ensure adequate fluids.
	Administer alimentation therapy as prescribed.	To provide nutrients not provided orally.
Decreased cardiac output related to effects of toxin and anoxia on heart muscle	Assess vital signs; monitor for symptoms of dysrhythmias.	To detect tachycardia, hypertension, or signs of heart failure.
	Administer prescribed therapy.	To improve cardiac output.
	Provide standby emergency equipment and be prepared to resuscitate and provide life support.	To provide life support.
Hyperthermia related to effect of toxin	See inside back cover.	
Potential for injury related to effect of toxin on multiple organ systems	Provide continuous supervision. Use padded side rails and headboard on bed and padded tongue blade; remove dentures.	To protect patient from injury in convulsions.
	Maintain quiet, nonstimulating environment to reduce seizures. Minimize physical handling of patient during acute stage. Take vital signs and perform any procedures while patient is in a sedated state.	To minimize convulsions precipitated by environmental stimuli.
	Monitor patient closely for anaphylactic reaction to antitoxin therapy. Also monitor for signs of internal trauma and hemorrhage.	To provide life support if necessary.
Urinary retention related to motor neuron changes	Monitor urinary output or maintain indwelling catheter.	To relieve urinary retention.
	Provide for bladder retraining.	To return to preillness pattern of elimination.
Constipation related to motor neuron changes	Administer enemas as prescribed.	To prevent patient from straining to defecate.
	Ensure adequate fluid intake.	To prevent hard stools.

NURSING DIAGNOSIS	NURSING INTERVENTIONS	RATIONALE
Impaired physical mobility related to muscle spasms	Position sedated patient in proper alignment.	To maintain proper body alignment and to prevent foot drop.
	Administer range of motion exercises, and supervise gradually increasing movement during convalescence.	To prevent contractures.
	Turn frequently during convalescence. Place on air mattress or lamb's wool.	To avoid pressure sores.
	Inspect skin.	To detect beginning pressure areas.
	Provide all ADL care for sedated patients.	
Potential for infection: (patient) related to impaired functional state	Assess vital signs.	To detect signs of secondary infection.
	Use aseptic technique for all invasive procedures.	To prevent secondary infection.
	Administer active and passive immunization as prescribed (Chapter 13).	To provide immediate antitoxin to patient and to prevent future infections.

5 EVALUATE

PATIENT OUTCOME	DATA INDICATING THAT OUTCOME IS REACHED
Patient demonstrates normal respiratory pattern, oxygen intake, and blood gas levels	Chest is expanding normally. Patient is breathing on own without mechanical assistance. There are no periods of cyanosis or labored breathing or signs of pulmonary complications, such as pneumonia. Respiratory rate is normal. Skin color is good. Blood gas levels are normal.
Airway is patent and aspiration of secretions is avoided	Cough and gag reflex are normal or tracheal tube is clear of secretions.
Adequate fluid and nutrition intake is maintained; oral intake improves	Skin turgor is good; skin and mucous membranes are moist; weight is maintained at preillness level. Urinary output is equal to input. Patient is able to eat a regular diet during convalescence.
Circulation is maintained	Heart rate is normal, without tachycardias or dysrhythmias. Blood pressure is normal.
Body temperature is maintained within normal range; comfort and safety are maintained	See inside back cover.
Patient is not injured	Fractures, hemorrhages, or anaphylaxis do not occur.

➜ ➜ ➜

PATIENT OUTCOME	DATA INDICATING THAT OUTCOME IS REACHED
Urine is eliminated and patient resumes normal voiding pattern	Urine output equals fluid intake. Patient is able to empty bladder completely without assistance.
Patient returns to normal pattern of bowel elimination	Stools are soft. Abdomen is soft and not distended. Bowel movements occur at preillness intervals without aid of laxatives or enemas.
Patient maintains comfort, function, and skin integrity and demonstrates increasing strength and movement	Contractures and prolonged muscle weakness are not present. Mobility returns. There are no decubiti. Skin is warm and moist with good color.
Patient is free of secondary infection; patient and family are protected against tetanus for the future	Temperature is normal; no signs of pneumonia or urinary tract infection. WBC count is normal. Spinal pressure decreases to normal. There is no acidosis. Serum iron and serum enzyme levels are normal. Blood platelet count is normal. Prothrombin time is normal. Prothrombin levels are normal. Patient's family is immunized for tetanus.

PATIENT TEACHING

1. Tetanus is a severe disease with a very high fatality rate. **It is preferable to prevent this condition.**
2. Teach the public the dangers of tetanus and the advantages of initiating immunization at 2 to 3 months of age and adhering to the recommended immunization schedule (see inside front cover). (See Patient Teaching Guide: Immunization page 304.)
3. Remind adults to receive tetanus toxoid vaccine every 10 years in the absence of a wound.
4. Refer persons with skin injuries for tetanus prophylaxis (see Chapter 13).

CHAPTER 12

Nosocomial Infections

Nosocomial describes infections that are hospital acquired in contrast to community acquired. An infection classified as nosocomial is not present nor is the microorganism incubating (unless the organism was acquired during a previous hospitalization) at the time of admission to an inpatient health care facility. Symptoms of the nosocomial infection need not be present during the hospitalization but may become evident after discharge.

Any infectious disease that is transmitted directly or indirectly from person to person has the potential for becoming a nosocomial infection. Infections that develop in a hospital from microorganisms present in normal flora or from normally nonpathogenic microorganisms in the hospital environment and that invade and colonize in a susceptible patient are also considered nosocomial. Infections occurring in newborns that are acquired during birth from an infected mother are also classified as nosocomial.

A community-acquired infection is one that is present or incubating at the time of hospital admission. The known incubation period of a disease is used to determine whether an infection that becomes symptomatic during or after hospitalization is hospital or community acquired. A disease occurring in the hospital with an unknown incubation period is generally classified as nosocomial.

Extent. Reported occurrences of nosocomial infections in the United States range from 3% to 15.5% of hospital discharges, depending on the type of hospital, type of patients, and completeness of the reporting system. On the average, 5% to 7% of people who are admitted to a general hospital acquire a nosocomial infection.[135] The extent of nosocomial infections in hospital personnel is thought to be high, especially for TB and hepatitis.

Nosocomial infection studies report on body sites and the hospital services where infections occur most frequently. The National Nosocomial Infections Surveillance System reported that in 1984, 38.5% of all nosocomial infections involved the urinary tract, 16.6% involved surgical wounds, 17.8% involved the lower respiratory tract, 7.5% were primary bacteremias, 5.8% were cutaneous infections, and 13.8% were other types. Most infections (64%) were caused by a single pathogen, with *E. coli*, *Pseudomonas aeruginosa*, enterococci, and *Staphylococcus aureus* most often implicated.[20]

ETIOLOGY

Certain interacting agent, host, and environmental characteristics of hospitals contribute to the risk for nosocomial infections. A large number of individuals (patients, families, and personnel) are brought together in one small environment. Some of these individuals have community-acquired, overt or subclinical infections. Taking care of patients requires close contact with body fluids and excretions, which increases the risk of transmission of pathogens from person to person and to the hospital environment. Thus a greater variety of microorganisms of greater virulence is likely to be present in hospitals. The increase in antibiotic-resistant strains of bacteria in hospitals is an example of this phenomenon. Hospitals also contain a wide range of potential reservoirs for microorganism growth such as infusion liquids, foods, biologic materials, and equipment.

Patients, already weakened by existing disease or treatment, are susceptible to invasion and infection by normal flora microorganisms, opportunistic organisms in the environment, and pathogens. Exposure to invasive diagnostic and treatment technologies further increases opportunities for microorganism invasion. Treatments that result in immunosuppression compromise patient resistance and further increase the risk for infection.

Nosocomial infections are transmitted according to the same chain of transmission as described in Chapter 1.

CONTROL

Control of nosocomial infections, as with community-acquired infections, relies on efforts to break the chain of transmission at one or more of its links. The point of the chain most amenable to control varies with the microorganism and disease process. (See the box at right for general hospital procedures for control.)

Hospital infection control also requires systematic monitoring and complete reporting to the hospital infection control committee of *all* infections occurring in the hospital. In addition, select infections must be reported to the local health authority. These infections are identified in the tables in each disease section in this book and inside front cover.

The Joint Commission for Hospital Accreditation requires that hospitals have an effective infection-control program in order to qualify for accreditation. The program must contain the following components:

- Infection-control committee.
- Systematic surveillance of nosocomial infections.
- Employee health program.
- Isolation policies.
- In-service education on infection control for employees.
- Regular procedures for environmental sanitation.
- Microbiology laboratory.
- Implementation of accepted infection control procedures in patient care.

URINARY TRACT INFECTIONS[1,138]

The urinary system, except for the distal urethra, is normally sterile.[1,138] Endogenous or exogenous microorganisms enter the system from devices that enter it or have contact with it. Approximately 75% of nosocomial urinary tract infections have been preceded by urologic implementation, including catheterization. The organisms most frequently associated with urinary

---

CONTROL OF NOSOCOMIAL INFECTIONS

Agent

Sterilization and disinfection of inanimate reservoirs and vehicles of transmission

Reservoir

Antibiotic treatment of patients and employees
Limitation of visitors that may be infected
Policies that encourage ill employees to stay home

Portal of exit and mode of transmission

Isolation procedures and secretion and excretion precautions
Handwashing between patients by personnel
Proper handling of specimens
Environmental air control, sanitation, proper waste disposal, and proper laundry practices

Portal of entry

Protective isolation of high-risk patients
Sterile techniques
Recommended procedures that minimize organism invasion (see recommendation for each body system discussed in this chapter)

Susceptible host

Nursing procedures that minimize stasis of body fluids (i.e., coughing, turning, ambulating), that prevent compromise in body defenses (i.e., skin and mucous membrane care, hydration, nutrition), and that improve immunologic status (i.e., active and passive immunization of patients and employees)

---

tract infections are gram-negative organisms usually found in the colon, including *E. coli, Klebsiella, Proteus, Enterobacter,* group D *Streptococcus, Pseudomonas,* and *Candida.* They are frequently introduced from the hands of health personnel at the time of catheterization. Bacteriuria increases the risk for septicemia and nephritis and should be treated.

Criteria for Classification

Urinary tract infections meeting the following Centers for Disease Control (CDC) criteria are classified as nosocomial:

- Asymptomatic bacteriuria with colony counts greater than 100,000 organisms/ml urine where patient had had a previous negative culture at a time when the patient was not receiving antibiotics; or colony counts of a new organism greater than 100,000/ml even if patient had previous positive cultures of a different organism.

- Symptomatic urinary tract infection (fever, dysuria, costovertebral angle tenderness, suprapubic tenderness) with onset after admission and a prior negative urinalysis or present urinalysis with one or both of the following:

    Colony counts greater than 10,000 microorganisms/ml of midstream urine specimen.

    Pyuria greater than 10 WBCs per high-power field in an uncentrifuged specimen.

Urinary System Alterations that Increase Risk for Infection

- Obstructions: urethral strictures, calculi, tumors, blood clots.
- Trauma: injury to abdomen, ruptured bladder.
- Congenital anomalies: polycystic kidneys, exstrophy of bladder, horseshoe kidney.
- Disorders of other systems: abdominal or gynecologic surgery, rectovesicular fistula, meningomyelocele, spina bifida.
- Acute or chronic renal failure.
- Postpartum state.
- Aging changes, particularly in the female.

Procedures that Increase Risk

- Urethral catheterization.

    Indwelling (continuous): risk increases greatly after 7 days. A closed system is superior to an open system in delaying colonization of urine.
- Disconnecting a closed system increases the risk.

    Straight catheterization: less risk than with indwelling catheter. Intermittent urethral catheterization, using clean technique and performed by the patient, has less risk than indwelling catheterization.
- External (condom) catheter can cause urinary tract infections, but the risk is less than with urethral catheterization.
- Suprapubic catheterization: risk for infection may be lower than for urethral catheterization.
- Ureteral catheterization: microorganisms from urethral colonization or contaminated instruments increase the risk for urinary tract infection.
- Irrigations: irrigation equipment and solutions have great potential for contamination. Frequent disconnection of system further increases risk for infection.
- Urethral dilation: the procedure may introduce bacteria and produce tissue trauma.
- Cystometrography: same risks as those with urethral catheterization.
- Cystoscopy: septicemia may result if urine is not sterile before the procedure.

- Transurethral resection of the prostrate: bacteremia may result if urine is not sterile before the procedure.
- Operative procedures on the bladder and kidneys: microorganisms introduced at the time of the procedure or from a subsequent wound infection increase the risk for a urinary tract infection
- Urinary diversion procedures: chronic infections are common as a result of colonization of bacteria at the stomal site.

Recommendations for Prevention

1. Avoid unnecessary catheterization.
2. Use aseptic techniques for insertion of devices and for opening the drainage system.
3. Use closed indwelling catheter system in preference to an open system.
4. Decrease the duration of indwelling catheters.
5. Use external catheter for males who can empty bladder but cannot control micturition.
6. Use clean-catch midstream method of collecting urine specimens in preference to catheterization.
7. Use straight rather than indwelling catheter whenever possible.
8. Use smallest catheter possible to minimize trauma.
9. Avoid leg bags in acute care setting.
10. Obtain specimens by aspirating urine from catheter or sampling port rather than by disconnecting catheter from drainage tubing.
11. Use silicone catheters rather than latex for long-term catheterization.
12. Anchor the catheter to stabilize and reduce irritation of the urethra.
13. Maintain a continual downward flow of urine.
14. Routinely empty drainage bags, but do not change unless entire closed system is changed. The addition of disinfecting agents in the bag is still controversial.
15. Use a separate, clean measuring container for each patient.
16. Gently and regularly clean perineum. Meatal care with antimicrobial agents has not been found to be helpful and in some cases has produced infection.
17. Avoid irrigations unless obstruction is anticipated. Use continuous irrigation in a closed system in preference to intermittent irrigation in an open system.
18. Persons with chronic catheterization should receive antibiotic treatment only for clinically apparent pyelonephritis, epididymitis, or bacteremia.

SURGICAL WOUND INFECTIONS[1,74]

The intact integumentary system provides the first line of defense against the invasion of microorganisms; and any disruption in the integrity of the system increases the risk for infection. The risk is increased with the extensiveness and severity of the disruption of the skin integrity and the length of time until the disruption is repaired. Repair and healing are further influenced by host factors such as age, nutrition, and circulation status. Postoperative wound infections vary substantially by hospital, suggesting that hospital practices and surgical skill may also greatly affect the occurrence. The incubation period for surgical wound infections is 3 to 8 days after the operation, suggesting that many infections are acquired in the operating suite.

Criteria for classification. A surgical wound is classified as the site of a nosocomial infection if it drains purulent material with or without a positive culture for bacteria.

Surgical Variables that Increase Risk for Infection

- Class of operation. (The risk for infection increases from class I to class IV procedures.)

   Class I (clean wound): no break in sterile technique; no inflammation; the GI, respiratory, urinary, and genital tracts are not entered.

   Class II (clean, contaminated wound): GI, GU, or respiratory tract is entered with no spillage of contents; minor breaks in technique; operations involving the biliary tract, appendix, vagina, and oropharynx are included in this category.

   Class III (contaminated wound): acute inflammation without pus encountered; spillage from a hollow viscus occurs; trauma from a clean source.

   Class IV (dirty): pus or perforated viscus is encountered; trauma from a dirty source; organisms causing infection present before surgery.

- Duration of preoperative stay: prolonged presurgery hospitalization increases the risk for microbial colonization in or on the patient before the surgery.
- Location of the surgery: infection increases if surgery is in body areas with impaired circulation or in areas with microorganisms already present.
- Surgical technique: delayed wound closure, excess tissue trauma, improper suture tension, excess blood loss, and presence of a drain increase the risk.
- Presence of bacteria at closure: the single most common agent causing postoperative wound infections is S. aureus, which is part of the normal flora for some people and has been found in the respiratory passages of 21% of operating suite personnel. Other gram-negative bacteria, accounting for 60% of infections, are transient on the hands of hospital employees and may be transmitted after surgery as well as in the operating suite.

Alterations in the Host that Increase Risk for Infection

- Impaired immune response.
- Age (newborns and elderly individuals).
- Diabetes mellitus with accompanying degenerative blood vessel changes.
- Corticosteroids, which reduce inflammatory response.
- Chemotherapy, which decreases immune response.
- Neurologic deficits causing loss of sensation and potential tissue pressure and anoxia.
- Infection elsewhere in the host.
- Malnutrition resulting in inadequate nitrogen for tissue repair.
- Obesity.
- Presence of S. aureus on patient, particularly in the anterior nares.

Recommendations for Prevention

1. Surveillance and classification: all surgical procedures should be classified and recorded; and surveillance should be maintained on all postsurgical infections by classification. Surgeons should be apprised of their infection rates.
2. Preoperative preparation: the preoperative hospital stay should be as short as possible. Preexisting bacterial infections, excluding those for which the operation is performed, should be treated and controlled. Malnourished patients should receive oral or parenteral hyperalimentation before elective surgery. The patient should be bathed the night before elective surgery with an antiseptic soap. Hair should not be removed unless it will interfere with the procedure. If hair removal is necessary, it should be done immediately before surgery. Hair should be clipped or removed with depilatories rather than shaved. Skin preparation includes scrubbing with a detergent solution followed by application of an antiseptic solution.* The patient should be completely covered with sterile drapes.
3. Postoperative wound care: use aseptic technique in dressing changes. A drain for an infected wound should be placed in an adjacent stab

---

*Tincture of chlorhexidine, iodophors, or tincture of iodine are among the preferred antiseptic solutions.

wound and attached to a closed suction system. Dressings should be changed if wet or if patient has signs of infection. Exudate should be cultured. Personnel must wash hands before and after caring for a surgical wound.

4. Prophylactic antibiotics: parenteral antibiotic prophylaxis should be started immediately before operations that are associated with a high risk of infection. They should be discontinued promptly after the surgery.

Some Common Practices that are not Useful for Preventing Surgical Wound Infections

- Routine microbiologic sampling of operating room air and surfaces.
- Use of tacky or antiseptic mats at door entrances.

BACTEREMIA AND SEPTICEMIA[1]

Vascular System Alterations that Increase Risk for Infection

- Thrombophlebitis caused by mechanical or chemical irritation from IV cannula or infusate.
- Decreased blood volume.
- Circulatory stasis caused by immobility or pressure.
- Immunosuppression of host.
- Vascular changes associated with diabetes, collagen diseases, and other chronic diseases.

Procedures that Increase Risk for Cannula-Related Infection

- Type of cannula used for IV therapy (plastic cannulas generally associated with higher rate of infection than steel "scalp vein" cannulas).
- Method of insertion: cutdown has greater infection risk than percutaneous insertion.
- Duration over 48 to 72 hours.
- Purpose of the cannula: CVP lines are associated with high risk for infection.
- Microbial contamination of infusion fluid: rare and usually caused by gram-negative bacteria.

Recommendations for Prevention of Secondary Bacteremia

1. Prevention of original underlying infection.
2. Early recognition and treatment of underlying surgical wound, urinary tract, and pulmonary infections.

Recommendations for Prevention of Primary Bacteremias Induced by Intravenous Catheters

1. Wash hands before insertion.
2. Use sterile gloves and antiseptic hand wash for cutdowns or central lines.
3. Use upper extremity veins; lower extremity veins develop phlebitis more readily.
4. Use an antiseptic preparation before venipuncture (in declining order of preference: tincture of iodine, chlorhexidine, iodophors, 70% alcohol); avoid quaternary ammonium compounds and hexachlorophene.
5. Use plastic catheters for cannulation of central veins and steel needles for IV infusions.
6. Secure catheter and apply sterile dressing.
7. Inspect daily.
8. Insert new cannula every 48 to 72 hours.
9. Change dressing and apply antibiotic ointment every 48 hours.
10. Change IV tubing every 48 hours and after blood products or lipid emulsions.
11. Avoid irrigations or blood drawing.

LOWER RESPIRATORY TRACT INFECTIONS[1,4]

As many as 1% to 2% of hospitalized patients develop nosocomial bacterial pneumonias, with 30% of those infected persons dying even with adequate antimicrobial therapy. Certain factors contribute to the risk for pneumonia in hospitalized patients.

- The integrity of normal respiratory defense mechanisms may be disrupted, thus permitting the invasion of oropharyngeal normal flora microorganisms into the lung alveoli.
- Medical diagnostic and treatment procedures may introduce microorganisms from the oropharynx or from the equipment or solutions into the lower respiratory tract.
- Ill persons with altered respiratory clearance mechanisms are susceptible to rapid oropharyngeal colonization of pathogens from the hospital environment, equipment, or the patient's normal flora. The pathogens that frequently colonize in hospitalized patients and are most often associated with nosocomial pneumonia are *Klebsiella*, *S. aureus*, *Pseudomonas*, *E. coli*, *Enterobacter*, *S. pneumoniae*, and *H. influenzae*. Opportunistic organisms such as *Candida*, *Aspergillus*, cytomegalovirus, and *Pneumocystis carinii* cause pneumonia in immunocompromised hosts.
- Microbial invasion of lung alveoli can occur from one of three routes: aspiration from the oropharynx, inhalation of aerosolized droplets or gas containing suspended organisms, or lymphohematogenous spread.

Aspiration is probably the most frequent route in nosocomial pneumonia.

Criteria for Classification

The criteria used by the Hospital Infections Branch of the Centers for Disease Control for classifying nosocomial pneumonia are as follows:

- Purulent sputum developing 48 hours or more after admission, or increased production of purulent sputum with recrudescence of fever in a patient hospitalized with pulmonary disease; plus one of the following:
- Cough, fever, and pleuritic chest pain, or
- Infiltration seen on chest roentgenography or physical findings of infection

An infection present on admission can be classified as nosocomial if it is related to a previous hospitalization.

Host Factors that Increase the Risk for Nosocomial Pneumonia

- Airway obstruction caused by tumors, foreign bodies, edema, fluid, or chronic obstructive pulmonary disease.
- Impairment of mucociliary defenses as a result of dehydration, inhalation of chemical irritants, viral infection, or anticholinergic drugs.
- Impaired immunologic function.
- Traumatic injury to respiratory tract or surgery to abdominal or thoracic cavity.
- Altered swallowing, clearing, or coughing caused by central nervous system disorders; alcoholism; depressed levels of consciousness; dysphagia; nasogastric tubes; anesthesia, sedation, or medications that alter the cough reflex; immobilization.
- Oropharyngeal colonization of bacteria. (This increases with length of hospital stay, prolonged intubation, and preceding antibiotic therapy.)
- Smoking.

Procedures That Increase Risk for Infection

- Large-volume nebulizers: the major source of aerosolized bacteria; humidifiers do not have the same risk.
- Any device or airway that may carry bacteria from the oropharynx to the lower respiratory tract including nasogastric tubes and endotracheal tubes.
- Ventilation equipment including intermittent positive pressure machines.
- Administration of oxygen or anesthesia.
- Pulmonary function testing.
- Bronchoscopy.
- Surgical procedures, including lung biopsy and tracheostomy.

Recommendations for Prevention of Nosocomial Pneumonia Associated with Respiratory Care Equipment

1. Use sterile, adequately disinfected, or disposable breathing circuits (mouthpieces, tubing, cannulae) that come in contact with the patient.
2. Replace circuitry for patients on continuous assisted or controlled ventilation and on intermittent therapy every 24 to 48 hours. Remove fluid buildup in the tubing.
3. Use high-efficiency bacterial filters on ventilators and intermittent positive pressure machines between the machine and the patient. Use in-line filters to prevent contamination of internal parts of anesthesia machines and ventilators from patient's exhaled air.
4. Change, sterilize, or disinfect aerosol-producing equipment between patients and every 24 hours for the same patient. Do not use spinning disc nebulizers.
5. Use sterile solutions in fluid reservoirs, dispensed under aseptic conditions. Fill water reservoirs at the time needed, not in advance. Unused portions should be discarded every 24 hours at the time the reservoir is sterilized or replaced.
6. Do not add to fluid levels in nebulizers or humidifiers. If additional fluid is needed, empty reservoir and fill with sterile water.
7. Use sterile medications in single-use vials for nebulization.
8. For suctioning, use sterile catheter and sterile glove. Change suction catheter after each use. Use intermittent rather than continuous suctioning.

Recommendations for Prevention of Nosocomial Pneumonia Associated With Patient Risk Factors

High-risk surgical patients and patients with impaired chest function should receive:

1. Preoperative and postoperative therapy to treat any underlying infection.
2. Preoperative instruction to discontinue smoking.
3. Preoperative and postoperative instruction and therapy to encourage and stimulate postoperative deep breathing, coughing, movement in bed and early ambulation.
4. Postoperative interventions to remove secretions and stimulate coughing (i.e. percussion, postural drainage).
5. Postoperative pain control.

CHAPTER 13

Therapeutic Procedures

IMMUNIZATIONS

Immunization is the action of artifically stimulating an immune response in a host. Two methods are available. The first method is **active immunization,** in which an antigen in the form of a vaccine is injected. The second method is **passive immunization,** in which antibodies, produced in another host, are injected in the form of immune globulins, antitoxins, or antisera. Refer to Chapter 1 for a full discussion of antibodies.

Chapters 4, 6, 7, and 11 describe diseases for which vaccines, immune globulins, antitoxins, and antisera are available, as well as the recommendations for the use of these immunizations. The recommended schedules for routine active immunization of infants, children, and adults are presented inside the front cover, and general clinical considerations for immunization are presented here.

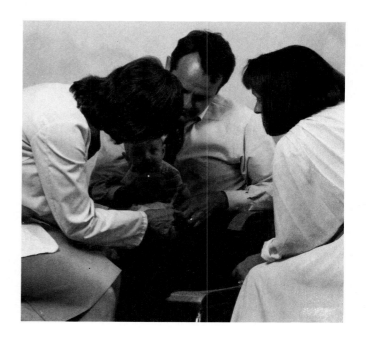

IMMUNIZATION RECOMMENDATIONS FOR HEALTH CARE WORKERS

Hepatitis B	Rubella	Diphtheria
Measles	Poliomyelitis	Influenza*
Mumps	Tetanus	Pneumococcal disease*

*For those with chronic diseases and/or other personal risks

Table 13-1

CLINICAL CONSIDERATIONS FOR COMMONLY ADMINISTERED IMMUNIZATIONS

	Tetanus	Diphtheria	Pertussis	Measles (Rubeola)	Mumps	Rubella
Vaccine	Toxoid (detoxified toxin)	Toxoid (detoxified toxin)	Killed vaccine	Live attenuated virus Single dose	Live attenuated virus Single dose Give combined as MMR	Live attenuated virus Single dose
Recommendations	Ideally begin at 2-3 mo		Do not give pertussis after 7 yr	Must be given on or after 15 mo; earlier during epidemics	All persons over 12 mo with no history of mumps (includes adults)	All persons over 12 mo with no evidence of immunity (includes adults)
Major adverse reactions	Rare: neurologic reactions including neuritis and transverse myelitis		Convulsions; loss of consciousness	Rare: central nervous system reactions (encephalitis)	Rare: encephalomyelitis	In older children and adults, transient arthralgias and arthritis 2 wks after immunization
Less severe reactions	Fever within 24-48 h; soreness, swelling, and redness at injection site; lump may persist for weeks but gradually disappears; may also have urticaria and malaise		Thrombocytopenia	Anorexia, malaise, rash, and fever within 7-10 days	Brief, mild fever	Mild rash lasting 1 or 2 days after immunization
Passive immunization	Immune globulin following injury for those without active immunization	Antitoxin for unimmunized contacts with an active case	Hyperimmune pertussis globulin for active cases	When active immunization is contraindicated in exposed person, give immune globulin	Not recommended	Not recommended

Data from CDC.[16,18,25,33,35,39,47]

RECOMMENDATIONS FOR ROUTINE IMMUNIZATIONS OF HIV-INFECTED CHILDREN

	HIV Infection	
Vaccine	Asymptomatic	Symptomatic
DTP	Yes	Yes
OPV	No	No
IPV*	Yes	Yes
MMR	Yes	Yes
HbCV	Yes	Yes
Pneumococcal	No	Yes
Influenza	No	Yes

*Inactivated Polio Vaccine
Data from CDC[29]

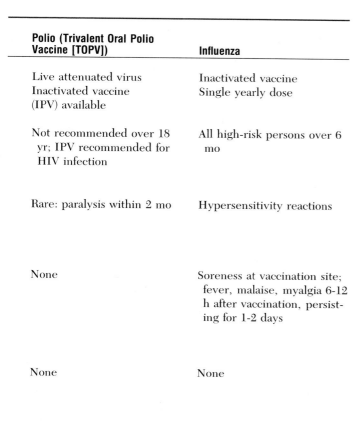

Polio (Trivalent Oral Polio Vaccine [TOPV])	Influenza
Live attenuated virus Inactivated vaccine (IPV) available	Inactivated vaccine Single yearly dose
Not recommended over 18 yr; IPV recommended for HIV infection	All high-risk persons over 6 mo
Rare: paralysis within 2 mo	Hypersensitivity reactions
None	Soreness at vaccination site; fever, malaise, myalgia 6-12 h after vaccination, persisting for 1-2 days
None	None

CLINICAL CONSIDERATIONS FOR ACTIVE AND PASSIVE IMMUNIZATION

Active immunization

Vaccines used for active immunization are prepared from bacteria or viruses, or their derivatives, that have been modified to stimulate antibody production without causing disease. Modification is accomplished by inactivation or killing of the organism or by alteration of the organism so it retains its antigenicity while losing its virulence (attenuated).

Inactivated vaccines must be given in multiple first doses to stimulate an adequate antibody response, and a periodic booster must be given to maintain serum antibody levels. Attenuated vaccines stimulate lifetime antibody levels with one administration.

Routine immunizations are given according to a schedule that facilitates administration at a time earliest in life when the vaccine will be effective. The health care provider administering the immunization should fully inform the patient or parent of the reason for the immunization, the schedule, side effects that may occur, and actions to take in the event of side effects. Informed consent must be obtained (Table 13-1).

Passive immunization

Active immunization is preferred to passive in most situations. Passive immunization with serum antitoxins prepared in animals or with human immune globulins is recommended only for those situations for which active immunization procedures have not been developed; exposure has already occurred, leaving insufficient time for active immunization; or concurrent active and passive immunization is required for immediate and future protection.

The use of human immune globulins for passive immunization is preferred to use of serum antitoxins from animals. The risk for anaphylaxis-like reactions and serum sickness is greater when prepared animal sera are used. Anaphylaxis-like reactions affect principally the cardiovascular and respiratory systems, producing dyspnea, asthma, respiratory decompensation, and possible death. These reactions occur in minutes to a few hours after administration of the serum, and they range from mild to severe. The much more common serum sickness reactions develop in 7 to 12 days after injection of the serum, producing mild to severe symptoms of fever, urticaria, or arthralgia. The severity of the symptoms depends on the type of serum and the route of administration (IV administration leads to more severe reactions). Individuals previously sensitized to the serum may react within 1 to 3 days of receiving the serum.

Multiple dose vaccines

Some vaccines must be administered in more than one dose for full protection. If the intervals between doses are longer than recommended, there is usually not a reduction in final antibody levels. It is therefore unnecessary to restart an interrupted series or to add extra doses.

Simultaneous administration of certain vaccines

Most of the widely used vaccines can be safely and effectively administered simultaneously. Inactivated vaccines can be administered simultaneously at different sites unless the person is known to have experienced past side effects to one or more of the vaccines. In that case the vaccines should be administered on separate occasions. An inactivated vaccine and a live attenuated virus vaccine can be administered simultaneously at different sites.

Hypersensitivity to vaccine components

Vaccine antigens produced in systems or with substrates that contain allergenic substances may cause hypersensitivity reactions and possible anaphylaxis. Antigens grown in eggs of chickens or ducks should not be given to anyone with a history (or questionable history) of allergy to eggs. Influenza vaccine antigens, although produced from viruses grown in eggs, are highly purified and are associated with only rare hypersensitivity reactions. Influenza vaccine should not be administered to anyone with a history of an anaphylactic reaction to eggs.

No hypersensitivity reactions have been reported from administration of live attenuated measles, mumps, or rubella (MMR) vaccine prepared from viruses grown in cell cultures.

Some vaccines that are derived from organisms grown in bacteriologic media frequently produce local or systemic reactions that are not allergenic. These vaccines—including cholera; diphtheria, pertussis, and tetanus (DPT); plague; and typhoid—should not be given to persons who have a history of serious side effects from the vaccine.

Vaccines that contain preservatives or trace amounts of antibiotics, as indicated on the package insert, should not be given to any person with a history of hypersensitivity to those substances.

Contraindications for immunization

1. Altered immunity: immunosuppressed persons should not receive live attenuated virus vaccines because of the risk for multiplication of the virus within those persons. Also, individuals living in the same household with an immunocompromised person should not be given oral polio vaccine (OPV) because vaccine viruses are excreted and may be transmitted to other persons. Inactivated vaccines, such as the influenza vaccine, are safe for HIV-infected persons.
2. Severe febrile illnesses: although the presence of mild illnesses does not preclude vaccination, immunization should be deferred for those with severe febrile illnesses.
3. Pregnancy: attenuated virus vaccines, particularly MMR, should not be given to pregnant women or women who may become pregnant within 3 months of the vaccination. OPV and yellow fever vaccines may be given if there is a high risk for acquired infection. There is no contraindication for administration of inactivated viral vaccines, bacterial vaccines, or toxoids to pregnant women. Influenza vaccine can be given safely.
4. Recent administration of immune globulin: live attenuated virus vaccines should not be administered within 3 months of passive immunization. Similarly, immunoglobulins should not be ad-

RECOMMENDATIONS FOR TETANUS PROPHYLAXIS IN WOUND MANAGEMENT

	Clean minor wounds		All other wounds	
History of tetanus immunization	Toxoid (detoxified toxin; Td)*	Tetanus immune globulin (TIG)	Toxoid (detoxified toxin Td)*	Tetanus immune globulin (TIG)
Uncertain history or < three doses	Yes	No	Yes	Yes
Three or more doses†				
Last dose within past 5 yr	No	No	No	No
Last dose 5-10 yr ago	No	No	Yes	No
Last dose over 10 yr ago	Yes	No	Yes	No

Data from Centers for Disease Control.[18]

*For children under 7 years, administer DTP (or DT if pertussis vaccine is contraindicated).

†If only three doses of fluid toxoid have been administered, a fourth dose of toxoid, preferably an absorbed toxoid, should be given.

ministered for at least 2 weeks after a vaccine has been given. These precautions reduce the risk that high serum levels of immunoglobulins would prevent the development of active acquired immunity.

5. All adverse reactions to vaccines must be reported to the local or state health authority, since the passage in 1988 of the Vaccine Adverse Event Reporting System (CDC, October 19, 1990).[55]

6. DPT or single-antigen pertussis vaccine is contraindicated if any of the following events occurred after the patient received a vaccine containing pertussis antigen:

- Allergic hypersensitivity
- Fever of 40.5° C (105° F) or higher within 48 hours
- Collapse or shocklike state within 48 hours
- Persistent, inconsolable crying lasting 3 hours or more or an unusual, high-pitched cry occurring within 48 hours
- Convulsion(s) with or without fever occurring within 3 days of receipt of pertussis vaccine
- Encephalopathy (with generalized or focal neurologic signs and/or alterations in consciousness) occurring within 7 days
- Children with a history of seizure or other neurologic disorders should be evaluated before vaccine administration

ISOLATION PROCEDURES

Isolation procedures are designed to prevent the spread of microorganisms among hospitalized patients, personnel, and visitors. Most of the infectious diseases discussed in this chapter have the potential for being transmitted to others. For infections that can be transmitted, the recommended hospital isolation category precautions are specified in each chapter with nursing interventions. These recommendations were published in 1983 by the Centers for Disease Control (CDC).[15]

The 1983 CDC guidelines provide for two isolation systems: one based on revised categories of isolation and a new system based on disease-specific isolation precautions. The disease-specific isolation system differs from the category system by specifying only the necessary precautions to interrupt the transmission of each disease. Only a single instruction card is used, on which specific precautions may be checked or written.

The category system specifies seven categories of isolation based on the major modes of transmission of infectious diseases. Each disease has been assigned to one of the categories. Precautionary procedures have been specified for each category. Color-coded, cate-

gory-specific instruction cards are available for use with this system.

Hospitals may choose one of these systems, modify one, or develop their own system. The CDC recommendations are not meant to restrict hospitals or medical and nursing personnel from requiring more stringent precautions. Nurses are advised to follow isolation procedures that are operative within their facility and to use the material presented here for reference and clarification. The isolation precautions given here may also require modification for patients who need constant care or emergency intervention.

Hospital policy usually designates the personnel responsible for placing a patient on isolation precautions and the personnel who have ultimate authority to make decisions regarding isolation precautions when conflicts arise. All personnel are responsible for complying with isolation precautions to protect themselves, co-workers, patients, and visitors.

Recent research on AIDS transmission (see Chapter 8) has led the CDC to publish recommendations for prevention of human immunodeficiency virus (HIV) transmission in health care settings. The CDC now recommends that all health personnel consistently use "universal blood and body-fluid precautions" with **all** patients because the infectious status of patients is rarely known.[24] This is particularly applicable to hepatitis, syphilis, HIV, and many other blood-borne infections. Portions of these universal precautions are reproduced in the box on page 286. Universal precautions are also summarized inside the front cover of this book. Category-specific recommendations are also reproduced in the box on page 287.

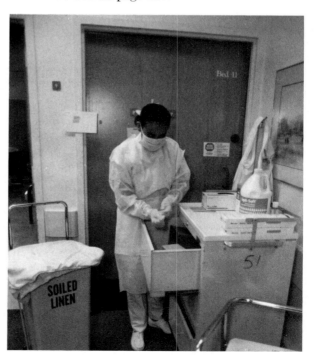

UNIVERSAL BLOOD AND BODY FLUID PRECAUTIONS

1. All health care workers should routinely use appropriate barrier precautions to prevent skin and mucous membrane exposure when contact with blood or other body fluids of any patient is anticipated. Gloves should be worn for touching blood and body fluids, mucous membranes, or nonintact skin of all patients, for handling items or surfaces soiled with blood or body fluids, and for performing venipuncture and other vascular access procedures. Gloves should be changed after contact with each patient. Masks and protective eyewear or face shields should be worn during procedures that are likely to generate droplets of blood or other body fluids to prevent exposure of mucous membranes of the mouth, nose, and eyes. Gowns or aprons should be worn during procedures that are likely to generate splashes of blood or other body fluids.

2. Hands and other skin surfaces should be washed immediately and thoroughly if contaminated with blood or other body fluids. Hands should be washed immediately after gloves are removed.

3. All health care workers should take precautions to prevent injuries caused by needles, scalpels, and other sharp instruments or devices during procedures; when cleaning used instruments; during disposal of used needles; and when handling sharp instruments after procedures. To prevent needlestick injuries, needles should not be recapped, purposely bent or broken by hand, removed from disposable syringes, or otherwise manipulated by hand. After they are used, disposable syringes and needles, scalpel blades, and other sharp items should be placed in puncture-resistant containers for disposal; the puncture-resistant containers should be located as close as practical to the use area. Large-bore reusable needles should be placed in a puncture-resistant container for transport to the reprocessing area.

4. Although saliva has not been implicated in HIV transmission, to minimize the need for emergency mouth-to-mouth resuscitation, mouthpieces, resuscitation bags, or other ventilation devices should be available for use in areas in which the need for resuscitation is predictable.

5. Health care workers who have exudative lesions or weeping dermatitis should refrain from all direct patient care and from handling patient-care equipment until the condition resolves.

6. Pregnant health care workers are not known to be at greater risk of contracting HIV infection than health care workers who are not pregnant; however, if a health care worker develops HIV infection during pregnancy, the infant is at risk of infection resulting from perinatal transmission. Because of this risk, pregnant health care workers should be especially familiar with and strictly adhere to precautions to minimize the risk of HIV transmission.

From Centers for Disease Control.[24]

Implementation of universal blood and body-fluid precautions for **all** patients eliminates the need for use of the isolation category of "Blood and Body Fluid Precautions" previously recommended by CDC for patients known or suspected to be infected with blood-borne pathogens. Isolation precautions (e.g., enteric and "AFB") should be used as necessary if associated conditions, such as infectious diarrhea or tuberculosis, are diagnosed or suspected.

Precautions for invasive procedures

In this document, an invasive procedure is defined as surgical entry into tissues, cavities, or organs or repair of major traumatic injuries in (1) an operating or delivery room, emergency department, or outpatient setting, including both physicians' and dentists' offices; (2) cardiac catheterization and angiographic procedures; (3) a vaginal or cesarean delivery or other invasive obstetric procedure during which bleeding may occur; or (4) the manipulation, cutting, or removal of any oral or perioral tissues, including tooth structure, during which bleeding occurs or the potential for bleeding exists. The universal blood and body-fluid precautions listed above, combined with the precautions listed below, should be the minimum precautions for **all** such invasive procedures.

1. All health care workers who participate in invasive procedures must routinely use appropriate barrier precautions to prevent skin and mucous membrane contact with blood and other body fluids of all patients. Gloves and surgical masks must be worn for all invasive procedures. Protective eyewear or face shields should be worn for procedures that commonly result in the generation of droplets, splashing of blood or other body fluids, or the generation of bone chips. Gowns or aprons made of materials that provide an effective barrier should be worn during invasive procedures that are likely to result in the splashing of blood or other body fluids. All health care workers who perform or assist in vaginal or cesarean deliveries should wear gloves and gowns when handling the placenta or the infant until blood and amniotic fluid have been removed from the infant's skin and should wear gloves during post delivery care of the umbilical cord.

2. If a glove is torn or a needlestick or other injury occurs, the glove should be removed and a new glove used as promptly as patient safety permits; the needle or instrument involved in the incident should also be removed from the sterile field.

CATEGORY-SPECIFIC ISOLATION SYSTEM

Strict isolation

Strict isolation is an isolation category designed to prevent transmission of highly contagious or virulent infections that may be spread by both air and contact.

Specifications for strict isolation

1. Private room is indicated; door should be kept closed. In general, patients infected with the same organism may share a room.
2. Masks are indicated for all persons entering the room.
3. Gowns are indicated for all persons entering the room.
4. Gloves are indicated for all persons entering the room.
5. Hands must be washed after touching the patient or potentially contaminated articles and before taking care of another patient.
6. Articles contaminated with infective material should be discarded or bagged and labeled before being sent for decontamination and reprocessing.

Diseases requiring strict isolation

Diphtheria, pharyngeal
Lassa fever and other viral hemorrhagic fevers, such as Marburg virus disease*
Plague, pneumonic
Smallpox*
Varicella (chickenpox)
Zoster, localized in immunocompromised patient or disseminated

Contact isolation

Contact isolation is designed to prevent transmission of highly transmissible or epidemiologically important infections (or colonization) that do not warrant Strict Isolation.

All diseases or conditions included in this category are spread primarily by close or direct contact. Thus masks, gowns and gloves are recommended for anyone in close or direct contact with any patient who has an infection (or colonization) that is included in this category. For individual diseases or conditions, however, 1 or more of these 3 barriers may not be indicated. For example, masks and gowns are not generally indicated for care of infants and young children with acute viral respiratory infections; gowns are not generally indicated for gonococcal conjunctivitis in newborns; and masks are not generally indicated for patients infected with multiply-resistant microorganisms, except those with pneumonia. Therefore some degree of "over-isolation" may occur in this category.

Specifications for contact isolation

1. Private room is indicated. In general, patients infected with the same organism may share a room. During outbreaks, infants and young children with the same respiratory clinical syndrome may share a room.
2. Masks are indicated for those who come close to patient.
3. Gowns are indicated if soiling is likely.
4. Gloves are indicated for touching infective material.
5. Hands must be washed after touching the patient or potentially contaminated articles and before taking care of another patient.
6. Articles contaminated with infective material should be discarded or bagged and labeled before being sent for decontamination and reprocessing.

Diseases or conditions requiring contact isolation

Acute respiratory infections in infants and young children, including croup, colds, bronchitis, and bronchiolitis caused by respiratory synctial virus, adenovirus, coronavirus, influenza viruses, parainfluenza viruses, and rhinovirus
Conjunctivitis, gonococcal in newborns
Diptheria, cutaneous
Endometritis, group A *Streptococcus*
Furunculosis, staphylococcal in newborns
Herpes simplex, disseminated, severe primary or neonatal
Impetigo
Influenza, in infants and young children
Multiply-resistant bacteria, infection, or colonization (any site) with any of the following:
  1. Gram-negative bacilli resistant to all aminoglycosides that are tested. (In general, such organisms should be resistant to gentamicin, tobramycin, and amikacin for these special precautions to be indicated.)
  2. *Staphylococcus aureus* resistant to methicillin (or nafcillin or oxacillin if they are used instead of methicillin for testing).
  3. *Pneumococcus* resistant to penicillin.
  4. *Haemophilus influenzae* resistant to ampicillin (beta-lactamase positive) and chloramphenicol.
  5. Other resistant bacteria may be included if they are judged by the infection control team to be of special clinical and epidemiologic significance.
Pediculosis
Pharyngitis, infectious, in infants and young children
Pneumonia, viral, in infants and young children
Pneumonia, *Staphylococcus aureus* or Group A *Streptococcus*
Rabies
Rubella, congenital and other
Scabies
Scalded skin syndrome, staphylococcal (Ritter's disease)
Skin wound or burn infection, major (draining and not covered by dressing or dressing does not adequately contain the purulent material) including those infected with *Staphylococcus aureus* or group A *Streptococcus*
Vaccinia (generalized and progressive eczema vaccinatum)

*A private room with special ventilation is indicated.
From Centers for Disease Control.[15]

Continued.

CATEGORY-SPECIFIC ISOLATION SYSTEM—cont'd

Respiratory isolation

Respiratory isolation is designed to prevent transmission of infectious diseases primarily over short distances through the air (droplet transmission). Direct and indirect contact transmission occurs with some infections in this isolation category but is infrequent.

Specifications for respiration isolation

1. Private room is indicated. In general, patients infected with the same organism may share a room.
2. Masks are indicated for those who come close to the patient.
3. Gowns are not indicated.
4. Gloves are not indicated.
5. Hands must be washed after touching the patient or potentially contaminated articles and before taking care of another patient.
6. Articles contaminated with infective material should be discarded or bagged and labeled before being sent for decontamination and reprocessing.

Diseases requiring respiratory isolation

Epiglottis, *Haemophilus influenzae*
Erythema infectiosum
Measles
Meningitis
    Haemophilus influenzae, known or suspected
    Meningococcal, known or suspected
Meningococcal pneumonia
Meningococcemia
Mumps
Pertussis (whooping cough)
Pneumonia, *Haemophilus influenzae*, in children (any age)

Tuberculosis isolation (AFB isolation)

Tuberculosis isolation (AFB isolation) is an isolation category for patients with pulmonary TB who have a positive sputum smear or a chest x-ray that strongly suggests current (active) TB. Laryngeal TB is also included in this isolation category. In general, infants and young children with pulmonary TB do not require isolation precautions because they rarely cough, and their bronchial secretions contain few AFB, compared with adults with pulmonary TB. On the instruction card, this category is called AFB (for acid-fast bacilli) Isolation to protect the patient's privacy.

Specifications for tuberculosis-isolation (AFB isolation)

1. Private room with special ventilation is indicated; door should be kept closed. In general, patients infected with the same organism may share a room.
2. Masks are indicated only if the patient is coughing and does not reliably cover mouth.
3. Gowns are indicated only if needed to prevent gross contamination of clothing.
4. Gloves are not indicated.
5. Hands must be washed after touching the patient or potentially contaminated articles and before taking care of another patient.
6. Articles are rarely involved in transmission of TB. However, articles should be thoroughly cleaned and disinfected or discarded.

Enteric precautions

Enteric precautions are designed to prevent infections that are transmitted by direct or indirect contact with feces. Hepatitis A is included in this category because it is spread through feces, although the disease is much less likely to be transmitted after the onset of jaundice. Most infections in this category primarily cause gastrointestinal symptoms, but some do not. For example, feces from patients infected with "poliovirus" and coxsackieviruses are infective, but those infections do not usually cause prominent gastrointestinal symptoms.

Specifications for enteric precautions

1. Private room is indicated if patient hygiene is poor. A patient with poor hygiene does not wash hands after touching infective material, contaminates the environment with infective material, or shares contaminated articles with other patients. In general, patients infected with the same organism may share a room.
2. Masks are not indicated.
3. Gowns are indicated if soiling is likely.
4. Gloves are indicated if touching infective material.
5. Hands must be washed after touching the patient or potentially contaminated articles and before taking care of another patient.
6. Articles contaminated with infective material should be discarded or bagged and labeled before being sent for decontamination or reprocessing.

CATEGORY-SPECIFIC ISOLATION SYSTEM—cont'd

Diseases requiring enteric precautions

Amebic dysentery

Cholera

Coxsackievirus disease

Diarrhea, acute illness with suspected infectious etiology

Echovirus disease

Encephalitis (unless known not to be caused by enteroviruses)

Enterocolitis caused by *Clostridium difficile* or *S. aureus*

Enteroviral infection

Gastroenteritis caused by

　Campylobacter species

　Cryptosporidium species

　Dientamoeba fragilis

　Escherichia coli (enterotoxic, enteropathogenic, or enteroinvasive)

　Giardia lamblia

　Salmonella species

　Shigella species

　Vibrio parahaemolyticus

　Viruses—including Norwalk agent and rotavirus

　Yersinia enterocolitica

　Unknown etiology but presumed to be an infectious agent

Hand, foot, or mouth disease

Hepatitis, viral, type A

Herpangina

Meningitis, viral (unless known not be caused by enteroviruses)

Necrotizing enterocolitis

Pleurodynia

Poliomyelitis

Tyhoid fever (*Salmonella typhi*)

Viral pericarditis, myocarditis, or meningitis (unless known not be caused by enteroviruses)

Drainage/secretion precautions

Drainage/secretion precautions are designed to prevent infections that are transmitted by direct or indirect contact with purulent material or drainage from an infected body site. This newly created isolation category includes many infections formerly included in Wound and Skin Precautions, Discharge (lesion), and Secretion (oral) Precautions, which have been discontinued. Infectious diseases included in this category are those that result in the production of infective purulent material, drainage, or secretions, unless the disease is included in another isolation category that requires more rigorous precautions. For example, minor limited skin, wound, or burn infections are included in this category, but major skin, wound, or burn infections are included in Contact Isolation.

Specifications for drainage/secretion precautions

1. Private room is not indicated.
2. Masks are not indicated.
3. Gowns are indicated if soiling is likely.
4. Gloves are indicated for touching infective material.
5. Hands must be washed after touching the patient or potentially contaminated articles and before taking care of another patient.
6. Articles contaminated with infective material should be discarded or bagged and labeled before being sent for decontamination and reprocessing.

Diseases requiring drainage/secretion precautions

The following infections are examples of those included in this category provided they are not (a) caused by multiply-resistant microorganisms, (b) major draining (and not covered by a dressing or dressing does not adequately contain the drainage) skin, wound, or burn infections, including those caused by *S. aureus* or group A *Streptococcus*, or (c) gonococcal eye infections in newborns. See Contact Isolation if the infection is one of these three.

Abscess, minor limited

Burn infection, minor limited

Conjunctivitis

Decubitus ulcer, infected, minor or limited

Skin infection, minor or limited

Wound infection, minor or limited

CHAPTER 14

Patient Teaching Guides

Patient education is important in all areas of nursing care. An understanding of a disorder and its therapy is crucial for the patient's recovery. Education of patients with infectious diseases is doubly important. For example, education must aim at protecting or restoring the individual's health, and teaching must stress the necessity for halting transmission of the infectious agent.

This dual objective poses a special challenge for nurses. The majority of infections are treated on an outpatient basis, and in some cases the patient's initial visit offers the only opportunity for teaching.

Compliance with treatment for infections is often a problem. Patients often stop therapy when their symptoms disappear, assuming they are cured before the prescribed therapy is completed. This can result in re-infection or a superinfection that is more difficult to eradicate. Some infections—most notably sexually transmitted diseases (STDs)—can be asymptomatic, only briefly symptomatic, or have a long incubation period. For patients with a poor understanding of their disease, the lack of symptoms provides little incentive for compliance.

Controlling the spread of infectious agents also relies on compliance of another sort. Without a clear understanding of the way a disease is transmitted, patients may fail to follow instructions. For example, the mistaken belief that STDs are transmitted in sperm has led some people to the risky practice of having unprotected genital contact early during intercourse and using a condom only during the ejaculatory phase.

The need to teach patients about the risk they pose to others, while maintaining a nonjudgmental attitude, can present a dilemma for nurses. The idea of an infected person being "unclean" is pervasive in most cultures. Education aimed at preventing disease transmission reinforces this view. Thus the nurse is faced with both offering the patient reassurance and emphasizing the risk the patient presents to others.

This chapter provides written materials to help reinforce patient teaching and compliance. They can be photocopied and used as handouts for patients or their caregivers. Although handouts do not replace direct teaching, they provide basic information on infections, including how patients can protect themselves and others against infection.

The handouts are designed to be used singly or in combination. For example, a patient with a confirmed diagnosis of an STD may be given 'Facts About Sexually Transmitted Diseases,' 'About Condoms,' and 'Facts abut HIV Infection and AIDS. (We strongly recommend that all sexually active patients receive the latter three handouts.)

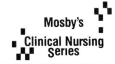

Facts About Sexually Transmitted Diseases

Gonorrhea

Neisseria gonorrhoeae is the bacterium that causes gonorrhea, or "clap." It is often symptomless, expecially in women. When symptoms do occur, they appear 2 to 14 days after exposure in men, and 7 to 12 days in women. Women may have painful urination and a vaginal discharge. Men have painful urination and a puslike discharge from the urinary opening. Rectal gonorrhea can cause anal discomfort and a rectal discharge, and the stool may be coated with pus. Infection of the throat (called **gonococcal pharyngitis**) is often symptomless, but some patients develop a sore throat. Babies born to mothers with gonorrhea, may develop an eye infection (neonatal ophthalmitis), which can cause blindness if not treated.

Complications of untreated gonorrhea can be serious. In men, painful infection or abscesses involving the testicles and sperm duct can cause sterility. Pelvic inflammatory disease (PID), or salpingitis, in women usually requires hospitalization and can also cause sterility. Occasionally, the bacteria spread through the bloodstream, causing disease elsewhere in the body.

Gonorrhea can be completely cured with antibiotics. There are several different courses of treatment, some involving only one injection of an antibiotic, some consisting of oral antibiotics for 7 days, and some requiring a combination of injections and oral drugs. If an oral antibiotic is prescribed, take it exactly as ordered, for as long as you are supposed to. Do not have sexual contact until you have finished treatment and the infection is cured. If symptoms persist after completing the medication, return to your doctor. You may require treatment with a different antibiotic.

Chlamydia and nongonococcal urethritis

These diseases are caused by a bacterium called *Chlamydia trachomatis* and can cause symptoms similar to gonorrhea. Like gonorrhea, *Chlamydia* is often symptomless in women. Men usually have burning during urination and a clear or puslike discharge. Women may have a vaginal discharge, burning on urination, and pain similar to menstrual cramps. The symptoms usu-

ally appear 5 to 10 days after exposure. Untreated infection can lead to the same serious complications as gonorrhea, including blindness in newborns.

Treatment consists of taking an oral antibiotic for 7 to 10 days. Be sure to take the antibiotic exactly as prescribed, for as long as prescribed. Do not have sexual contact until you have finished therapy and are completely cured.

Syphilis

Syphilis is caused by an organism called *Treponema pallidum.* The organism rapidly travels through the blood and invades the bones, brain, heart, and other organs. Untreated syphilis can cause serious disability. There are four stages that mark the progression of this disease: primary syphilis, secondary syphilis, latent syphilis, and tertiary (late) syphilis. Treatment at early stages will stop the progression to later stages.

A chancre, the sign of primary syphilis, usually appears within 4 weeks of exposure. The chancre starts as a small red pimple or blister that soon becomes an ulcer. It is not painful, but a clear fluid oozes from the ulcer. This fluid contains many organisms. One or more chancres can appear anywhere on the body exposed to the infection—on the penis, vulva, anus, rectum, inside the vagina, or on the lips or mouth. Even without treatment, the chancres disappear in about 4 to 6 weeks. Without treatment, however, many organisms continue their destructive path through the body.

In secondary syphilis, skin rashes appear 6 to 12 weeks after infection. The rashes may come and go on different parts of the body or they may be persistent. Swollen lymph nodes in the groin, armpit, and neck are common, as are fever and other flulike symptoms.

The latent stage begins about 1 year after exposure. Skin rashes sometimes erupt, but by the second year, all symptoms usually disappear. This stage can last a few years. In the tertiary stage (about 3 to 10 years after exposure), a type of ulceration called a **gumma** develops on the skin, bone, or internal organs. Heart, brain, and nervous system complications are common at this stage.

Untreated syphilis, even in the absence of chancres, can be transmitted sexually and to the

PATIENT TEACHING GUIDE

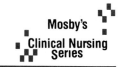

fetus. Infections can cause serious malformations and even death to the fetus.

Often a single dose of penicillin injected into a muscle will cure early syphilis. For syphilis that has been present for over 1 year, several injections are necessary. Do not have sexual contact until you have finished treatment. See your doctor in 3 months after treatment to ensure that you are cured.

Genital herpes

Genital herpes is caused by the herpes simplex virus. About 4 to 7 days after exposure, a small cluster of blisters appears on the external genitals, around the anus, or inside the vagina. The blisters, which may be very painful and itchy, form ulcers. The tissue around the ulcers is very red and inflamed. After a few days, the ulcers crust over, and by about the tenth day, they heal. Some people have swollen lymph nodes, fever, and flulike symptoms.

If you are pregnant, tell your doctor if you have ever been infected with herpes. Babies born to mothers with active herpes can be infected during passage through the birth canal. This can cause serious, life-threatening infection in newborns. For this reason, cesarean delivery may be performed.

Unfortunately, the virus stays inside the body, and herpes nearly always recurs, although subsequent attacks are milder. Treatment with an antiviral drug (acyclovir) for 7 to 10 days helps lessen the symptoms and speeds healing of the ulcers. Do not have sexual contact while the herpes is active. Tell your sex partner(s) that you have herpes because there is a chance you can transmit the virus, even between attacks.

Genital warts

Genital warts (also called **venereal warts** or **condylomata acuminata**) are caused by papilloma viruses. The warts appear 1 to 20 months (within an average of 4 months) after exposure. They begin as small, soft, moist, red or pink swellings and quickly develop into the taglike pendulum-shape typical of warts. Often they grow in clusters and have a texture similar to cauliflower. Genital warts can appear on the outer genitals (penis or vulva) and around the anus or inside the urinary opening, vagina, or rectum.

Genital warts are removed by cauterization or freezing (cryosurgery) or surgery. In some cases drugs are applied directly to the warts to kill the virus. Genital warts are not easily cured, and repeated treatments are often necessary. Do not have unprotected sex while the warts are present.

Trichomoniasis

Trichomoniasis is caused by the protozoa *Trichomonas vaginalis.* In women this STD causes a heavy greenish yellow, frothy discharge with a strong odor. Irritation and soreness in the genital area and pain on urination are common. Many women are symptomless carriers of *Trichomonas* for a long period, although symptoms can appear suddenly. Most men are symptomless but can carry and transmit the disease.

The drug metronidazole, which is taken orally in one large dose or in smaller doses for 7 days, cures the infection completely. Both the woman and her sexual partner(s) must be treated. Do not have sexual contact until treatment is completed.

Protecting yourself in the future

To protect yourself from getting an STD, you have three choices: (1) complete abstinence from sex; (2) having a totally monogamous relationship, and (3) using a condom correctly from start to finish. Abstinence is not acceptable to many people, and for this reason learn to use a condom and use one every time you have sex. There is no way to be certain if your partner is sexually active with others.

If you get an STD during pregnancy, seek treatment immediately. If you are treated for an STD, make sure that your sexual partner is treated also to avoid being reinfected.

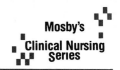
FACTS ABOUT HIV INFECTION AND AIDS

HIV infection and AIDS: the difference

AIDS (which is an abbreviation for acquired immune deficiency syndrome) is caused by the human immunodeficiency virus, or HIV. HIV weakens the body's natural defenses, making the person more susceptible to infections.

HIV infection. Most people have absolutely no symptoms for several months or even years after they are infected with HIV. Some people have a mild, temporary illness early in the infection, consisting of fatigue, fever, and swollen glands—much like mononucleosis. Later, the person has repeated bouts of viral and fungal infections, such as herpes and *Candida* (thrush or yeast infections).

AIDS. AIDS occurs when an HIV-infected person becomes seriously ill with Kaposi's sarcoma (a rare form of cancer), *Pneumocystis* pneumonia, widespread severe bacterial or fungal infections, or brain disease.

How is HIV infection diagnosed?

A positive result on both of two blood tests (ELISA and Western blot) confirms infection with HIV.

Who gets the AIDS virus?

Anyone—women, men, and children—can get the AIDS virus. It is not a "gay disease" or a "drug addict's disease." All it takes is being exposed one time!

People are at greatest risk for getting the AIDS virus if (1) they or their sexual partner have sex with homosexual males, bisexual males, intravenous (IV) drug users, male or female prostitutes, or many different people; (2) they shoot IV drugs and share "works" (e.g., needles, syringes, and cookers); (3) they have gotten other sexually transmitted diseases; or (4) they had a blood transfusion or were given blood products between 1978 and March 1985). Babies born to infected mothers can also have the AIDS virus.

How the AIDS virus is transmitted

There are only two ways of getting the AIDS virus: (1) by having direct sexual contact with someone who is already infected or (2) by getting infected blood into your bloodstream.

How can the AIDS virus get in your bloodstream? This can occur by shooting IV drugs and sharing "works" (e.g., needles, syringes, and cookers) with someone who is infected, by getting a blood transfusion or blood products that are infected with the AIDS virus, by body fluids from an infected person entering your body through a wound and by the mother's blood to the fetus during pregnancy.

You **cannot** get the AIDS virus through casual contact with an infected person. The virus is **not** spread through the air, so you can't get it if an infected person coughs or sneezes. You **can't** get the virus by shaking hands, hugging, or kissing. And you **can't** get AIDS from a toilet seat, swimming pool, or sharing food with an infected person.

Protecting yourself from sexual exposure

Next to total abstinence, the only protection against the AIDS virus is using condoms plus contraceptive foam or jelly containing nonoxynol-9. Learn to use a condom correctly, and use a condom every time. The AIDS virus can also be transmitted during oral sex, so you must use a condom for all activity that involves penetration of any part of the body. Ask for information about correct use of condoms.

If someone close to you has HIV infection

Your friend or family member needs your help now, more than any other time. Be supportive and try to keep a positive attitude. Encourage the person to seek professional counseling to help him or her cope. A good diet, plenty of sleep, and avoiding stress are important. Any risky activities that could make the HIV infection worse. If the person has a drug or alcohol problem, encourage him or her to get help to quit.

You can be physically affectionate with an HIV infected person without worrying about getting the virus yourself. Hugging, stroking each other and dry kissing (avoid deep, wet, or "French" kissing) are safe. Do not share personal items that might carry small amounts of blood—things like toothbrushes and razors.

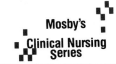

HIV Testing

What are the HIV tests?

HIV antibody tests can tell if you have HIV antibodies in your blood. HIV tests are performed on a small amount of blood drawn from a vein in the arm. Two laboratory tests are used. The blood is tested first with the ELISA test. If the results are negative—no further testing is done. If the results of the ELISA are positive, the Western blot test is performed. If this test is positive, the person is considered infected with HIV.

Who should be tested?

Anyone who believes they have been exposed to HIV or whose life style puts them at risk for exposure should be tested. HIV is passed from one person to another through sexual contact and through the blood. People are considered to be "high risk," meaning they are more likely to be infected, if (1) they have sex with homosexual males, bisexual males, intravenous (IV) drug users, male or female prostitutes, or many different partners; (2) their sexual partner has had sex with someone in this group; (3) they shoot drugs and share "works" (e.g., needles, syringes, and cookers); (4) they have gotten other diseases from having sex; (5) they had a blood transfusion or were given blood products between 1978 and March 1985. An unborn child whose mother has the AIDS virus can also be infected.

Will anyone find out about my test?

There are two procedures for HIV testing: confidential testing and anonymous testing. **Confidential testing** is like any other medical test—the results become part of your medical record. Insurance companies and employers may obtain a copy of your medical record, with the results of your HIV antibody test. Some states allow **anonymous testing,** in which the person does not give a name. Each person is assigned a code number, and you must give the code to find out the test results. With anonymous tests, the decision to tell anyone—even a doctor—is up to the individual.

What does a negative test mean?

If your test results are negative, it means no HIV antibodies were found in your blood. How-

ever, it takes about 4 to 12 weeks after a person is infected for HIV antibodies to form. This means that a person recently infected can have a negative HIV test. If you are in a "high risk" category or suspect you may have been exposed to the AIDS virus, you may want to be tested again 6 months after your last exposure. Even if your test is negative, you and your partner(s) should protect yourself during sex by always using condoms **from start to finish.** You should not shoot drugs, but if you do, you should never share works with anyone.

What if the test is positive?

A positive HIV test does not mean that you necessarily have AIDS now, but you could have it in the future. We do not know whether everyone infected with HIV eventually develop AIDS. We know that some people have had HIV infection for several years and have not developed AIDS. It seems that by taking very good care of themselves—both physically and emotionally—many of these people are leading normal, productive lives for many years with the HIV infection.

The main thing is not to panic. HIV infection is only part of your total life picture. Take care of your health, see your doctor regularly, seek emotional support from a trained counselor, protect yourself and others from further exposure to the AIDS virus, and continue with productive, satisfying activities.

Who should you tell?

Tell your doctor and dentist, so they will be able to give you the best possible care. You should also tell your current and past sex partner(s) and encourage them to get tested. Discuss with them how you can protect each other. And if you have used IV drugs, you should tell anyone with whom you have shared "works."

It is important to have people to help you cope—friends, relatives, or other people who are HIV positive. But you should choose with care the people you tell. In spite of the tremendous efforts made in recent years to educate the public, there are still many people with misconceptions about HIV infection and AIDS.

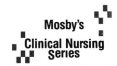

When Your HIV Test is Positive

A positive HIV test does not mean that you have AIDS. It means that you are infected with the HIV virus and must take steps to protect your health and prevent transmission.

Your medical care

Your positive test is only part of the picture—your overall health counts for a great deal. Your doctor may suggest drugs or other treatment that can help you stay healthy and avoid other infections. Drugs, such as AZT, are proving beneficial in slowing the progress of HIV infection. And a great deal of research is under way to find other treatments and, hopefully, a cure. You should be alert for changes in your body because HIV-positive people are more susceptible to other infections. See your doctor if a sudden acute illness occurs or if you notice a change (e.g., fever, pain, cough, shortness of breath, bleeding, or an unusual skin condition).

The importance of a healthy life style

The better you care for your body, the better your body can fight the HIV infection. A nutritious diet and adequate rest are essential. Exercise is important because it strengthens your body, increases your energy and stamina, and makes you feel better mentally. Do not abuse alcohol or use IV drugs because they can make the HIV infection worse and you will be more likely to develop AIDS. Alcohol and drugs can also impair your judgment, and you might take risks you ordinarily would not. If you have a problem with drugs or alcohol, get help to quit.

Coping

Coping with a diagnosis of HIV can be difficult. Many people feel they are all alone, that no one can understand what they are going through. **But help is out there—you don't have to face this alone.** Seek professional help from a trained counselor, psychologist, or psychiatrist. These professionals can provide emotional support and guidance in helping you cope with the variety of social problems that HIV-positive people may face. Friends and family members can be valuable in helping you cope. Share information about HIV infection and AIDS with these people so they can better help you.

How can you protect others?

Most people would not deliberately place their friends, sex partner(s), or even total strangers in jeopardy by exposing them to the AIDS virus.

Sex. The only sure way to protect your sexual partner(s) is to not have sex. It is safe to hug, cuddle, masturbate each other (as long as the skin isn't broken), rub, or "dry kiss." If you have sex, here are ways to minimize the chance of spreading the infection: (1) Use a latex condom **from start to finish,** with a birth control foam or jelly that contains nonoxynol-9. (2) Do not do anything that might cause a tear, abrasion, or bleeding (such as anal intercourse). (3) Use only a water-based lubricant, such as K-Y Jelly. Do not use saliva or oily lubricants, such as petroleum jelly or vegetable oil. (4) Avoid oral sex. (5) Avoid deep, wet, or French kissing.

Drug Use. If you shoot drugs, please get help to quit because drugs can make your HIV infection worse. Until you quit: (1) do not share 'works' with anyone else, (2) never use works that someone else has used, and (3) if you reuse your own works, clean them with bleach and water between uses.

Women. Do not get pregnant, because there is a strong chance you could pass the virus to your unborn baby. Babies with the AIDS virus usually die before age 2 years. Pregnancy may also make the HIV infection worse, and some women have become very sick and even died during pregnancy. If you already have a baby, do not breastfeed because you could pass the virus to your baby in your milk.

Personal items. Even during normal use, some personal items may carry small amounts of blood that can be passed on to other people if you share them. Items such as toothbrushes, razors, and sex toys should not be shared.

Donations. Do not donate blood, sperm, or body organs.

The following toll-free numbers can supply important information: National AIDS Hotline at 1-800-342-AIDS, AIDS Information Line at 1-800-551-2728, Drug Abuse Helpline at 1-800-338-6745, and Outreach Inc. Hotline at 1-800-441-2437.

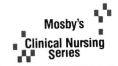

Mosby's
**Clinical Nursing
Series**

About Condoms

Condoms ("rubbers") were once used mainly for birth control. Today, condoms are an important weapon in preventing the spread of AIDS and other sexually transmitted diseases (STDs). Total abstinence from sex is the only completely safe method of preventing AIDS and STDs. Condoms are the next best way to be safe—but only if they are used correctly. If you are sexually active, learn how to use condoms and **always use them from start to finish!**

Buying and storing condoms

There are many brands and styles of condoms on the market. Whether you choose plain or fancy condoms is up to you—as long as you **buy only condoms made of latex.** You should also use a contraceptive foam or jelly that contains nonoxynol-9. In addition to being a spermicide, nonoxynol-9 may kill the AIDS virus on contact and gives extra protection against other STDs. Applying a nonoxynol-9 spermicide foam or jelly on the outside of the condom will give you protection in case the condom breaks. (Some condoms are packaged with nonoxynol-9 jelly, but the amount is too small to protect against the AIDS virus so you should use the foam or jelly even with these kinds of condoms.) Other instructions include:

- Store condoms in a cool, dry place away from sunlight and heat.
- If the package is damaged, don't use the condom because it may also be damaged.
- Do not use a condom that is brittle, discolored, or sticky because these are signs of age. An old condom can break easily.

Using condoms correctly

- Handle condoms carefully to prevent puncture.
- Always use a condom **from start to finish.** Even the briefest sexual contact can result in infection.
- If you use a lubricant, be sure it is water-based, such as K-Y Jelly. Lubricants that contain petroleum (e.g., Vaseline) or oil weaken the latex and may cause the condom to break.
- Before sexual contact, apply the nonoxynol-9 contraceptive foam or jelly on the outside of the condom and intravaginally or rectally.

- If a condom breaks, replace it immediately. If ejaculation occurs with a broken condom, use additional nonoxynol-9 to reduce the risk of getting an infection.
- Never reuse a condom!
- The penis must be erect to put on a condom correctly.
- Hold the tip of the condom with one hand (see diagram below). With the other hand, slip the rolled-up portion over the head of the penis and unroll the condom down the shaft of the penis. A space should be left at the tip to collect semen, but be sure the tip is not filled with air, since this could cause the condom to break.
- After ejaculation, the penis should be withdrawn while still erect.
- Hold the base of the condom during withdrawal to prevent accidental slipping. Wrap the used condom in tissue and discard.

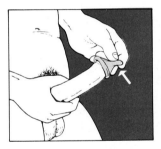

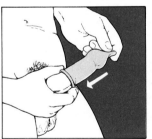

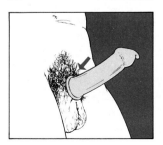

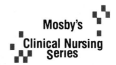

Mosby's
**Clinical Nursing
Series**

Hepatitis

Hepatitis is a viral infection of the liver. Different viruses cause hepatitis, but they all produce a very similar illness that usually starts with flu-like symptoms, progressing suddenly to loss of appetite, fatigue, fever, and nausea and vomiting. Smokers notice a sudden distaste for cigarettes. A rash and aching joints sometimes occur. Between 3 and 10 days later, the urine becomes dark and jaundice (yellowish skin and eyes) appears. Most people feel better at this point, even though the jaundice becomes worse. The jaundice worsens for 1 to 2 weeks, then begins to fade over 2 to 4 weeks. Hepatitis usually resolves completely, but occasionally complications develop, including chronic hepatitis, liver cirrhosis, or even liver failure.

How hepatitis is spread

Hepatitis A. The hepatitis A virus is transmitted in feces. Outbreaks of hepatitis A occur mainly from contaminated water and food. In some developing countries, hepatitis A is widespread because of poor sanitation. However, in the United States most infections result from eating raw shellfish or from oral contact with food or other matter contaminated with feces from an infected person.

Hepatitis B. The hepatitis B virus is mostly spread by sexual contact with an infected person or by blood-to-blood contact—that is, either by transfusion or by drug users sharing needles. People at greatest risk for hepatitis B infection are homosexual men, heterosexual men and women with multiple sex partners, and intravenous (IV) drug users and their sex partners. Also at risk are dialysis patients and hospital personnel who are in contact with blood. The hepatitis B virus can also be spread by chronic carriers—people who are infected but do not become ill.

Hepatitis non-A, non-B. Little is known about these oddly named viruses that cause hepatitis. One such virus has recently been named hepatitis C. Hepatitis C, similar to hepatitis B, is spread through blood transfusions, contact with contaminated blood or needles, and possibly by sexual contact. Other non-A, non-B viruses are transmitted, similar to hepatitis A, through fecal-oral routes.

Hepatitis-type illnesses can also be caused by other viruses, such as the Epstein-Barr virus (which causes mononucleosis) and the cytomegalovirus.

Prevention

Hepatitis A is prevented through good personal hygiene and avoiding the eating of raw shellfish. An injection of immune globulin may be given to household contacts of a person who has hepatitis A. Immune globulin is also recommended for anyone planning to travel to an area where hepatitis A is widespread.

The best way of preventing hepatitis B is by reducing your risk of exposure as much as possible by not having anal intercourse, not having multiple sex partners, and not sharing needles. Hepatitis B vaccine is recommended for people who are high risk—staff and patients in dialysis units, health care personnel who are exposed to blood, homosexual or bisexual men, prostitutes, IV drug users, and staff and residents of correctional facilities and long-term care institutions. Vaccination is also given to people whose sexual partners have hepatitis B.

Treatment

There is no specific treatment for hepatitis. Until you begin to feel better, rest and try to maintain a good diet. Remember that hepatitis is a liver infection, and alcohol and most drugs are processed by your liver. Therefore it is essential that you avoid all alcohol and drugs (except those drugs your doctor says to take) to prevent serious complications. You can safely return to work after the jaundice disappears and you feel recovered.

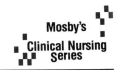
Tuberculosis

Tuberculosis (TB) is caused by *Mycobacterium tuberculosis,* a bacterium that is transmitted by inhaling moist secretions coughed into the air by an infected person. Although TB is an infection in the lungs, the bacteria does enter the bloodstream and infect other parts of the body. TB infection progresses in stages, the primary stage and a secondary stage, with a latency stage sometimes intervening between the two.

During the primary stage, the bacteria reside in tissue in the lungs and elsewhere in the body. During this stage, most people have no symptoms. The body's natural defenses are activated to produce antibodies to fight the infection. If the body's defenses are successful, the bacteria are walled off within a capsule, and the infection doesn't progress. The person is now in latency stage. However, the bacteria are still alive and can escape and become active later. This can happen if the body's immune system becomes impaired by illness, poor nutrition, certain drugs, or infection with AIDS.

The secondary stage (active stage) begins several months after the primary stage if the body's defenses were not successful. Bacteria begin destroying body tissue, particularly lung tissue. Symptoms include a slight fever, weight loss, fatigue, and night sweats. TB in the lungs causes a chronic cough that is initially dry but eventually produces sputum that contains blood and pus. Symptoms will also appear in other areas of the body where the bacteria have spread.

Diagnosing TB

A skin test is given when a person is suspected of having TB or has been exposed to people with TB. A positive test detects antibodies against the mycobacterium. Antibodies are detectable 4-12 wks after exposure and will produce a positive test for the remainder of a person's life. A positive test does not indicate active disease—only the presence of antibodies.

The most widely used test, the **Mantoux test,** consists of injecting a solution containing a small amount of bacteria just under the skin on the inside of the forearm. A skin reaction consists of a rash, blisters, or swelling around the injection site. An early reaction is not significant. Swelling in 48 to 72 hours may indicate a positive reaction, depending on the size of the swelling. If a skin test is positive, further procedures are necessary to determine whether the TB is active. The only way to diagnose active TB is by laboratory examination of a sputum specimen to detect live mycobacteria. Chest x-rays may show an area of lung disease. To diagnose TB of other organs, a small sample from the infected area is examined.

Treatment

Treatment of TB consists of taking a combination of drugs for 9 to 12 months (or longer), depending on the extent of the TB. Isoniazid and rifampin are nearly always prescribed, and other drugs may also be added. **It is important that you take the drugs exactly as your doctor orders, and for as long as necessary.** If you do not finish the treatment, the TB can reappear and may be even harder to treat.

Avoid alcohol while taking isoniazid and rifampin because this can cause serious liver problems. Take both drugs on an empty stomach with a full glass of water. If stomach upset is a problem, take them with a small amount of food. Avoid taking antacids that contain magnesium or aluminum within 1 hour of taking isoniazid, since this can interfere with drug absorption. Rifampin can make oral contraceptives less effective, so if you are on the pill, use another method of birth control. Rifampin gives a reddish or brownish color to urine, saliva, sputum, stools, sweat, and tears and will discolor soft contact lenses. Other possible side effects are dizziness, stomach upset, diarrhea, or rash.

Report to the doctor blurred vision, eye pain, chills, joint pain and swelling, breathing difficulty, fever, weakness, vomiting, or yellowing of the skin or eyes.

Preventing the Spread of TB

TB is not extremely contagious, but you need to protect close contacts. Bacteria is spread by coughing, so cover your nose and mouth and dispose of soiled tissues properly and wash hands thoroughly. Good room ventilation helps to reduce the amount of bacteria in the air. Sometimes household members are required to take antituberculosis drugs for 6 to 9 months (as a precaution).

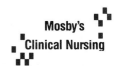

Food Safety

Food contaminated with bacteria, viruses, or parasites can cause illness. The following tips are designed to help you guard against contaminated food. **Wash hands with soap before and after handling food.** Most food contamination happens at home.

Commercially packaged food

The U.S. government has strict standards aimed at protecting the consumer from improperly canned and packaged foods. Even so, contaminated foods occasionally find their way to the grocery shelves. Observe the following guidelines and remember: **if in doubt, throw it out! Do not even taste a small amount.**

- Do not buy containers that appear to have been opened or have broken seals on jar lids.
- Do not buy or use cans that have bulging ends, leaks, or rust.
- Do not use food that shows spoilage, such as mold, an off-color, or an off-odor. A can that spurts liquid when opened is unsafe.
- Be sure to refrigerate after opening a jar if the label so instructs.

Home canned foods

Home canning requires following very precise methods of preparing the food, using the proper kind of jars, and sealing the jars carefully. Nonacid foods are especially susceptible to the bacteria responsible for botulism. (Note: nonacid foods include all vegetables, tomatoes, meat, poultry, and fish.) Pressure canning using 10 pounds of pressure at 240° F is the only method recommended for nonacid foods. The botulism bacteria does not cause an odor, a change in color or texture, or the formation of gas. **Never taste home canned nonacid food before first cooking!** To cook nonacid home canned foods, vigorously boil in an uncovered pot (vegetables for 3 to 5 minutes, meat, poultry, and fish for 10 minutes).

Meat and poultry

Salmonella and other bacteria may be present in raw meat and poultry. Any kitchen equipment that comes in contact with raw meat or poultry should be washed thoroughly before it is used with other foods.

- Use hot water and detergent to wash utensils that have touched raw meat or poultry before using the equipment with other food.
- When cutting raw meat or poultry, use a non-porous cutting board (plastic, marble, or glass) and wash it immediately.
- Keep meat refrigerated at 35 to 40° F. Ground meats are very perishable and should be cooked (or frozen) within 24 hours after purchase. Roasts will keep for 3 or 4 days without freezing. Poultry should be eaten within 2 days. Before cooking, check the odor of meats and poultry. Do not risk it if there is an unpleasant smell. Wash hands between handling raw meat and other foods and **cook** all meat.

Pork

Pork may contain a parasite that causes trichinosis. The only way to destroy the parasite is to cook pork thoroughly until the meat is white or greyish all the way through or registers 137° F on a meat thermometer.

Eggs

Eggs may be infected with *Salmonella* or other bacteria. Never use an egg that has an unpleasant odor or that has a cracked shell. Only eat eggs that have been cooked. Refrigerate eggs and prepared food that contains eggs (mayonnaise and other salad dressings) until ready to serve.

Milk and dairy products

Milk and other dairy products made from raw (unpasteurized) milk have caused TB. Buy only pasteurized dairy products.

Fish and shellfish

Because of environmental pollution, hepatitis has been caused by eating raw oysters, and several types of bacterial food poisoning can occur from eating raw shellfish or fish. Avoid eating any uncooked fish and shellfish.

Travel outside the U.S.

Travelers to developing countries should not drink local water nor eat uncooked vegetables. Fruits that require peeling are safe, but peel them yourself. Do not eat food from street vendors.

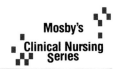

Infections Spread by Insects

Many people view insects as nuisances whose main jobs seem to be spoiling picnics or surprising the unwary. But some insects also pose a serious threat to humans because they carry infectious diseases. The following tips will help you avoid disease-carrying insects.

Fleas

Fleas live on the skin of both domestic and wild animals, piercing the skin to suck blood. Flea control is not always easy for pet owners. Fleas proliferate in hot weather, so during the warm weather months, use flea powder or spray on your pets and their sleeping areas weekly. Severely infested pets may need to be dipped. If the house becomes infested with fleas, spray or powder the rugs and upholstery, then vacuum the following day. Most flea poisons do not kill flea eggs, you will need to repeat the process every 5 days for a few times to get all the fleas. Flea eggs hatch 1 to 12 days after they are laid.

Ticks

Ticks feed on the blood of livestock, deer, coyotes, dogs, and other animals. These insects can carry typhus, Rocky Mountain spotted fever, and Lyme disease. Ticks attach to the skin, gripping so firmly that pulling on the tick to remove it often severs the head, leaving it under the skin. The life cycle of ticks involves engorging on a host, dropping off to wait on nearby vegetation, and hopping on as another animal passes by. In this way, ticks find their way to humans and pets.

Ticks can live nearly anywhere, as long as there is grass, weeds, trees, or other vegetation. During warm-weather months, apply a good insect repellent to all exposed skin. In areas with a high tick population, take special precautions before walking in woods or fields. Be sure your legs and feet are well-covered—wear long pants tucked into socks or boots. Check your body for ticks after being in high-vegetation areas. Remove ticks with tweezers.

Lice

Lice live on the skin, particularly areas covered with hair, and feed on blood. These tiny parasites are difficult to see with the naked eye, but can be found by searching for the tiny eggs (called **nits**), which are visible as greyish, transparent dots that cling to hair or are found in clothing or bedding. Lice cause intense itching and can transmit typhus, and relapsing fever.

Head lice ("cooties") can infest the scalp, eyebrows, eyelashes, and beard. They are common in schoolchildren and are spread by sharing combs, hats, and other personal items. Pubic lice ("crabs") inhabit the genital area and are transmitted by sexual contact and in bedding and clothes. Body lice actually live in the seams of clothing, rather than on the skin. Bites and itching from body lice are common on the shoulders, abdomen, and buttocks.

Lice are easily eradicated by applying special products called **pediculicides,** which are available without prescription as shampoos, creams, and lotions. Treatment consists of applying the pediculicide for 2 days according to the directions on the label and then repeating the treatment 10 days later to destroy any surviving nits. To avoid reinfection, everything that might be contaminated should be washed or dry-cleaned.

Mosquitos

Mosquitos are carriers of numerous diseases, including malaria, yellow fever, dengue fever, and encephalitis. Most of these diseases are limited to the tropics and subtropics. Community-wide mosquito control efforts in the Southern United States have eliminated malaria and yellow fever as a major threat in this country. However, several cases of encephalitis, a life-threatening brain infection, are reported every year from various parts of the United States.

Mosquitos require warm weather and water for breeding. While there is little one can do about the temperature, eliminating all standing water will deprive these insects of breeding areas. Flower pots and other containers should be turned upside down to prevent water from collecting. While outdoors, wear long sleeves and apply insect repellent to all exposed areas of skin. Keep screens repaired to discourage mosquitos from getting indoors. In heavily infested areas, mosquito netting over the bed may be necessary. Stay indoors during the evening hours when mosquitos feed.

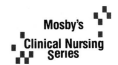
Collecting a clean-catch urine specimen

A clean-catch urine specimen is needed to diagnose infections of the kidney, bladder, and urinary tract. Laboratory tests will be made to identify the cause of the infection so that the right treatment can be prescribed.

What is a "clean-catch" specimen? Bacteria normally inhabit the genital area around the urinary opening. Usually these bacteria do not cause any problems, but the laboratory tests will not be accurate if these bacteria appear in the urine specimen. The clean-catch method keeps these bacteria from contaminating the urine specimen.

Follow these instructions very carefully:

Men

- You were given a sterile cup for the urine specimen and three sealed wipes for cleaning. Remove the plastic wrap from the cup, taking care not to touch the rim or inside of the cup. Write your name, date, and the time on the outside of the cup.
- Using a cloth with soap and water, wash the head of the penis. If you are not circumcised, pull back the foreskin and wash well. Rinse with water.
- Open the sealed packages containing the sterile wipes. Wipe across the urinary opening **once** with each pad.
- Start urinating and stop. Position the sterile cup to catch the stream and begin urinating again. (Be careful not to touch the rim or inside of the cup.)
- When you have provided the amount of urine specified, stop urinating and remove the cup.
- Discard the wipes in the trash. Follow instructions about where to take the specimen.

Women

This procedure is somewhat awkward (some women say it would help to have three hands), but it really can be done. However, you need to plan ahead, so read through these instructions in advance. Obtaining a clean-catch specimen is much easier if you do it sitting on a toilet.

- You were given a sterile cup for the urine specimen and three sealed wipes for cleaning. Remove the plastic wrap from the cup, taking care not to touch the rim or inside of the cup. Write your name, date, and the time on the outside of the cup.
- Using a cloth with soap and water, wash the entire genital area—the vulva, labia, and inside the labia around the urinary opening. Rinse well with water.
- Open the sealed packages so that you can remove each wipe with one hand.
- With the fingers of one hand, separate the inner labia so that the urinary opening is exposed. From here on out, you will need to keep the labia separated so be sure you are positioned securely enough to manage this.
- Use the first pad to wipe **once** down one side of the urinary opening, wiping front to back. Use the second pad to wipe once down the other side of the urinary opening. Use the third pad to wipe once directly over the urinary opening.
- Start urinating and stop. Place the cup under you to catch the urine when you restart the stream (Take care not to touch the cup rim against you.)
- Start urinating again, stopping when you have provided the specified amount.
- Discard the wipes in the trash. Follow instructions about where to take the specimen.

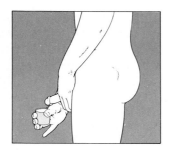
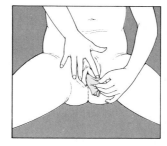
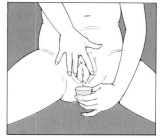

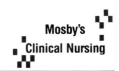
Fever

Fever—a temperature of 100.4° F (38° C) or above—is usually a sign of infection. A person with a fever may be flushed, irritable, tired, and complain of aching. Fever may start with chills, which are caused by the body temperature rising. Sweating often occurs with high temperatures and when the fever "breaks"—a sign that the temperature is decreasing. Some infections produce little or no fever so a normal temperature by itself does not necessarily mean that no infection is present.

Fever should always be watched carefully. Although most of the time fever is an expected reaction to infection, a very high fever is dangerous because it can cause convulsions, especially in children. Therefore it is important to know how to take a temperature correctly, what you can do to help reduce the fever, and when to call the doctor.

The most accurate reading is done with an oral temperature. However, taking an oral temperature requires cooperation so do not attempt this method with young children or anyone who is not conscious and cooperative. A regular thermometer can also be used under the arm. Authorities advise against taking temperatures rectally, even in children.

Although 98.6° F is considered the "normal" oral temperature, a healthy person's temperature actually ranges from about 97° F to 99.5° F during a 24-hour period. Underarm temperature is 1° or 2° lower than oral readings.

Mercury thermometers

A mercury thermometer is a glass tube with a bulb at one end that contains mercury. A scale on the tube shows degrees of temperature, with an arrow marking the normal point of 98.6° F. The bulb is placed under the tongue or in the armpit. As the mercury is heated, it rises up the tube to a point that shows the person's temperature. To read a thermometer, hold it at eye level in good light and rotate it slowly until you see the thin sliver line of mercury.

Never leave a child alone, even for a minute, with a mercury thermometer! Injury can occur from broken glass, and mercury is a poison.

- First, clean the thermometer with soap and then rinse it with cool tap water. Hot water will cause the thermometer to break. Hold the thermometer at the end opposite the mercury bulb and shake it a few times to make the mercury go below the arrow.
- To take an oral temperature, place the bulb of the thermometer under the tongue as far toward the back as possible. Have the person close his or her mouth and hold the thermometer in place for 4 to 5 minutes.
- To take an underarm temperature, place the bulb of the thermometer snuggly in an armpit and have the person keep the upper arm clasped tightly to the side, with the elbow bent and the lower arm folded across the chest. Leave the thermometer in place for 10 minutes.
- After you're done, wash the thermometer again with soap and cool water and shake it to return the mercury to the bulb.

Managing a fever

Rest and plenty of liquids are needed when someone is running a fever. Encourage the person to drink water and juice to prevent dehydration. Try to make the person as comfortable as possible—extra covers during the chill stage, and sponging with a cool wet cloth when the person feels hot. Keep the room air cool or use a fan.

Infants and children. Children can run a fever very suddenly. A feverish child's temperature should be taken every hour. Never give children aspirin unless your doctor says it is okay because giving aspirin with some viral infections may cause a serious complication called **Reye's syndrome.** Your doctor may suggest an aspirin substitute, such as acetaminophen (Tylenol). **Call the doctor immediately if the child's temperature reaches 102° F or over.** High fevers can lead to convulsions very quickly, especially in children under 5 years.

Teenagers and adults. A moderate amount of fever is actually beneficial, so unless the fever is high (above 100.4° F) or headache or other pain is present, it is not necessary to take aspirin or an aspirin substitute to bring down fever. However, you should call the doctor if the temperature exceeds 102° F or lasts longer than 24 hours.

PATIENT TEACHING GUIDE

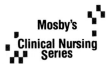
Mosby's
Clinical Nursing
Series

Facts about your prescription

Your doctor has prescribed one or more drugs to treat an infection. It is important that you take the drugs exactly as prescribed, for as long as needed. Even if you feel better, **don't stop taking the drug before you are supposed to!** This could cause the infection to reappear, and it is sometimes harder to get rid of the second time.

MEDICATION INFORMATION FORM

Here is some information about the medication your doctor prescribed:

Name of Drug: _____
                 (generic and brand)

Dose: _____

When to take: _____

Special instructions for taking: _____

_____

Cautions:

Do not take on an empty stomach _____

Do not take with milk or antacids _____

Avoid alcohol _____

Avoid sun exposure while taking _____

Take with food _____

Drink plenty of fluids _____

May cause drowsiness _____

Do not take while pregnant _____

Do not take while breastfeeding _____

Do not take with these other drugs: _____

_____

_____

Side effects: _____

_____

Cease taking medicine and call your doctor if any of the following occur:

_____

_____

Doctor's Phone Number _____

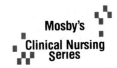
Mosby's
Clinical Nursing
Series

Immunizations

Diphtheria, tetanus, pertussis, polio, measles, mumps, and rubella can be killers. All infants and children should be vaccinated against these infections. People at risk for certain kinds of infections need additional immunizations. Protect yourself and your family by keeping immunizations up to date.

Before getting any immunizations, be sure to tell the nurse or doctor if you or your child is allergic to eggs or has any illness. Certain vaccines cannot be given during pregnancy or to people who have immune disorders, such as lymphoma, leukemia, and AIDS.

DTP protects children against diphtheria, tetanus, and pertussis. Children need a total of five doses (DTP-1, DTP-2, etc.).

TD (diphtheria and tetanus) is given after age 14 years.

OPV is oral polio vaccine, and children need a total of four doses (e.g., OPV-1 through OPV-4).

IPV is injectable polio vaccine for adults and persons with immune disorders who need polio immunization.

MMR immunizes against measles, mumps, and rubella. Two doses (MMR-1 and MMR-2) are needed for protection. Adults are sometimes given the measles vaccine by itself.

Haemophilus vaccine protects against a type of meningitis that particularly affects children.

HB vaccine is recommended for anyone who is at risk for hepatitis B. Usually a series of three doses is given. People who have already been exposed to hepatitis need one dose of hepatitis B immune globulin, followed by three doses of HB vaccine.

BCG protects against TB. This vaccine is sometimes recommended for people who travel to areas where this infection is widespread or who are at risk of being exposed to TB.

Recommended immunizations for children

Age	Vaccines
2 months	DTP-1, OPV-1
4 months	DTP-2, OPV-2
6 months	DTP-3
12 months	MMR-1 in urban areas or where measles outbreaks have occurred
15 months	DTP-4, OPV-3, and MMR-1 if not given at 12 months *Haemophilus* B vaccine
4-6 years	DTP-5, OPV-4, and MMR-2 before starting kindergarten or first grade
14-16 years	TD

Adolescents and young adults

Between 14 and 16 years, immunization against tetanus and diphtheria (TD vaccine) is needed. The TD vaccine is given in three doses for previously vaccinated persons. (Otherwise, a booster is given.) The first and second doses are 8 weeks apart, and the third dose is 6 to 12 months after the second dose. After that, a single TD booster is needed every 10 years.

Recent outbreaks of measles among young adults have pointed to the need for revaccination. Colleges and other post-high school educational institutions are now requiring proof of two doses of measles vaccine. Anyone who has not had both doses will need to be vaccinated, either with the MMR vaccine or the measles vaccine.

Adults over 25 years

A TD booster is needed every 10 years. People over age 65 years should also be vaccinated against influenza and pneumonia.

People with special risks

Chronic illnesses. People with blood clotting diseases (hemophilia) and dialysis patients should be vaccinated against hepatitis. Vaccines for influenza and pneumonia are recommended for people with any chronic health problem.

Life style risks. Homosexually active men and people who inject drugs are at high risk for hepatitis B infection.

Travelers. Travelers outside the U.S. may need to update their immunizations. Adults may need a polio vaccine or other immunizations.

Immigrants, refugees, and foreign students. Many countries do not routinely immunize. As a result, persons entering the United States may be more susceptible to these infections and should be immunized.

Residents of institutions. Outbreaks of hepatitis, TB, and other infectious diseases can occur in correctional facilities and institutions for the mentally retarded.

Side effects of vaccines

Vaccines are carefully tested for both effectiveness and safety before they are approved. Some soreness, redness, and swelling at the injection site can be expected with most vaccines. Usually these symptoms are very mild and disappear after 1 or 2 days. Call the doctor immediately if any of the following symptoms occur after vaccination; fever of 100° F or more, severe headache, swelling of the mouth and throat, difficulty breathing, wheezing, fainting, or seizures.

CHAPTER 15

Antiinfective Agents

Antibiotics, strictly defined, are substances produced by one living organism that may kill another living organism. **Antimicrobial** is a more generic term that applies to any substance—either natural or synthetic—that suppresses the growth of other microorganisms and may eventually destroy them. Many of the "antibiotics" are actually synthetic; however, they retain the classification of antibiotic because of their effect. Antimicrobial drugs may be described as either **bacteriostatic,** that is, they inhibit the growth of an organism, or **bactericidal** (or **fungicidal, amebicidal,** etc.), meaning that they destroy (or kill) the organism. The terms are often used interchangeably, since a drug that is bacteriostatic to one microorganism at a specific concentration may be bactericidal in higher concentrations or to other organisms. Infections that are treated with antimicrobial drugs often recur unless the body's own defense mechanisms are capable of eradicating the infection.

The treatment of infectious disease is based on the type of infecting organism, the location and severity of the infection, and the sensitivity (or susceptibility) of the organism to specific drugs. The goal of drug treatment is to eradicate the infecting organism by directly destroying it or suppressing growth so the body's own defenses are able to control the disease.

The number or range of organisms against which a drug is effective is referred to as its **spectrum** of activity. Often drugs are referred to as **broad-spectrum** antibiotics or **narrow-spectrum** antibiotics, referring to their effectiveness against a broad or narrow range of organisms.

A side effect common to most antimicrobials following prolonged or repeated administration is inhibition of normal flora, leading to overgrowth of nonsusceptible organisms. Secondary infection as a result of this overgrowth of bacteria or fungi is called a **superinfection.**

Dosing of antimicrobials is extremely varied. The infecting organism and the severity and location of the infection all influence the dose and route of administration. The age, size, and health of the host also are important considerations when determining antimicrobial doses. Doses given in this chapter are only very general guidelines. More specific dosages are provided, when available, with the discussion of specific infections.

GENERAL NURSING CONSIDERATIONS FOR ALL ANTIMICROBIAL DRUGS

When it is possible, assist with the identification of the infecting organism by obtaining cultures **before** antimicrobial therapy is instituted. Cultures should be sent to the laboratory and processed as soon as possible. Administer antimicrobials at the prescribed times, even when it means waking a patient or disturbing routines. Around-the-clock administration at regular intervals is often necessary to maintain antimicrobial therapeutic plasma or tissue levels. Many drugs have side effects; some are minor whereas others are life-threatening. The nurse must monitor and evaluate the patient for side effects that may develop. Serum levels should be drawn at appropriate times (see box, page 306) and monitored. Observe for development of superinfections. Reinforce the importance of completing the full course of therapy, even though the patient may be symptomless, and instruct the patient to not take "leftover" drugs for new illnesses. Clients with drug allergies should be instructed how to protect themselves from receiving the drug by alerting health care providers and carrying identification of the allergy, such as wallet cards or bracelets.

SERUM DRUG LEVELS

The effects of some antibiotics are difficult to measure. Other antibiotics may have a narrow therapeutic index with either toxicity or lack of efficacy possible. To establish efficacy within safe ranges, a therapeutic range has been established for some antibiotics. The therapeutic range is the "safe range" in which serum levels are sufficient for desired drug effect but remain below the toxic level. Serum drug concentrations are used for adjustments of either dosage or dosing interval. Blood samples are often drawn to measure maximal drug concentration (peak level) and minimal drug concentration (trough level). Peak drug levels are drawn shortly following administration when serum levels are expected to be the highest. Exact timing is related to the route of administration. Peak levels are achieved immediately following IV administration and generally 30 to 60 minutes after IM or oral administration, but peak levels may vary significantly between drugs. Trough levels are drawn at the end of the dosing interval, immediately before the next dose is administered. The organism and site of infection also influence the desired concentration.

ANTIBACTERIALS

Antibacterial agents are commonly classified or grouped together based on their mechanism of action. Four primary mechanisms of antibacterial action are commonly recognized:

1. Inhibition of cell wall synthesis
2. Alteration of cell membrane permeability or active transport across the cell membrane
3. Inhibition of protein synthesis
4. Inhibition of nucleic acid synthesis

Dosages and route of administration are based on the sensitivity of the infecting organism to the antibiotic and the location and severity of infection. Because different organisms require different concentrations of antibiotic for effectiveness, general guidelines for administration of many antibiotics cannot be given. In general, therapy should continue for at least 48 hours after the patient becomes symptomless. With all antibiotics, therapy should continue for the prescribed length of time even after symptoms have subsided.

Penicillins

Penicillins are the most widely effective and widely used antibiotics. Penicillins and cephalosporins are two large groups of antibiotic drugs that share similar properties. These drugs are referred to as **beta-lactam drugs** because of their chemical structure, which includes a "beta-lactam" ring. Antibiotics in this class exert their antibacterial effect by inhibiting cell wall synthesis. Penicillin G, the prototype penicillin, was discovered in 1929 by Fleming. There are significant differences within the penicillins in degree of inactivation by gastric acids, protein binding, inactivation by penicillinase,

and spectrum of antimicrobial activity.

Resistance to many of the penicillins may occur by organisms producing an enzyme, beta-lactase (also called penicillinase), which inactivates some penicillins by breaking the beta-lactam ring in their structure. Penicillins that are resistant to these enzymes are called **penicillinase resistant.** Combinations of a penicillin with a beta-lactamase inhibitor are now available. The combination is thought to increase the effectiveness of penicillin by inhibiting the beta-lactamase enzyme.

The amidinopenicillins are a new group of penicillins, of which amdinocillin is the prototype. Because this drug binds with different receptors rather than other penicillins, it may be synergistic with penicillins.
Indications: Infections caused by penicillin-sensitive bacteria. Commonly used in the treatment of infections attributable to gonococci, spirochetes, *Actinomyces, Haemophilis, Pseudomonas, Staphylococcus aureus, Streptococcus pneumoniae,* group A streptococci, and *Serratia.* Penicillins have been used prophylactically in treating persons exposed to S. *pyogenes,* gonorrhea or syphilis, preventing recurrences of rheumatic fever, and preventing subacute bacterial endocarditis (in patients with valvular heart disease who are undergoing surgical or dental procedures).
Usual dosage: Varies (Table 15-1).
Precautions/contraindications: All penicillins are cross-sensitizing and cross-reacting.
Side effects/adverse reactions: The incidence of allergic reactions to the penicillins has been estimated to be as high as 5% to 10% in adults. Original sensitizing exposure may come from exposure to environmental mold and dermatophytes living on the skin, which are capable of producing penicillin-like molecules. Another source of exposure is from penicillin in the milk of cows

Table 15-1

PENICILLINS

Generic name	Trade names	Administration	Administration
Penicillin G	Pentids	200,000-400,000 U q 6-8 h	Oral
		5-40 million U/day in 4 divided doses	IM, IV
Penicillin V	Compocillin-V, Penicillin V, Pen-Vee, V-Cillin	200,000-400,000 U q 6-8 h	Oral
Penicillinase-resistant			
Methicillin	Staphcillin, Dimocillin	4-12 g/day in 4-6 divided doses	IM, IV
Nafcillin	Unipen, Nafcil, Nallpen	1-6 g/day in 4-6 divided doses	Oral
		2-12 g/day in 4-6 divided doses	IM, IV
Oxacillin	Prostaphlin, Bactocill	1-6 g/day in 4-6 divided doses	Oral
		1-12 g/day in 4-6 divided doses	IM, IV
Cloxacillin	Cloxapen, Tegopen	1-4 g/day in 4 divided doses	Oral
Dicloxacillin	Dynapen, Pathocil	1-2 g/day in 4 divided doses	Oral
Ampicillins			
Ampicillin	Ampicill, Omnipen, Polycillin, Totacillin	1-4 g/day in 4 divided doses	Oral
		1-12 g/day in 4-8 divided doses	IM, IV
Bacampicillin	Spectrobid	400 mg-1.6 g q 12 h	Oral
Amoxicillin	Amoxil, Larotid, Polymox, Trimox	250-500 mg q 8 h	Oral
Cyclacillin	Cyclapen	250-500 mg q 6 h	Oral
Extended spectrum			
Carbenicillin	Geopen, Pyopen	250-500 mg/kg/day in divided doses	IM, IV
	Geocillin	382-764 mg q 6 h	Oral
Ticarcillin	Ticar	50-300 mg/kg/day in 3-6 divided doses	IM, IV
Mezlocillin	Mezlin	100-350 mg/kg/day in 4-6 divided doses	IM, IV
Piperacillin	Pipracil		IM, IV
Azlocillin	Azlin	100-350 mg/kg/day in 4-6 divided doses	IV
Amidinopenicillins			
Amdinocillin	Coactin		IM, IV
Combined penicillin/beta-lactase inhibitors			
Amoxicillin/Clavulanic acid	Augmentin	500 mg/125 mg q 8 h	Oral
Ticarcillin/Clavulanic acid	Timentin	3.1 g q 4-8 h	IV
Ampicillin/Sulbactam	Unasyn	1-2 g/0.5-1 g q 6 h	IM, IV

being treated for mastitis. Allergic reactions may be immediate (e.g., pruritus, urticaria, asthma, rhinitis, laryngeal edema, and anaphylaxis), intermediate (e.g., rashes and fever), or delayed even after the antibiotic is stopped (e.g., serum sickness, rash, thrombocytopenia, and anemia). Anaphylactic reactions, although rare, most commonly occur following parenteral therapy. All penicillins are **cross-sensitizing,** which means that a patient allergic to any one penicillin may be allergic to other penicillins.

Penicillins are generally well-tolerated by most patients. Penicillins may produce gastrointestinal (GI) upset, local pain may accompany intramuscular (IM) injections, and sclerosing phlebitis may follow intravenous (IV) administration. High doses of ticarcillin, carbenicillin, mezlocillin, piperacillin, azlocillin, or nafcillin have been reported to cause bleeding abnormalities.

Many penicillins have a high sodium content, which may lead to electrolyte imbalances when high doses are administered. Hypokalemia has been reported in patients receiving azlocillin, mezlocillin, ticarcillin, pipracillin, and carbenicillin.

Ampicillin frequently causes skin rashes, some of which are not related to allergy.

Bone marrow depression with granulocytopenia, or interstitial nephritis may occur with the penicillinase-resistant penicillins.

Pharmacokinetics: Penicillins are primarily eliminated through the kidney. Nafcillin is least dependent on renal elimination, with about 80% of a dose excreted in the bile. Penicillin is also excreted in saliva and breast milk in roughly 3% to 15% of serum levels. Penicillin G and several other penicillin drugs may be either partially or totally inactivated by gastric acids with a pH of 2 or less. Absorption of most penicillins is affected by food.

Penicillins have been formulated to provide a prolonged action following IM administration. Procaine or benzathine salts are used for IM administration to maintain effective serum concentrations for up to 4 weeks as the result of slow, prolonged absorption from the injection site.

Interactions: Administration of probenecid blocks renal tubular excretion of penicillin and prolongs blood levels. Probenecid is sometimes administered with the penicillin for this effect. An increased incidence of breakthrough bleeding and pregnancy has been reported following the use of some penicillins in patients using oral contraceptives.

Nursing considerations: Penicillins (except amoxicillin) should not be administered at meal time but at least 1 hour before meals or 1 to 3 hours after meals to minimize inactivation by gastric acid. All patients should be monitored closely for signs of immediate or delayed al-

lergic reaction. When administering parenteral penicillins, emergency drugs for treating anaphylaxis should be immediately available. Caution women using oral contraceptives to use an alternate method of birth control during antibiotic therapy. Monitor patients at risk for electrolyte imbalance for signs of potassium imbalance, sodium imbalance, or water retention.

Cephalosporins

The cephalosporins are beta-lactam with activity similar to penicillins. They are bactericidal by interfering with the cell wall synthesis of bacteria. Cephalosporin antibiotics are classified as first, second, or third generation agents. This terminology, which was developed for marketing, does not necessarily follow the chronological development of the drugs, but it does follow their spectrum of antibacterial activity. As a patient progresses through first, second, and third generation cephalosporins, the effectiveness against gram-negative organisms generally increases whereas the effectiveness against gram-positive organisms decreases. Several second generation agents are also active against anaerobic organisms.

Indications: Treatment of cephalosporin-sensitive bacterial infections and surgical prophylaxis.

Usual dosage: Varies (Table 15-2).

Precautions/contraindications: Cross-reactivity with the penicillins has been reported rarely but is potentially serious when it occurs.

Side effects/adverse reactions: Allergic reactions and tissue irritation are similar in nature and incidence to penicillins. Renal toxicity has been reported with some of the early cephalosporins, especially when used concomitantly with an aminoglycoside antibiotic.

Pharmacokinetics: Many of the cephalosporins are poorly absorbed from the GI tract and therefore are administered parenterally. Cephalosporins are eliminated primarily by the kidney. Food may increase or decrease absorption, depending on which oral cephalosporin is used.

Interactions: Nephrotoxicity attributable to aminoglycosides may be potentiated. Oral anticoagulants may have an increased effect. Nausea and vomiting may occur if alcohol is consumed while the drug is in the body (the "Antabuse" reaction).

Nursing considerations: See penicillins.

Aztreonam

Aztreonam, a synthetic bactericidal agent that has a monocyclic beta-lactam nucleus, is structurally different from other beta-lactam antibacterials, which are bicyclic. This drug is the first of a new class of antibacterials known as *monobactams.*

Indications: Aztreonam is effective against a wide vari-

Table 15-2

CEPHALOSPORINS

Generic name	Trade names	Dosage range	Administration
First generation			
Cephalothin	Keflin	0.5-1 g q 4-6 h	IM, IV
Cefazolin	Ancef, Kefzol, Zolicef	0.5-1 g q 6-8 h	IM, IV
Cephapirin	Cefadyl	0.5-1 g q 4-6 h	IM, IV
Cephradine	Anspor, Velosef	500 mg q 12-24 h 12.5-25 mg/kg/day q 6 h	Oral IM, IV
Cephalexin	Keflet, Keflex, Keftab	250 mg-1 g q 6 h	Oral
Cefadroxil	Duricef, Ultracef	1-2 g/day q 12-24 h	Oral
Second generation			
Cefamandole	Mandol	0.5-1 g q 4-8 h	IM, IV
Cefuroxime	Ceftin, Kefurox, Zinacef	250-500 mg bid 0.75-1.5 g q 8 h	IM, IV
Cefonicid	Monocid	1 g q 24 h	IM, IV
Cefoxitin	Mefoxin	1-2 g q 6-8 h	IM, IV
Cefaclor	Ceclor	250-500 mg q 8 h	Oral
Cefotetan	Cefotan	1-2 g q 12 h	IM, IV
Ceforanide	Precef	0.5-1 g q 12 h	IM, IV
Cefmetazole	Zefazone	2 g q 6-12 h	IV
Third generation			
Cefotaxime	Claforan	1-12 g/day q 6-12 h	IM, IV
Ceftriaxone	Rocephin	1-2 g once a day	IM, IV
Moxalactam	Moxam	2-4 g/day q 8-12 h	IM, IV
Cefoperazone	Cefobid	1-2 g q 12 h	IM, IV
Ceftizoxime	Cefizox	1-2 g q 8-12 h	IM, IV
Ceftazidime	Fortaz, Tazidime	0.25-2 g q 8-12 h	IM, IV
Cefixime	Suprax	400 mg/day	Oral

ety of gram-negative aerobic bacteria, including most strains of *Enterobacter, Escherichia coli, Haemophilus influenzae, Serratia marcescens, Klebsiella pneumoniae, Proteus mirabilia,* and *Pseudomonas aeruginosa.*
Usual dosage: 0.5 to 2 g every 8 to 12 hours, depending on the type of infection. It is administered either IM or IV.
Precautions/contraindications: Prolonged or increased serum levels may occur in patients with reduced renal function. Safety and efficacy of use in infants and children has not been established.
Side effects/adverse reactions: Adverse effects are uncommon. Hypersensitivity reactions, including anaphylaxis may occur. Local reactions that may occur include phlebitis following IV administraton and swelling or discomfort following IM administration. Systemic reactions include GI disturbances and rash.
Pharmacokinetics: Primarily excreted through the kidneys with a small amount recovered in the feces.
Interactions: Beta-lactamase-inducing antibiotics (e.g., cefoxitin and imipenem) may result in an antagonistic effect and should not be administered concurrently. Aztreonam and aminoglycosides are synergistic against some strains of bacteria.
Nursing considerations: When preparing solutions, vigorously shake the container **immediately** after adding the diluent. When administering IM, inject deeply into a large muscle mass; do not mix with local anesthetics.

Table 15-3

ERYTHROMYCINS

Generic name	Trade names	Dosage range	Administration
Erythromycin	E-Mycin, Ery-Tab, Eryc	250-500 mg q 6-12 h	Oral
Erythromycin estolate	Ilosone	250-500 mg q 6-12 h	Oral
Erythromycin stearate	Eramycin, Ethril, Erypar	250-500 mg q 6-12 h	Oral
Erythromycin ethylsuccinate	E.E.S., Pediamycin, Wayamycin, Eryped	400-800 mg q 6-12 h	Oral
Erythromycin lactobionate	Erythrocin Lactobionate	15-20 mg/kg/day	IV
Erythromycin gluceptate	Ilotycin Gluceptate	15-20 mg/kg/day	IV

PSEUDOMEMBRANOUS COLITIS

Pseudomembranous colitis (also called antibiotic-associated colitis) has been reported following administration of many antibiotics, including penicillins, cephalosporins, erythromycin, chloramphenicol, lincosamides, tetracyclines, streptomycin, and cotrimoxazole. This syndrome is characterized by abdominal pain, fever, and diarrhea with mucus and blood; it may be lethal. It is not related to dosage, can follow oral or parenteral administration, and may occur several weeks after discontinuance of antibiotic therapy. In most cases the primary cause is a toxin associated with *Clostridium difficile*. Vancomycin is effective in the treatment and may be lifesaving. Oral metronidazole and bacitracin also may be effective treatment.

Intravenous doses may be administered either by bolus injection over 3 to 5 minutes or as an infusion lasting 20 to 60 minutes. Closely monitor patients who have had an immediate reaction to penicillins or cephalosporins.

Erythromycin

Erythromycin exerts its antibacterial effect by interfering with protein synthesis. The base form of erythromycin is destroyed in stomach acid and therefore must be administered with an enteric coating.

Indications: Infections caused by erythromycin-sensitive bacteria, including diphtheria, *Mycoplasma pneumoniae*, and *Legionella* infections. Erythromycin is also used as a substitute for penicillin in patients allergic to penicillin.

Usual dosage: Varies (Table 15-3).

Precautions/contraindications: Erythromycin should be used with caution in patients with impaired hepatic function. Erythromycin estolate and ethylsuccinate are contraindicated in the presence of liver disease.

Side effects/adverse reactions: Impaired liver function and jaundice have been reported following use of erythromycin estolate and ethylsuccinate but the effects appear to be reversible upon discontinuation. GI disturbances, including nausea, cramping, anorexia, and diarrhea are common with oral administration. Discomfort at the site of infusion and phlebitis are commonly associated with parenteral administration. Reversible hearing loss can occur with high doses. Pseudomembranous colitis may occur (see box above).

Pharmacokinetics: Erythromycin is concentrated in the liver and eliminated in the bile, with a small amount eliminated by the kidneys.

Interactions: Increased effects of digoxin, carbamazepine (Tegretol), xanthines, and oral anticoagulants may occur, most commonly from altered metabolism. Erythromycins may antagonize the effects of chloramphenicol or lincomycin.

Nursing considerations: Do not administer concurrently with chloramphenicol or lincomycin. Monitor for jaundice or other signs of liver dysfunction with erythromycin estolate and ethylsuccinate. When oral forms are used, instruct the patient to take the drug on an empty stomach (i.e., 1 hour before or 2 hours after meals). Erythromycin estolate, ethylsuccinate, and enteric-coated tablets may be taken without regard to meals. Oral doses should be taken with a full glass of water. Monitor for symptoms of GI intolerance.

Table 15-4

LINCOSAMIDES

Generic name	Trade name	Dosage range	Administration
Lincomycin	Lincocin	500 mg q 6-8 h	Oral
		600 mg q 12-24 h	IM
		600 mg-1 g q 8-12 h	IV
Clindamycin	Cleocin	150-450 mg q 6 h	Oral
		900 mg q 8 h	IM, IV
		10% applied twice daily	Topical

Lincosamides

The lincosamides, which include lincomycin and clindamycin, exert their effect by inhibiting bacterial protein synthesis. Lincomycin resembles erythromycin in its spectrum of activity. Clindamycin is the more commonly used of the two drugs because it has a broader spectrum of antibacterial activity, with fewer adverse effects.

Indications: Infections caused by erythromycin-sensitive bacteria.

Usual dosage: Varies (Table 15-4).

Precautions/contraindications: Use cautiously in patients with impaired renal or hepatic function.

Side effects/adverse reactions: Rash occurs in about 10% of patients, and mild GI effects are common. Pseudomembranous colitis may occur. Hepatic and renal dysfunction have been reported, usually associated with prolonged therapy.

Pharmacokinetics: Administration with food impairs absorption of lincomycin but not clindamycin. Both drugs are greater than 60% protein bound and are eliminated primarily via hepatic metabolism. A significant amount of the drugs can be found in breast milk.

Interactions: Lincosamides have a neuromuscular blocking effect that may enhance the effect of other neuromuscular blocking drugs.

Nursing considerations: Oral lincomycin should be administered on an empty stomach either 1 hour before or 2 hours after meals.

Chloramphenicol

Chloramphenicol is a broad-spectrum antibiotic that exerts its effect by inhibiting bacterial protein synthesis. Because of the serious blood disorders that may occur with chloramphenicol therapy, its use is reserved for serious infections when less dangerous agents are ineffective or contraindicated.

Indications: *Salmonella* infections, *H. influenzae* meningitis or laryngotracheitis, and susceptible gram-negative bacteremia.

Usual dosage: Chloramphenicol (Chloromycetin), 12.5 to 25 mg every 6 hours, oral or IV. Chloramphenicol is ineffective when given IM.

Precautions/contraindications: Monitor blood studies before and every 2 days during therapy for bone marrow depression. Impaired renal or hepatic function may lead to higher than anticipated serum drug levels. Serum drug levels should be monitored during therapy if possible.

Side effects/adverse reactions: Serious and sometimes fatal blood disorders have been reported, including aplastic anemia (estimated occurrence of 1:40,000), hypoplastic anemia, thrombocytopenia, and granulocytopenia. The development of these blood disorders is not related to the dose or duration of therapy. A toxic reaction, referred to as the "gray baby syndrome," has occurred when administered to premature or newborn babies, with up to a 40% fatality rate. GI disturbances, including nausea, vomiting, and diarrhea, occasionally develop. Rashes and fever may occur with use of the drug but are uncommon.

Pharmacokinetics: Chloramphenicol is well-absorbed from the GI tract. It is eliminated by the kidneys, with about 10% excreted in unchanged form and 90% as metabolites.

Interactions: Chloramphenicol may increase the effects of phenytoin, tolbutamide, chlorpropamide, and warfarin.

Nursing considerations: Administer the oral medication at least 1 hour before or 2 hours after meals. The IV drug should be administered over at least 1 minute. Monitor the patient and alert him or her to report to a physician signs of blood disorders, including sore throat, fever, extreme fatigue, or unusual bleeding or bruising. Complete blood cell counts (CBC) should be monitored during therapy.

Tetracyclines

The tetracyclines exert their antibacterial effect by inhibiting bacterial protein synthesis.

Indications: Infections caused by a variety of gram-positive bacteria, gram-negative bacteria, spirochetes,

Table 15-5

TETRACYCLINES

Generic name	Trade names	Dosage range	Administration
Short duration			
Tetracycline	Achromycin, Panmycin	1-2 g/day in 2-4 divided doses	Oral
	Sumycin, Tetralan	250 mg q 24 h	IM
		250-500 mg q 12 h	IV
Chlortetracycline	Achromycin	3% ointment	topical
		1 cm ribbon, 10 preparation	ophthalmic
Oxytetracycline	Terramycin, Uri-Tet	250 mg q 24 h	IM, Oral
Intermediate duration			
Demeclocycline	Declomycin	150-300 mg q 6-12 h	Oral
Methacycline	Rondomycin	150 mg q 6 h	Oral
Longer duration			
Doxycycline	Vibramycin, Doxychel,	200 mg 1st day, then 100 mg/day	Oral
	Doxy Caps, Doryx	100-200 mg/day	IV
Minocycline	Minocin	100 mg q 12 h	IV, Oral

Leptospira, chlamydiae, mycoplasmae, amebae, and some rickettsiae.

Usual dosage: Varies (Table 15-5).

Precautions/contraindications: Tetracyclines should not be administered to pregnant women or children under the age of 6 years to avoid bone and tooth discoloration and dysplasia.

Side effects/adverse reactions: GI upset and diarrhea may occur from direct irritation or altered gut flora. IV administration can cause severe hepatic and pancreatic injury. Tetracyclines are readily bound to newly formed bones and teeth, leading to brownish discoloration and possibly dysplasia. Systemic administration may lead to photosensitivity. Enterocolitis and pseudomembranous colitis may occur.

Pharmacokinetics: Absorption following oral administration is variable. Calcium and aluminum salts tend to impair absorption. Elimination is primarily through the kidney.

Interactions: A nonabsorbable complex is formed, leading to reduced absorption if given in combination with calcium, magnesium, or aluminum-containing antacid preparations and also iron-containing products.

Nursing considerations: Oral preparations should be taken on an empty stomach with a full glass of water to avoid esophageal or gastric irritation. Avoid dairy products or laxatives containing aluminum, calcium, or magnesium for 1 hour after or 2 hours before taking tetracyclines. Inform patients that the drug may cause photosensitivity and instruct them to avoid direct sunlight as much as possible and to use sunscreen.

Aminoglycosides

The aminoglycoside antibiotics are effective against a wide range of bacteria, but their use is limited primarily to the treatment of serious gram-negative infections attributable to the toxicity of these drugs. The aminoglycosides exert their bactericidal effects by interfering with protein synthesis. An oral forms of aminoglycosides (Neomycin) are not significantly absorbed and are used to suppress GI flora in preparation for abdominal surgery or for reducing ammonia-forming bacteria in the treatment of hepatic coma.

Indications: Parenteral administration for treatment of gram-negative infections caused by *E. Coli*, *Proteus*, *Pseudomonas*, *Klebsiella*, *Enterobacter*, and *Serratia* organisms. Streptomycin is used as an antitubercular drug. Oral forms (Neomycin) are used to suppress GI flora in preparation for abdominal surgery and for reducing ammonia-forming bacteria in the treatment of hepatic coma. Paromomycin is used in the treatment of intestinal amebiasis.

Usual dosage: Varies (Table 15-6).

Precautions/contraindications: Not used for long-term therapy because of the high incidence of ototoxicity and nephrotoxicity. Dehydration and advanced age increase the risk of toxicity. May aggravate muscle weakness, especially in patients with neuromuscular disorders such as myasthenia gravis.

Side effects/adverse reactions: Aminoglycosides are associated with nephrotoxicity and ototoxicity even at conventional doses. Renal damage may be evidenced by decreased creatinine clearance levels, cells or casts in urine, oliguria, proteinurea, or increased serum

Table 15-6

AMINOGLYCOSIDES

Generic name	Trade names	Dosage range	Administration
Amikacin	Amikin	15 mg/kg/day in 2-3 doses	IM, IV
Gentamycin*	Garaycin	1 mg/kg q 8 h	IM, IV
Kanamycin	Kantrex, Klebcil	15 mg/kg/day	IM
		1 g q 4-6 h	Oral
Neomycin	Mycifradin,	15 mg/kg/day in 4 doses	IM
	Neobiotic	1 g q 4-6 h	Oral
Netilmicin	Neo-IM, Netromycin	3-6.5 mg/kg/day	IM, IV
Paromomycin	Humatin	10 mg/kg q 8 h	Oral
Streptomycin		1-4 g/day	IM
Tobramycin*	Nebcin	1 mg/kg q 8 h	IM, IV

*Also available in cream, ointment and solution forms for ophthalmic and topical use.

BUN or creatinine levels. The renal damage may be reversible. The drugs are toxic to the eighth cranial nerve, causing both auditory and vestibular damage. The damage may appear as high-frequency hearing loss, tinnitus, or vertigo. Onset of deafness may occur several weeks after administration has been stopped and may be irreversible. High doses may be neurotoxic and exhibit a neuromuscular blocking effect.

Pharmacokinetics: Oral forms are not significantly absorbed, whereas absorption is rapid and complete following IM administration. Excretion of the unchanged drug is through the kidney and is markedly reduced in the presence of decreased renal function.

Interactions: The potential for ototoxicity or nephrotoxicity is enhanced when administered with other aminoglycosides or other nephrotoxic agents, such as amphotericin B, bumetanide, cephalosporins, cyclosporin, ethacrynic acid, furosemide, and vancomycin.

Nursing considerations: Doses should be reduced in patients with reduced renal function or in the elderly. Assessment of renal function and hearing and vestibular function should be done before and during high-dose or long-term therapy (>10 days). IV administration should be over a period of 30 to 60 minutes to reduce the possibility of toxic serum levels. Patients should be well-hydrated and instructed to report any hearing loss, tinnitus, or dizziness. Peak and trough serum drug levels should be monitored.

Spectinomycin

Spectinomycin (Trobicin) is an aminocyclitol antibiotic related to the aminoglycosides. Its antibacterial action results from inhibition of protein synthesis. The drug is indicated only for treatment of gonorrheal infections using a single IM dose of 2 to 4 g. The dose should be administered deep in the gluteal muscle (2 g at each in-

jection site). Pain at the injection site, and occasionally fever, chills, urticaria, or nausea may occur.

Vancomycin

Vancomycin inhibits bacterial cell wall synthesis.

Indications: Parenteral forms used in the treatment of serious staphylococcal infection or endocarditis not responsive to other antibiotic treatment. Oral therapy is used in the treatment of staphylococcal enterocolitis and antibiotic-associated pseudomembranous colitis from *Clostridium difficile*. Vancomycin is increasingly being used for the treatment of infections attributable to penicillinase strains of staphylococci.

Usual dosage: Vancomycin (Vancocin) 500 mg every 6 hours, over at least 60 minutes when administered IV, or given orally.

Precautions/contraindications: IM administration is not used because pain and necrosis may result. Reduced doses are needed in the presence of renal impairment.

Side effects/adverse reactions: Thrombophlebitis and pain may occur following IV administration. If IV administration is too rapid, a sudden fall in blood pressure—with or without development of a rash over the face, neck, chest, and upper extremities—may occur. This is not an allergic reaction but is most likely the result of histamine release and resolves after administration is completed. Nephrotoxicity and ototoxicity may occur similar to the aminoglycoside antibiotics.

Pharmacokinetics: Oral doses are very poorly absorbed.

Interactions: There is an increased chance of nephrotoxicity if administered with other nephrotoxic antibiotics.

Nursing considerations: The IV dose should be given over 1 to 2 hours in a dilute solution of at least 100 ml fluid for each 500 mg. Renal and auditory function should be monitored, especially in patients over 60 years or in patients with already impaired renal function. Monitor blood pressure closely during IV infusion. Serum levels should be monitored and dosages adjusted accordingly.

Fluoroquinolones

Ciprofloxacin and norfloxacin are synthetic broad-spectrum antibacterial agents. They work through inhibition of protein synthesis.

Indications: Because of poor bioavailability and low serum concentrations, norfloxacin is approved only for treatment of urinary tract infections. Ciprofloxacin is indicated for both urinary and systemic infections.

Usual dosage: Norfloxacin (Noroxin), 400 mg every 12 hours. Ciprofloxacin (Cipro) 250 to 750 mg every 12 hours. Both drugs are only administered orally.

Precautions/contraindications: Use with caution in patients with known or suspected CNS disorders or with a predisposition to seizures. Reduced dosages may be needed in patients with diminished renal function.

Side effects/adverse reactions: CNS stimulation, including tremors, restlessness, light-headedness, and seizures, may occur with use of ciprofloxacin. Nausea, vomiting, or diarrhea may occur with use of either drug.

Pharmacokinetics: Both drugs are well-absorbed and eliminated primarily through the kidney, with an increased half-life in the presence of decreased renal function. Food may decrease the absorption of norfloxacin. The rate of absorption of ciprofloxacin is delayed by the presence of food in the stomach, but the overall absorption is not altered.

Interactions: Antacids containing magnesium or aluminum hydroxide may interfere with ciprofloxacin absorption. Theophylline levels may be increased because of reduced theophylline clearance in patients taking fluoroquinolones.

Nursing considerations: Norfloxacin tablets should be taken 1 hour before or 2 hours after meals. Ciprofloxacin may be taken with or without meals. Patients should be well-hydrated. Patients taking theophylline should be monitored for signs of toxic effects and have serum theophylline levels monitored.

Metronidazole

Metronidazole is effective against a variety of anaerobic bacteria and protozoa. It works by interfering with protein synthesis.

Indications: Anaerobic infections, prophylaxis during colorectal surgery, antibiotic-associated pseudomembranous colitis, amebiasis, and trichomoniasis.

Usual dosage: For metronidazole (Flagyl, Metryl, Satric) the oral dose is 500 to 750 milligrams 3 or 4 times daily, the parenteral dose is 7.5 mg/kg every 6 hours.

Precautions/contraindications: Reduced doses may be needed in patients with liver disease.

Side effects/adverse reactions: Nausea, anorexia, vomiting, diarrhea, and other GI disturbances, as well as dry mouth and a "metallic" taste, are common side effects. Nausea and vomiting may occur if alcohol is consumed while the drug is in the body (Antabuse reaction). Darkened urine may occur, which is of no clinical significance. High cumulative doses have been associated with seizures or peripheral neuropathy. Pseudomembranous colitis may occur.

Pharmacokinetics: Food intake delays but does alter total absorption. Elimination is primarily through the kidneys.

Interactions: Metronidazole may potentiate oral anticoagulants. Concurrent use with phenobarbital and phenytoin may increase metabolism of metronidazole and reduce effectiveness unless the dosage is increased.

Nursing considerations: Administering the oral form with meals may reduce GI disturbances. Monitor for signs of nervous system toxicity, particularly dizziness, vertigo, incoordination, confusion, weakness, or numbness or paresthesia of an extremity. Warn patients not to consume alcohol.

Sulfonamides and Trimethoprim
Sulfonamides

The sulfonamides are bacteriostatic drugs. They competitively antagonize para-aminobenzoic acid (PABA), which is essential for folic acid synthesis. Microorganisms that require endogenous folic acid are therefore susceptible to the sulfonamides.

Indications: The sulfonamides have a broad spectrum of activity; however, they are most often used in the treatment of urinary tract infections or in topical preparations.

Usual dosage: Varies (Table 15-7).

Precautions/contraindications: In patients with porphyria, these drugs may precipitate an attack. Photosensitivity can occur.

Side effects/adverse reactions: Nausea, vomiting, abdominal pain, photosensitivity, rashes, pruritus, and exfolaitive dermatitis can occur. Cross-sensitivity can occur in patients sensitive to carbonic anhydrase inhibitors, thiazides, furosemide, bumetanide, and the sulfonylurea hypoglycemic agents. Sulfonamides can cause blood disorders, including anemia, granulocytopenia, and thrombocytopenia. The drugs can rarely precipitate in the urine, causing crystalluria, hematuria, or obstruction.

Pharmacokinetics: Sulfonamides are readily absorbed from the GI tract and eliminated mainly through the kidneys.

Table 15-7

SULFONAMIDES AND TRIMETHOPRIM

Generic name	Trade names	Dosage range	Administration
Sulfadiazine	Microsulfon	2-4 g/day in 3-6 doses	Oral
Sulfacytine	Renoquid	250 mg q 6 h	Oral
Sulfisoxazole	Gantrisin	4-8 g/day in 4-6 doses	Oral
		100 mg/kg/day in 2-4 doses	SC, IM, IV
Sulfamethoxazole	Gantanol Urobak	1 g twice daily	Oral
Sulfamethizole	Proklar	0.5-1 g 3-4 times/day	Oral
Multiple sulfonamides*			
Trisulfapyrimidines	Triple Sulfa Neotrizine Terfonyl	2-4 g/day in 3-6 doses	Oral
Trimethoprim	Proloprim Trimpex	200 mg/day	Oral
Trimethoprim/ Sulfamethoxazole (SMZ)	Bactrim TMP-SMZ Comoxol Cotrim Sulfatrim Septra	80 mg TMP/400 mg SMZ to 160 mg TMP/ 800 mg SMZ q 12 h	IV, Oral

*Multiple sulfonamides provide the same therapeutic effect as the total sulfonamide content but reduces the risk of precipitation in the kidneys.

Interactions: Sulfonamides may displace highly-protein-bound drugs, such as oral anticoagulants, anticonvulsants, and oral antidiabetic agents, from protein binding sites, resulting in higher serum levels and increased therapeutic effects. There is increased potential for toxic effects when administered with hepatotoxic or bone marrow-suppressing drugs.

Nursing considerations: Instruct the patient to take each dose on an empty stomach with a large glass of water. If GI upset occurs, instruct the patient to take the drug with food. To minimize precipitation in urine, encourage patients to drink large amounts of liquids. Caution patients to avoid or minimize exposure to sunlight and to use sun screens when outside.

Trimethoprim

Trimethoprim blocks the production of folic acid at a site different from that of the sulfonamides.
Indications: Treatment of urinary tract infections.
Usual dosage: Varies (Table 15-7).
Precautions/contraindications: Use with caution in patients with renal or hepatic impairment.
Side effects/adverse reactions: Rash, pruritus, exfoliative dermatitis, and GI disturbances can occur. Trimethoprim rarely causes bone marrow depression, which is usually associated with large doses or prolonged administration.

Pharmacokinetics: Well-absorbed after oral administration, with primary elimination through the kidneys.
Interactions: May increase the effect of phenytoin because of inhibition of metabolism.
Nursing considerations: The tablets should be protected from light.

Trimethoprim/Sulfamethoxazole

The combination of trimethoprim and sulfamethoxazole results in a dual block of folate synthesis, which provides a synergistic effect with increased activity and antibacterial spectrum. The drug combination is used primarily to treat urinary tract infections and otitis media in children. See individual drugs for profile and nursing considerations. The IV form should be administered over 60 to 90 minutes and must be diluted and used within 2 hours of mixing.

URINARY ANTIBACTERIALS
Cinoxacin

Cinoxacin is a synthetic organic acid related to nalidixic acid, which inhibits replication of bacterial DNA.
Indications: Treatment of urinary tract infections caused by susceptible organisms.
Usual dosage: Varies (Table 15-8).

Table 15-8

URINARY ANTIBACTERIALS

Generic name	Trade names	Dosage range	Administration
Cinoxacin	Cinobac	1 g/day in 2-4 divided doses	Oral
Methenamine			
Hippurate	Hiprex, Urex	1 g 2 times/day	Oral
Mandelate	Mandameth Mandelamine	1 g 4 times/day	Oral
Nalidixic acid		1 g 4 times/day	Oral
Nitrofurantoin	Furadantin Furan Macrodantin Nitrofan	50-100 mg 4 times/day	Oral
Norfloxacin	Noroxin	400 mg q 12 h	Oral

Precautions/contraindications: Toxicity may occur in patients with reduced renal function as a result of decreased renal elimination and increased serum drug levels.

Side effects/adverse reactions: Most common side effects involve GI or genitourinary (GU) disturbances, including nausea, vomiting, diarrhea, abdominal cramps, and perineal burning.

Pharmacokinetics: Cinoxacin is completely absorbed following oral administration. The drug is partially metabolized in the liver, with the metabolites and remaining active drug eliminated in the urine.

Interactions: Probenecid will reduce renal elimination of cinoxacin, which decreases the urine concentration and increases the systemic levels.

Nursing considerations: Caution the patient that the drug may cause dizziness or cause the eyes to be more photosensitive.

Methenamine

Methenamine is hydrolyzed to ammonia and formaldehyde, which is bactericidal. However, the drug does not release formaldehyde in the serum. Methenamine is available as acid salts (mandelate and hippurate) to promote a low urinary pH.

Indications: Suppression or elimination of bacterial urinary tract infections.

Usual dosage: Varies (Table 15-8).

Precautions/contraindications: Do not administer to patients with severe renal failure or dehydration. Not for use in liver disease because the drug promotes ammonia production.

Side effects/adverse reactions: Large doses can cause bladder irritation. Other adverse effects include GI symptoms, stomatitis, and rash.

Pharmacokinetics: Methenamine and related salts are readily absorbed from the GI tract, with up to 25% sub-

ject to hepatic metabolism. Generation of urinary formaldehyde depends on urinary pH and volume and the duration of urine retention in the bladder.

Interactions: Drugs that will increase the urinary pH (e.g., bicarbonate and acetazolamide) will reduce effectiveness.

Nursing considerations: Administer with food to minimize GI upset and encourage fluids to ensure adequate urine flow. Have the patient avoid or limit alkanizing foods, such as citrus fruits and milk products.

Nalidixic acid

Nalidixic acid is similar to cinoxacin but may produce more GI effects. See the discussion of cinoxacin for a more complete presentation.

Nitrofurantoin

This drug interferes with bacterial carbohydrate metabolism and may also disrupt cell wall synthesis. The action of nitrofurantoin is increased in an acid pH.

Indications: Treatment of urinary tract infections of susceptible bacteria.

Usual dosage: Varies (Table 15-8).

Precautions/contraindications: Renal impairment (creatinine clearance <40 ml/min), anuria, or oliguria reduce effectiveness of treatment and greatly increase toxicity.

Side effects/adverse reactions: Fever, rash, eosinophilia, and pulmonary infiltrates can occur. Pulmonary reactions may be acute or chronic and are manifested by dyspnea, chest pain, cough, fever, and chills. The pulmonary damages may be reversible or permanent. Hemolysis can occur in patients with a glucose 6-phosphate dehydrogenase (G-6-PD) deficiency.

Pharmacokinetics: The drug is well-absorbed following oral administration. When administered with meals, absorption is enhanced. Nitrofurantoin and its metabo-

Table 15-9

SYSTEMIC ANTIFUNGAL DRUGS

Generic name	Trade names	Dosage range	Administration
Amphotericin B	Fungizone	0.25-1.5 mg/kg/day	IV
Fluconazole	Diflucan	100-200 mg/day	IV, Oral
Fluctyosine	Ancobon	50-150 mg/kg/day in 4 divided doses	Oral
Griseofulvin	Fulvicin Grifulvin Grisactin	0.5-1 g microsize or 0.33-0.75 g ultramicrosize	Oral
Ketoconazole	Nizoral	200-400 mg once a day	Oral
Miconazole	Monostat IV	200-3,600 mg/day in 3 divided doses	IV
		20 mg	Intrathecal
		200 mg	Intrabladder
Nystatin	Mycostatin	500,000-1,000,000 U 3 times/day	Oral

lites are excreted into the urine, where therapeutic levels are achieved. Serum and tissue levels do not reach therapeutic levels following oral administration in patients with normal renal function.

Interactions: Probenecid can reduce renal clearance and increase serum levels, possibly to toxic levels.

Nursing considerations: Administer the medication with meals to improve absorption and minimize GI disturbances. Monitor the patient for signs of pulmonary changes and instruct them to report the development of any symptoms to their physician.

Norfloxacin

See fluoroquinolone antimicrobials, page 314.

ANTIFUNGAL DRUGS

Most fungi are resistant to the action of antibacterial drugs, whereas antifungal drugs generally have no effect on bacteria. Topical infections should be treated locally rather than with systemic therapy, which is associated with numerous adverse effects. The antifungal drugs available for systemic therapy are limited in both number and effectiveness. Therapy must continue for several weeks or months to prevent a recurrence of the infection. See Table 15-9 for dosage ranges for specific agents.

Amphotericin B

Amphotericin B, although highly toxic, is the most effective drug for treatment of systemic fungal infections. It is not absorbed following oral administration and must be given intravenously. Following IV administration, chills, fever, vomiting, and headache commonly occur. Aspirin, phenothiazines, antihistamines, antiemetics, and corticosteroids may be used to minimize or treat the adverse effects. The drug may impair renal

and hepatic function and produce anemia. Hypotension, electrolyte imbalances (especially hypokalemia), and occasionally neurologic symptoms accompany therapy. The toxic effects are usually reversible following discontinuance of drug therapy. The drug is administered as an IV infusion over 2 to 6 hours. Rapid infusion is not recommended.

Flucytosine

Flucytosine is effective against strains of *Candida* or *Cryptococcus*. The drug is well-absorbed following oral administration and is excreted in the urine. Drug accumulation may occur in patients who have diminished renal function, and dosages should be reduced in these patients. Before initiation of therapy, renal and hematologic status should be evaluated. The possibility that bone marrow depression can occur necessitates monitoring of marrow function during therapy. Other adverse reactions include GI disturbances, rash, and elevation of serum liver enzymes, BUN, and creatinine levels. To avoid nausea or vomiting, advise the patient to take the capsules over 15 minutes rather than all at once.

Griseofulvin

Griseofulvin is ineffective in *Candida* infections but is effective against *Microsporum, Epidermophyton* and *Trichophyton* infections. The drug is most commonly used for treatment of ringworm infections of the skin, hair, and nails. Serum levels may be increased by giving the medication with a meal of high-fat content. Side effects include headaches; rashes; GI disturbances; and, with long-term therapy, alterations in renal, hepatic, and hematopoietic function. The activity of oral anticoagulants is decreased. The drug may potentiate the effects of alcohol. Patients should be cautioned to minimize exposure to sunlight because photosensitivity may occur.

Ketoconazole

Ketoconazole is the first antifungal drug effective against systemic infections when administered orally and is generally well-tolerated. The drug is effective against a broad spectrum of fungi with less toxicity than amphotericin B. Side effects include GI disturbances and skin rashes. Ketoconazole blocks synthesis of adrenal steroids and androgens, which may lead to gynecomastia. High doses may cause liver dysfunction. An acid environment is needed for dissolution and absorption. Administration with food may minimize GI disturbances. Antacids and H_2 blockers should be given at least 2 hours after administration to avoid reduction in oral absorption. The patient should be instructed to notify the physician if signs of liver dysfunction (e.g., anorexia, jaundice, dark urine, and pale stools) occur. Nausea and vomiting may occur if alcohol is consumed while the drug is in the body (Antabuse reaction).

Miconazole

A variety of fungi are susceptible to miconazole; however, frequent side effects are seen. Side effects, including thrombophlebitis, rash, pruritus, nausea, vomiting, diarrhea, febrile reactions, anemia, thrombosytosis, hyponatremia, CNS toxicity, and hypersensitivity reactions occur. The drug may be antagonistic to the antifungal effects of amphotericin B. The effects of oral anticoagulants are enhanced when given concomitantly with miconazole. IV treatment should begin in a hospital with frequent monitoring of electrolyte, hematocrit, and lipids levels. The IV dose should be diluted with at least 200 ml of fluid and infused over 30 to 60 minutes.

Nystatin

Limited absorption, with no detectable blood levels following oral administration, makes nystatin useful in the treatment of oral, GI, or perineal infections. The drug is not useful for systemic infections. Nystatin is generally nontoxic and nonirritating, with few allergic reactions occurring.

ANTIVIRAL DRUGS

Because viruses are intracellular parasites, the drug treatment of viral infections is very difficult. The goal of drug therapy is to have the greatest effect on the virus-infected cells with minimal effect on other cells. Amantadine works by inhibiting penetration of the virus into cells, and the other antiviral drugs discussed inhibit intracellular synthesis.

Amantadine

Amantadine can be administered orally and is beneficial in institutional environments and high-risk groups.

Indications: Amantadine is used prophylactically for influenza A. Occasionally amantadine is used for short-term therapy of parkinsonism, in which it may influence the dopaminergic system.

Usual dosage: Varies (Table 15-10).

Precautions/contraindications: Reduced doses may be needed in patients with renal insufficiency and patients over 65 years. Use with caution in patients with seizure disorders.

Side effects/adverse reactions: Side effects include a variety of CNS effects, including headache, dizziness, insomnia, and convulsions. Nausea, vomiting, and anorexia can also occur.

Pharmacokinetics: The drug is readily absorbed from the GI tract. It is not metabolized and is eliminated through the kidneys.

Interactions: Atropine-like effects may occur rarely when anticholinergic drugs are used concurrently.

Nursing considerations: Amantadine is used only for prophylaxis. Use for 2 to 3 days before and 6 to 7 days after influenza A infection reduces the duration and severity of symptoms. There may be some therapeutic effect if administered within 18 hours of the onset of symptoms. Advise patients to use caution while driving or performing other tasks requiring mental alertness, since the drug can cause CNS effects, including blurred vision.

Acyclovir

Acyclovir has been shown to reduce the frequency, duration and severity of initial and recurrent herpes infections. It does not eliminate the infection. The drug should not be used for suppression of recurrent disease in individuals with mild symptoms.

Indications: Treatment of herpes simplex virus type 1 and 2, and vericella zoster (shingles) infections.

Usual dosage: Varies (Table 15-10).

Precautions/contraindications: When administered by rapid administration, acyclovir crystals can develop in the renal tubules.

Side effects/adverse reactions: Nausea, vomiting, diarrhea, headache, dizziness, fatigue, and rash may occur.

Pharmacokinetics: Absorption of oral acyclovir is slow and incomplete. Elimination is through the kidneys.

Interactions: Zidovudine and acyclovir administered together may result in severe drowsiness and lethargy.

Nursing considerations: Treatment may not reduce shedding of the virus. Caution patients to avoid sexual intercourse when visible herpes lesions are present because of the risk of infecting intimate partners. Avoid rapid bolus injections by infusing over at least 1 hour to reduce renal damage. Encourage fluids and ensure adequate hydration to prevent drug precipitation in the renal tubules following IV administration.

Table 15-10

ANTIVIRAL DRUGS

Generic name	Trade names	Dosage range	Administration
Amantadine	Symmetrel Symadine	200 mg/day in 1 or 2 doses	Oral
Acyclovir	Zorivax	200 mg q 4 h, 5 times/day	Oral
		5-10 mg/kg q 8 h	IV
Ganciclovir	Cytovene	5-6 mg/kg/day	IV
Ribavirin	Virazole	190 µg/L of air for 12-18 h/day	aerosol
Vidarabine	Vira-A	10-15 mg/kg/d infused over 12-24 h	IV
Zidovudine (azidothymidine [AZT])	Retrovir	100-200 mg q 4 h	Oral
		1-2 mg/kg q 4 h	IV

Ganciclovir

Subclinical or latent cytomegalovirus (CMV) infection is common. When the patient is immunocompromised, as are chemotherapy or transplant patients or those who have AIDS, activation and dissemination of the infection is common. Ganciclovir enters cells infected with CMV and inhibits replication. The dosage and duration of therapy with ganciclovir is limited by its potent toxicity and side effects.

Indications: Cytomegalovirus infection in immunocompromised patients.

Usual dosage: Varies (Table 15-10).

Precautions/contraindications: Toxicity is increased in renal insufficiency.

Side effects/adverse reactions: Granulocytopenia, thrombocytopenia, renal impairment, fever, rash, and abnormal liver function test can occur.

Pharmacokinetics: Ganciclovir is eliminated through the kidneys and is not metabolized.

Interactions: There is increased toxicity when administered with other cytotoxic drugs.

Nursing considerations: The IV dose should be administered over 1 hour. Neutrophil and platelet counts should be monitored every 2 days initially and reduced to every week with continued therapy.

Ribavirin

Respiratory syncytial virus (RSV) infections are inhibited by ribavirin. The mechanism of the inhibitory action is not known.

Indications: Treatment of hospitalized infants and children with severe respiratory infections attributable to RSV.

Usual dosage: Varies (Table 15-10).

Precautions/contraindications: The drug should be used only in patients when the infection is severe enough to require hospitalization. Because the drug may accumulate in respiratory equipment and interfere with effective ventilation, it should not be used in patients requiring mechanical ventilation.

Side effects/adverse reactions: Rash, conjunctivitis, or worsening of respiratory status can occur.

Pharmacokinetics: Ribavirin, administered by aerosol, is absorbed through the respiratory tract. Accumulation, metabolism, or excretion following inhalation is not well-understood.

Interactions: None reported.

Nursing considerations: Infants and children with severe RSV infections require close monitoring of respiratory and fluid status. Closely follow manufacturer's guidelines for aerosol administration. The drug may precipitate or accumulate in ventilation apparatus, leading to respiratory difficulties.

Vidarabine

The antiviral mechanism of vidarabine has not been established, however, it is one of the least toxic of the antiviral agents. As with most antiviral drugs, therapy is not curative but aims at reducing the duration and severity of symptoms. The drug is most effective when used as early in the infection as possible, especially if used within 72 hours after the appearance of vesicular lesions.

Indications: Severe systemic herpes simplex infections and herpes zoster in immunosuppressed patients.

Usual dosage: Varies (Table 15-10).

Precautions/contraindications: Patients with renal impairment may need reduced dosages. Because of the large amount of fluid required with IV administration, fluid overload is possible in patients with cerebral edema or renal impairment.

Side effects/adverse reactions: GI disturbances occur but seldom are severe enough to stop therapy. Depression of blood cell formation can occur during therapy. CNS symptoms, including tremor, headache, hallucinations, confusion, and ataxia can occur.

Pharmacokinetics: Vidarabine is eliminated through the kidneys, mostly as active metabolites. The metabolite can accumulate in patients with reduced renal function.

Interactions: Allopurinol may interfere with vidarabine metabolism.

Nursing considerations: Monitoring of CBC is necessary during therapy. The total daily dose should be slowly infused over 12 to 24 hours. The drug has very low solubility. IV fluid for infusion may be prewarmed to aid in dissolving the drug, and an in-line membrane filter is necessary during infusion.

Zidovudine

Zidovudine has shown some promise in slowing the onset of Acquired Immunodeficiency Syndrome (AIDS) and AIDS-related complex (ARC). The drug has only been studied for a limited period of time. The full safety and efficacy of zidovudine has not been completely established.

Indications: Management of patients with HIV infection who have some evidence of impaired immunity.

Usual dosage: Varies (Table 15-10).

Precautions/contraindications: There is no data available on patients with impaired renal or hepatic function being treated with zidovudine but they may be at increased risk or need dosage adjustments. Use caution in patients with preexisting bone marrow suppression.

Side effects/adverse reactions: The most common adverse reaction to zidovudine is granulocytopenia and anemia, which may require transfusions or dosage modification. Headache, GI disturbances, insomnia, myalgias, and CNS symptoms are among the many undesirable effects that may occur during therapy.

Pharmacokinetics: Zidovudine is well-absorbed orally and metabolized in the liver, with renal elimination of the drug and metabolites.

Interactions: Administration with other cytotoxic, nephrotoxic, hepatotoxic, or bone marrow-suppressing drugs may increase the toxicity of zidovudine.

Nursing considerations: The patient's blood count should be closely monitored. Warn patients that the use of other medication may increase toxicity. The medication must be taken every 4 hours around-the-clock, even if it means disrupting sleep. Patients should be closely monitored for development of opportunistic infections or other complications of AIDS and ARC that may develop during therapy.

ANTIMALARIAL DRUGS

The use of antimalarial drugs varies with the type of malaria, drug resistance of the organisms, and whether suppression of symptoms or cure of disease is the goal. Specific antimalarial regimens are presented in Chapter 10 with the discussion of malaria.

Mefloquine

Mefloquine is a structural analog of quinine that acts as a blood schizonticide. The mechanism of action is not known.

Indications: Treatment of acute malaria infection caused by susceptible strains of *Plasmodium falciparum* and *P. vivax* and prophylaxis of *P. falciparum* and *P. vivax* malaria.

Usual dosage: Varies (Table 15-11 and Chapter 10).

Precautions/contraindications: Do not use concurrently with quinine or quinidine because ECG abnormalities or cardiac arrest may occur. Use caution when performing hazardous tasks or driving because dizziness and impaired balance can occur. In doses used to treat malaria, adverse reactions to the drug may not be distinguishable from symptoms of the disease itself.

Side effects/adverse reactions: Dizziness, myalgia, nausea, fever, vomiting, chills, diarrhea, rash, abdominal pain, and fatigue can all occur during therapy.

Pharmacokinetics: Mefloquine is highly protein bound and is concentrated on erythrocytes, the target cells in malaria. The drug has a long elimination half-life of about 3 weeks.

Interactions: Cardiac arrest or ECG abnormalities may occur during concurrent therapy with beta-adrenergic blockers. The risk of seizures is increased when combined with chloroquine treatment. Concomitant use with quinine or quinidine may lead to ECG abnormalities or cardiac arrest.

Nursing considerations: Do not administer on an empty stomach. Administer at least 8 ounces of water with the dose.

Quinine Sulfate

Quinine was at one time the only agent available for the treatment of malaria. Newer agents are now available that are more effective and less toxic.

Indications: Quinine is used as an adjunct in the treatment of chloroquine-resistant malaria and in the treatment of nocturnal recumbency leg cramps.

Usual dosage: Varies (Table 15-11 and Chapter 10).

Precautions/contraindications: Use cautiously in patients with cardiac disease. Quinine is related to the antiarrhythmic drug quinidine and may be arrhythmogenic. Do not administer to patients with a deficiency of G-6-PD, since hemolysis can result. (The enzyme deficiency is a sex-linked genetic disease found in dark-skinned people and those of Mediterranean descent.)

Side effects/adverse reactions: Repeated or high doses

Table 15-11

ANTIMALARIAL DRUGS

Generic name	Trade names	Dosage range	Administration
Mefloquine	Lariam	1250 mg in a single dose (treatment) 250 mg once/wk (prophylaxis)	Oral
Quinine sulfate	Quine, Qunite, Strema	650 mg q 8 h	Oral
Quinacrine	Atabrine	200 mg q 6 h for 5 doses then 100 mg 3 times/day (treatment) 100 mg/day (suppression)	Oral
4-aminoquinoline compounds			
Chloroquine phosphate	Aralen	300 mg/wk	Oral
Chloroquine HCL	Aralen HCL	160-200 mg, may be repeated in 6 h	IM
Hydroxychloroquine sulfate	Plaquenil Sulfate	310 mg/wk	
Primaquine phosphate		26.3 mg daily or 79 mg once/wk	Oral
Pyrimethamine	Daraprim	25 mg/wk	Oral
Sulfadoxine and pyrimethamine	Fansidar	2-3 tablets (acute attack) 1 tablet/wk or 2 tablets q 2 wks (prophylaxis)	Oral

can cause cinchonism (e.g., tinnitus, headache, nausea, and visual disturbances). Hemolysis can occur in patients with a G-6-PD deficiency. Hypersensitivity reactions, including rash, pruritus, flushing, edema, and asthma.
Pharmacokinetics: Quinine is rapidly and almost completely absorbed following oral administration and is metabolized in the liver.
Interactions: Aluminum-containing antacids may reduce or delay absorption of quinine. Oral anticoagulants may have increased effects. Quinine may increase the plasma levels of digoxin.
Nursing considerations: Administer with meals or food to minimize GI disturbances. Observe for symptoms of cinchonism.

Quinacrine

Quinacrine combines with DNA and interferes with its ability to replicate. The drug produces both suppressive and therapeutic action against malaria.
Indications: Malaria treatment and suppression. Treatment of giardiasis and cestodiasis.
Usual dosage: Varies (Table 15-11 and Chapter 10).
Precautions/contraindications: Use in patients with psoriasis or porphyria may precipitate a severe attack. Use with promaquine is contraindicated because of increased toxicity.
Side effects/adverse reactions: Blood abnormalities, visual disturbances, headache, dizziness, and GI and neuropsychiatric disturbances can occur.
Pharmacokinetics: The metabolism of quinacrine is un-

known. The half-life is about 5 days, and the drug tends to accumulate (increasing the risk of toxic effects) during long-term therapy.
Interactions: Nausea and vomiting may occur if alcohol is consumed while the drug is in the body.
Nursing considerations: Administer after meals with a full glass of water. Warn the patient that the drug may give the skin or urine a yellowish color that will leave when the drug is discontinued. When using high doses for treatment, administer the first five 200-mg doses with 1 g sodium bicarbonate.

4-Aminoquinoline Compounds

Chloroqine phosphate, chloroquine hydrochloride and hydroxychloroqine sulfate compose the 4-aminoquinolone compounds. The compounds interfere with DNA and protein synthesis.
Indications: Suppression and relief of *Plasmodium* species malaria. Chloroqine phosphate and chloroquine hydrochloride are also used for treatment of extraintestinal amebiasis.
Usual dosage: Varies (Table 15-11 and Chapter 10).
Precautions/contraindications: Irreversible retinopathy has occurred with long-term or high-dose therapy. Use in patients with psoriasis or porphyria may precipitate a severe attack.
Side effects/adverse reactions: GI disturbances, hypotension, headache, and blood abnormalities. Hemolysis may occur in patients with G-6-PD deficiency.
Pharmacokinetics: The drug is absorbed readily from the GI tract and persists in the body for a prolonged

period. Elimination is through the kidneys and is enhanced with urinary acidification.

Interactions: Kaolin or magnesium trisilicate may decrease absorption of 4-aminoquinoline compounds.

Nursing considerations: Monitor CBCs during prolonged therapy and administer with food to minimize GI disturbances. Side and adverse effects are most common with acute high-dose treatment. Suppression therapy is generally well-tolerated. It is not effective against resistant strains of *P. falciparum*. Weekly doses should be administered on the same day each week.

Primaquine Phosphate

Primaquine is structurally similar to the 4-aminoquinoline compounds but has different antimalarial actions.

Indications: The drug is used in the cure and prevention of *P. vivax* malaria.

Usual dosage: Varies (Table 15-11 and Chapter 10).

Precautions/contraindications: Do not administer with quinacrine. Hemolytic reactions may occur in patients deficient in G-6-PD.

Side effects/adverse reactions: GI disturbances can occur.

Pharmacokinetics: Rapidly absorbed, with a plasma half-life of about 7 hours.

Interactions: May potentiate toxicity of quinacrine.

Nursing considerations: Administer with food to minimize GI upset.

Pyrimethamine

Pyrimethamine is a folic acid antagonist. The drug is useful in malaria prophylaxis but is not recommended for treatment of acute attacks.

Indications: Prophylaxis of malaria attributable to susceptible strains of plasmodia and to toxoplasmosis.

Usual dosage: Varies (Table 15-11 and Chapter 10).

Precautions/contraindications: May precipitate hemolysis in the patient with G-6-DP deficiency.

Side effects/adverse reactions: Large doses may produce nausea, anorexia, vomiting, and blood abnormalities.

Pharmacokinetics: Absorption is good after oral administration. The half-life is several days, with suppressive concentrations sustained for approximately 2 weeks.

Interactions: None reported.

Nursing considerations: There is a wide variation in tolerance between individuals. Administer with food to minimize GI upset.

Sulfadoxine and Pyrimethamine

The combination of pyrimethamine with sulfadoxine produces a synergistic effect. Use of the combination results in a block of folic acid synthesis at two sequential steps. Severe reactions, including Stevens-Johnson syndrome and toxic epidermal necrolysis have oc-

curred. Information provided for each drug used individually applies to the combination.

A MEBICIDAL DRUGS

Amebicidal drugs may affect amoeba in the gut (intraintestinal or luminal) or ameba that have penetrated into the body tissues (systemic or extraintestinal) or both. When treating extraintestinal infections, an intraintestinal drug should also be used because of the nature of the disease. All amebicides are administered orally except emetine.

Paromomycin

Paromomycin is an amebicidal and bacterial aminoglycoside. The drug is used to treat chronic intestinal amebiasis and as adjunct therapy in hepatic coma. The drug is very poorly absorbed from the GI tract, and large doses can cause GI disturbances. The drug profile and nursing considerations are similar to other aminoglycosides and are covered on pages 312 to 313. Doses are administered with meals for 5 to 10 days.

Iodoquinol

Iodoquinol is effective against the trophozoites and cysts of *Entamoeba histolytica* in the large intestine.

Indications: Treatment of intraintestinal amebiasis.

Usual dosage: Varies (Table 15-12).

Precautions/contraindications: Use with caution in patients with thyroid disease. Optic neuritis, optic atrophy, and peripheral neuropathy have occurred during long-term therapy.

Side effects/adverse reactions: Pruritus, diarrhea, urticaria, skin eruptions, GI disturbances, fever, chills, vertigo, and thyroid enlargement can occur.

Pharmacokinetics: The drug is very poorly absorbed from the GI tract, increasing its effectiveness against intraintestinal amebiasis.

Interactions: Interference with thyroid function tests can occur and persist for up to 6 months after therapy is stopped.

Nursing considerations: Observe and monitor closely for adverse effects, especially optic changes. Administer the drug after meals for 20 days.

Metronidazole

Metronidazole possesses both antibacterial and amebicidal activity. The mechanism of its amebicidal activity is not known. The drug has both extraintestinal and intraintestinal effectiveness and is indicated for treatment of acute amebiasis and amebicidal liver abscess. Because of a high failure rate when used alone, it is usually combined with an intraintestinal drug. The drug profile and nursing considerations are covered on pages 306 to 315 with antibiotics.

Table 15-12

AMEBICIDAL DRUGS

Generic name	Trade names	Dosage range	Administration
Paromomycin	Humatin	25-35 mg/kg/day in 3 divided doses	Oral
Iodoquinol	Yodoxin	650 mg 3 times/day	Oral
Metronidazole	Flagyl	500-750 mg 3 times/day	Oral
	Protostat		
Emetine	Emetine	1 mg/kg/day up to 65 mg/day in 1 or 2 doses	SC, IM
Chloroquine	Aralen phosphate	1 g/day for 2 days, then 500 mg/day	Oral
	Aralen HCL	200-250 mg/day	IM

Emetine

Emetine is related to ipecac and can be extremely toxic. It is used only in the hospitalized patient with fulminating dysentery, not for treatment of mild symptoms. Therapy with another amebicides is needed to ensure elimination of the infection.

Indications: Emetine is used for symptomatic management of fulminating intraintestinal amoebic dysentery and is highly effective against extraintestinal amebiasis.

Usual dosage: Varies (Table 15-12).

Precautions/contraindications: Contraindicated in children, pregnant patients, those with heart or kidney disease, or those who have had a course of emetine therapy less than 2 months previously. Discontinue use if tachycardia, hypotension, or considerable weakness appears.

Side effects/adverse reactions: Toxic reactions can occur at any dose level. Nausea and vomiting with dizziness and headache are common. Aching, tenderness, muscle stiffness, weakness, and local reactions at the site of injection are frequently seen. The most serious adverse effects involve the heart, with ECG changes (e.g., T wave inversion, prolonged QT interval, and ST elevation) occurring in all patients treated with the drug. The ECG changes first appear about 7 days into the therapy, and it may take up to 6 weeks following therapy for the ECG to return to normal.

Pharmacokinetics: The drug is slowly eliminated from the body following parenteral doses. Subcutaneous (SC) and IM doses tend to accumulate primarily in the liver but also in the spleen, kidneys, and lungs. Emetine may be excreted in the urine for up to 60 days following administration.

Interactions: None reported.

Nursing considerations: Emetine is not administered orally because it produces nausea and vomiting. IV administration is contraindicated. The preferred route of administration is in the deep SC tissue, but the IM route is also used. Emetine requires strict medical supervision in the hospital. ECG should be monitored before and during therapy. Patients should be kept on complete bed rest during and for several days following administration.

Chloroquine

Chloroquine is indicated for the treatment of extraintestinal amebiasis. The drug profile and nursing considerations are covered on pages 320 to 322 with the antimalarials.

ANTHELMINTIC DRUGS

Many of the anthelmintic drugs interfere with a worm's neuromuscular junction or energy metabolism. The anthelmintic drugs carry significant toxicity and should not be used until a clear diagnosis has been made. Most of the drugs are contraindicated for patients with intestinal obstruction and ulcers and during pregnancy. Side effects and adverse reactions following administration of the drug may be attributable to death of the worm rather than the drug itself.

Mebendazole

Mebendazole inhibits glucose uptake in susceptible worms but does not affect blood glucose levels in the host. The drug has a wide spectrum of effectiveness with little toxicity.

Indications: Effective in treatment of whipworm (*Tricuris trichiura*), pinworm (*Enterobius vermicularis*), roundworm (*Ascaris lumbricoides*), common hookworm (*Ancylostoma duoenale*), and American hookworm (*Necator americanus*).

Usual dosage: Varies (Table 15-13).

Precautions/contraindications: Teratogenic in rats; do not use in pregnant patients.

Side effects/adverse reactions: Transient abdominal pain or cramps can occur in cases of massive infection. Fever has occurred.

Table 15-13

ANTHELMINTIC DRUGS

Generic name	Trade names	Dosage range	Administration
Diethylcarbamazine	Hetrazan	2 mg 3 times/day	Oral
Mebendazole	Vermox	one tablet morning and evening	Oral
Niclosamide	Niclocide	2 g/day for up to 7 days	Oral
Oxamniquine	Vansil	12-15 mg/kg in a single dose	Oral
Piperazine		3.5 g for 2 days *or* 65 mg/kg for 7 days	Oral
Praziquantel	Biltricide	3 doses of 20-25 mg/kg, between 4-6 h apart	Oral
Pyrantel pamoate	Antiminth	11 mg/kg, single dose	Oral
Quinacrine	Atabrine	200 mg, 4 doses 10 min apart *or* 300 mg, 3 doses 20 min apart followed by 100 mg 3 times/day for 3 days	Oral
Thiabendazole	Mintezol	22 mg/kg/dose twice/day up to 1.5 g/day	Oral

Pharmacokinetics: Poorly absorbed following oral administration; excretion is in the feces.

Interactions: Carbamazepine and phenytoin may reduce the serum level and possibly decrease effectiveness.

Nursing considerations: The tablets may be swallowed, chewed, or mixed with food. A repeat course of therapy (3 days) is recommended if the patient is not cured 3 weeks following treatment. Strict hygiene is needed to limit spread or reinfection.

Diethylcarbamazine

Unlike other antiparasitic drugs, diethylcarbamazine is a synthetic compound without any toxic metallic elements. The drug is highly specific for several common parasites.

Indications: Effective in the treatment of Bancroft's filariasis, river blindness (onchocerciasis), Roundworm (ascariasis).

Usual dosage: Varies (Table 15-13).

Precautions/contraindications: Administer carefully to avoid unwanted effects.

Side effects/adverse reactions: Headache, GI disturbances, skin rash, and malaise are among the side effects reported.

Interactions: None reported.

Nursing considerations: Administer the dose following meals.

Niclosamide

Niclosamide inhibits energy metabolism in the mitochondria of the tapeworm and renders the tapeworm susceptible to destruction as it passes through the gut.

Indications: Treatment of beef tapeworm (*Taenia saginata*), fish tapeworm (*Diphyllobothrium latum*), and dwarf tapeworm (*Hymenolepis nana*).

Usual dosage: Varies (Table 15-13).

Precautions/contraindications: Safety in children under 2 years has not been established.

Side effects/adverse reactions: GI disturbances are most common. Headache, dizziness, drowsiness, skin rashes, and pruritus can also occur.

Pharmacokinetics: Not established.

Interactions: None reported.

Nursing considerations: The tablets should be thoroughly chewed before swallowing. Administering the drug with a light meal may reduce GI disturbances. Some patients may require a laxative.

Oxamniquine

Indications: Treatment of *Schistosoma mansoni* infection.

Usual dosage: Varies (Table 15-13).

Precautions/contraindications: Epileptic-like seizures have occurred in patients, usually in patients with a prior history of seizures.

Side effects/adverse reactions: CNS disturbances, including dizziness, drowsiness, headache, and rarely seizures. GI disturbances can also occur.

Pharmacokinetics: Well-absorbed following administration, with most of the dose eliminated as inactive metabolites in the urine.

Interactions: None reported.

Nursing considerations: Use in patients with a prior history of seizures should occur under close medical supervision in a setting appropriate to treat seizures. Administration with food can improve tolerance.

Piperazine

Piperazine causes flaccid paralysis of the worm.

Indications: Treatment of pinworm (enterobiasis) and roundworm (ascariasis) infections.

Usual dosage: Varies (Table 15-13).
Precautions/contraindications: Avoid prolonged or repeated administration because of the development of neurotoxicity. Contraindicated in patients with significant renal or hepatic impairment or seizure disorders.
Side effects/adverse reactions: GI disturbances are most common. Hypersensitivity reactions, headache, vertigo, tremors, and other CNS or visual symptoms can occur.
Pharmacokinetics: The drug is readily absorbed from the GI tract. About 25% of the drug is metabolized, and it is primarily eliminated through the kidneys.
Interactions: None reported.
Nursing considerations: The drug should be administered at least 1 hour before or 2 hours after meals. Because pinworm infections spread easily, all family members in close contact with the patient should also be treated. Strict hygiene and disinfection of toilets, clothes, and linens are needed to prevent reinfection.

Praziquantel

Praziquantel increases permeability of the cell membrane in susceptible worms, resulting in a loss of intracellular calcium. This leads to contractions and paralysis of the worm's musculature.
Indications: *Schistosoma mekonqi, S. japonicum, S. mansoni, S. haematobium, Clonorchis sinensis, Opisthorchis viverrini* and infections attributable to liver flukes
Usual dosage: Varies (Table 15-13).
Precautions/contraindications: The drug appears in significant concentrations in breast milk. Nursing mothers should not nurse on the day of treatment and for the following 72 hours.
Side effects/adverse reactions: Malaise, headache, dizziness, GI disturbance, and skin reactions can occur but are infrequent and usually mild.
Pharmacokinetics: About 80% of the oral dose is absorbed with significant first-pass metabolism in the liver. The inactive metabolites are excreted in the urine.
Interactions: None reported.
Nursing considerations: Warn the patient that this drug may produce drowsiness, making driving or other duties requiring attention hazardous on the day of treatment. The tablets should be swallowed quickly with liquids and not chewed.

Pyrantel pamoate

Pyrantel pamoate is a neuromuscular blocking agent that causes spastic paralysis of the worm.
Indications: Treatment of roundworm (ascariasis) and pinworm (enterobiasis) infections.
Usual dosage: Varies (Table 15-13).

Precautions/contraindications: Contraindicated in the presence of hepatic disease.
Side effects/adverse reactions: Rash, headache, and GI disturbances are infrequent side effects.
Pharmacokinetics: Poorly absorbed from the GI tract.
Interactions: Piperazine is antagonistic.
Nursing considerations: The drug may be taken without regard to food or time of day.

Quinacrine

Quinacrine is effective in treating intestinal cestodes and giardiasis. Its effects are discussed under antimalarial drugs.

Thiabendazole

Indications: Treatment of threadworm (strongyloidiasis) infection, cutaneous larva migrans, and visceral larva migrans.
Usual dosage: Varies (Table 15-13).
Precautions/contraindications: Hypersensitivity reactions may occur.
Side effects/adverse reactions: Dizziness, drowsiness, GI disturbances, and hematuria are among the many side effects that can occur. Hypersensitivity reactions, including pruritus, fever, chills, angioedema, anaphylaxis, and erythrema multiforme can occur.
Pharmacokinetics: Rapidly absorbed from the GI tract.
Interactions: The serum levels of xanthines may be increased.
Nursing considerations: Take with food to avoid stomach upset.

ANTITUBERCULAR AGENTS

Drug treatment of tuberculosis is made difficult by two factors, relatively poor blood supply to the organism and rapid development of resistance by the organism. Because of the relatively poor blood supply to the organism, therapy must continue on a long-term basis to prevent recurrence. To prevent the development of resistance, two or three drugs are often given simultaneously. Isoniazid, rifampin, and ethambutol are the three most widely used antitubercular drugs. Streptomycin is occasionally used, as are a variety of other secondary drugs. The secondary drugs are used in retreatment regimens in patients whose infection did not respond to the initial treatment. The secondary agents include pyrazinamide, aminosalicylate, ethionamide, cycloserine, and capreomycin, and are generally less effective and more toxic. If therapy lasts less than 6 months, the relapse rate is high. Most therapy must be maintained for a period of at least 12 to 24 months to achieve reliable results. Recommendations for initial treatment regimens are discussed in Chapter 7.

Table 15-14

ANTITUBERCULAR DRUGS

Generic name	Trade names	Dosage range	Administration
Isoniazid	Laniazid	5 mg/kg up to 300 mg once/day	IM, Oral
Ethambutol	Myambutol	15 mg/kg once/day	Oral
Rifampin	Rifadin	600 mg once/day	Oral
	Rimactane		
Streptomycin		1 g/day	IM

Isoniazid

Isoniazid (also called INH for isonicotinic acid hydrazide) is bactericidal by interfering with lipid and nucleic acid synthesis. The drug acts only on actively growing bacilli.

Indications: Treatment and prophylaxis of tuberculosis caused by susceptible organisms. This drug is used in nearly all treatment regimens for tuberculosis.

Usual dosage: Varies (Table 15-14).

Precautions/contraindications: Severe and occasionally fatal hepatitis has occurred in patients receiving INH. The incidence of hepatitis increases with age and in patients who consume alcohol daily.

Side effects/adverse reactions: CNS disorders (most commonly peripheral neuropathy with symmetrical numbness and tingling of extremities), rash, fever, and hepatotoxicity. Children generally tolerate the drug with fewer side effects.

Pharmacokinetics: Absorption is complete following oral administration but may be delayed by food. Metabolism occurs in the liver, with elimination through the kidneys.

Interactions: Aluminum salts (in antacid preparations) may impair absorption. Enhanced effects of oral anticoagulants, some benzodiazepines, and hydantoins can occur. Daily ingestion of alcohol has been associated with an increased incidence of hepatitis.

Nursing considerations: Liver enzymes should be monitored during therapy, and the patients should be assessed for signs of hepatotoxicity, including anorexia, nausea, malaise, and weakness. Pyridoxine (B_6) is often administered to reduce or treat peripheral neuropathies. Patients should be advised to limit intake of alcohol while taking the drug and notify their physician if they develop weakness, fatigue, nausea and vomiting, yellowing of the skin, darkened urine, or numbness and tingling in the extremities.

Ethambutol

Ethambutol diffuses into the cells of tubercle bacilli and inhibits metabolism.

Indications: Treatment of pulmonary tuberculosis in conjunction with another drug.

Usual dosage: Varies (Table 15-14).

Precautions/contraindications: Reduced doses are needed in patients with renal failure. Not recommended for children under the age of 13 years.

Side effects/adverse reactions: A reduction of visual acuity and color discrimination can occur with use of the drug. The visual changes may be unilateral or bilateral and are usually reversible if the drug is discontinued.

Pharmacokinetics: Absorption is not affected by food. About 20% of the dose is metabolized in the liver, whereas the rest is eliminated by the kidney and, to a lesser extent, in the feces.

Interactions: Aluminum salts (in antacid preparations) may reduce or delay absorption.

Nursing considerations: Administer with food to reduce GI disturbances. Visual monitoring should be carried out during therapy. Because visual changes may be unilateral, both eyes should be checked for visual acuity and color discrimination.

Rifampin

Rifampin is always used in conjunction with other agents. The drug inhibits bacterial RNA polymerase activity in susceptible organisms.

Indications: Treatment of pulmonary tuberculosis in conjunction with another drug.

Usual dosage: Varies (Table 15-14).

Precautions/contraindications: Use with caution in patients with liver impairment or in patients who are taking other hepatotoxic drugs.

Side effects/adverse reactions: A "flu-like" syndrome has occurred in 20% to 50% of patients taking high doses of the drug on an intermittent schedule, but it is not likely to occur at recommended doses. Elevations of liver enzymes and hepatitis can occur. Skin reactions, GI disturbances, and increases in BUN and serum uric acid levels can occur.

Pharmacokinetics: Well-absorbed orally; absorption is impaired by food. Metabolism occurs in the liver, with renal elimination of the metabolites. Dosage reduction may be needed in patients with severe liver disease but not in patients with renal failure.

Interactions: Rifampin induces hepatic enzymes, which increases the metabolism of many drugs and may decrease their therapeutic effect. The combination of rifampin with INH may lead to a higher incidence of hepatotoxicity.

Nursing considerations: The patient should be monitored for signs of hepatotoxicity (see Nursing Considerations for INH). The medication should be administered 1 hour before or 2 hours after meals. Rifampin may cause a reddish-brown discoloration of the urine, stool, tears, saliva, and other body fluids; patients should be warned of this effect. Permanent discoloration of contact lenses can occur.

Streptomycin

Streptomycin is an aminoglycoside drug that is effective against susceptible strains of tuberculosis. It is discussed with the other aminoglycoside drugs. When used in the treatment of tuberculosis, therapy is combined with at least one additional medication.

References

1. Association for Practitioners in Infection Control: The APIC curriculum for infection control practice, Iowa, 1981, Kendall/Hunt Publishing Co.
2. Bass J: Treatment of streptococcal pharyngitis revisited, JAMA, 256(6):740-743, 1986.
3. Benenson A editor: Control of communicable diseases in man, ed 15, Washington, DC, 1990, The American Public Health Association.
4. Bennett J and Brachman P, editors: Hospital infections, ed 2, Boston, 1986, Little, Brown.
5. Berne R and Levy M: Physiology, ed 2, St. Louis 1988, CV Mosby.
6. Bisno A: Nonsuppurative postrep tococcal sequelae: rheumatic fever and glomulonephritis. In Mandell GL, Douglas RG Jr, and Bennett JE, editors: Principles and practice of infectious diseases, ed 2, New York, 1985, John Wiley & Sons.
7. Bisno A. Streptococcal pyogenes. In Mandell GL, Douglas GL Jr, and Bennett JE, editors: Principles and practice of infectious diseases, ed 2, New York 1985, John Wiley & Sons.
8. Bolan G: Syphilis in HIV-infected persons, AIDS Clinical Care, 2(2): 9-12, 1990.
9. Bowers A and Thompson J: Clinical manual of health assessment, ed 3, St. Louis, 1988, C.V. Mosby Company.
10. Brunell P: Chickenpox. In Wehrle PF, and Top Sr FW, editors: Communicable and infectious diseases, ed 9, St. Louis, 1981, CV Mosby.
11. Brunell P: Mumps. In Wehrle PF, and Top FW Sr, editors: Communicable and infectious diseases, ed 9, St. Louis, 1981, CV Mosby.
12. Carpenito L: Nursing diagnosis: application to clinical practice, ed 2, Philadelphia, 1987, JB Lippincott.
13. Centers for Disease Control: Guidelines for prevention and control of nosocomial infection, 1981, The Center.
14. Centers for Disease Control: Sexually transmitted diseases treatment guidelines 1982, MMWR, 31(35-S), Aug 20, 1982.
15. Centers for Disease Control: CDC guideline for isolation precautions in hospitals, HHS pub. no. (CDC) 83-8314, Atlanta, 1983, The Centers.
16. Centers for Disease Control: (1984, Sept. 28). Recommendations of the Immunization Practices Advisory Committee (ACIP): adult immunization MMWR 33(1S), Sept 28, 1984.
17. Centers for Disease Control: Recommendations of the Immunization Practices Advisory Committee (ACIP): meningococcal vaccines, MMWR 34(18), May 10, 1985.
18. Centers for Disease Control: Recommendation of the immunization practices advisory committee (ACIP): diphtheria, tetanus, and pertussis—guidelines for vaccine prophylaxis and other preventive measures, MMWR 34(27), July 12, 1985.
19. Centers for Disease Control: Chlamydia, MMWR 34(38), Aug 23, 1985.
20. Centers for Disease Control: Nosocomial infection surveillance, 1984, MMWR, 35(1SS), 1986.
21. Centers for Disease Control: Acute rheumatic fever—Utah, MMWR 36(8): 108-110, 115, Mar 6, 1987.
22. Centers for Disease Control: Revision of the CDC surveillance case definition for acquired immunodeficiency syndrome, MMWR 36 (1S): 1-15S, Aug 14, 1987.
23. Centers for Disease Control: Public Health Service guidelines for counseling and antibody testing to prevent HIV Infection and AIDS, MMWR 36(31): 509-515, Aug 14, 1987.
24. Centers for Disease Control: Recommendations for prevention of HIV transmission in health-care settings, MMWR 36(2S), Aug 21, 1987.
25. Centers for Disease Control: Recommendations of the Immunization Practices Advisory Committee (ACIP), Poliomyelitis prevention: enhanced-potency inactivated poliomyelitis vaccine-supplementary statement, MMWR, 36(48): 795-798, Dec 11, 1987.
26. Centers for Disease Control: Tuberculosis, final data-United States, 1986, MMWR 36(50-51): 518-520, Jan 1, 1988.
27. Centers for Disease Control: Recommendations of the Immunization Practices Advisory Committee: update—prevention of Haemophilus influenzae type b disease, MMWR 37(2), Jan 22, 1988.
28. Centers for Disease Control: Condoms for prevention of sexually transmitted diseases, MMWR 37(9): 133-137, Mar 11, 1988.
29. Centers for Disease Control: Recommendations of the Immunization Practices advisory Committee (ACIP): immunization of children infected with human immunodeficiency virus—supplementary ACIP statement, MMWR 37(12): 181-183, April 1, 1988.
30. Centers for Disease Control: Changing patterns of groups at high risk for hepatitis B in the United States, MMWR 37(28); 429-437, July 22, 1988.
31. Centers for Disease Control: Recommendations of the Immunization Practices Advisory Committee: use of BCG vaccines in the control of tuberculosis: a joint statement by the ACIP and the Advisory Committee for Elimination of Tuberculosis, MMWR 37(43): 663-675, Nov 4, 1988.
32. Centers for Disease Control: Recommendations of the Immunization Practices Advisory Committee: pneumococcal polysaccharide vaccine, MMWR 38(5), Feb 10, 1989.
33. Centers for Disease Control: Recommendations of the Immunization Practices Advisory Committee (ACIP): general recommendations on immunization, MMWR 38(13): 205-214, 219-27, April 7, 1989.
34. Centers for Disease Control: Prevention and control of tuberculosis in correctional institutions: recommendations of the Advisory Committee for the Elimination of Tuberculosis, MMWR 38(18): 313-320, May 12, 1989.
35. Centers for Disease Control: Recommendations of the Immunization Practices Advisory Committee (ACIP): mumps prevention, MMWR 38(22): 388-392, 397-399, June 9, 1989.
36. Centers for Disease Control:

Non-A, non-B hepatitis—Illinois, MMWR 38(31): 529-531, Aug 11, 1989.

37. Centers for Disease Control: 1989 sexually transmitted diseases treatment guidelines, MMWR 38(S-8): 1-43, Sept 1, 1989.

38. Centers for Disease Control: Lyme disease—United States, 1987 and 1988. Lyme disease—Canada, MMWR 38(39): 668-672, 677-678, Oct 6, 1989.

39. Centers for Disease Control: Measles prevention: recommendations of the Immunization Practices Advisory Committee (ACIP), MMWR 38 (S-9), Dec 29, 1989.

40. Centers for Disease Control: Progress toward achieving the 1990 objectives for the nation for sexually transmitted diseases, MMWR 39(4): 53-57, Feb 2, 1990.

41. Centers for Disease Control: Protection against viral hepatitis: recommendations of the Immunization Practices Advisory Committee (ACIP), MMWR 39(RR-2): 1-26, Feb 9, 1990.

42. Centers for Disease Control: Imported dengue—United States, 1988, MMWR 39(8): 127-133, Mar 2, 1990.

43. Centers for Disease Control: Recommendations for the prevention of malaria among travelers, MMWR 39(RR-3): 1-10, Mar 9, 1990.

44. Centers for Disease Control: Recommendations of the Immunization Practices Advisory Committee: supplementary statement—change in administration schedule of Haemophilus b conjugate vaccines, MMWR 39(14): 232-233, April 13, 1990.

45. Centers for Disease Control: Viral agents of gastroenteritis: public health importance and outbreak management, MMWR 39(RR-5), April 27, 1990.

46. Centers for Disease Control: Rocky Mountain spotted fever and human ehrlichiosis—United States, 1989, MMWR 39(17): 281-284, May 4, 1990.

47. Centers for Disease Control: Recommendations of the Immunization Practices Advisory Committee: prevention and control of influenza, MMWR 39(RR-7), May 11, 1990.

48. Centers for Disease Control: Screening for tuberculosis and tuberculous infection in high-risk populations and the use of preventive therapy for tuberculous infec-tion in the United States, MMWR 39(RR-8): 1-12, May 18, 1990.

49. Centers for Disease Control: Outbreak of multidrug-resistant tuberculosis—Texas, California, and Pennsylvania, MMWR 39(22): 369-372, June 8, 1990.

50. Centers for Disease Control: Tickborne diseases—Georgia, 1989, MMWR 39(23): 397-399, June 15, 1990.

51. Centers for Disease Control: Typhoid immunization: Recommendations of the Immunization Practices Advisory Committee (ACIP), MMWR 39 (RR-10): 1-5, July 13, 1990.

52. Centers for Disease Control: Clarification: vol 39, no RR-7, MMWR 39(27): 469, July 13, 1990.

53. Centers for Disease Control: Revised dosing regimen for malaria prophylaxis with mefloquine, MMWR 39(36): 630, Sept 14, 1990.

54. Centers for Disease Control: Summary of notifiable diseases United States 1989, MMWR 38(54), Oct 5, 1990.

55. Centers for Disease Control: Vaccine adverse event reporting system—United States, MMWR 39(41): 730-733, Oct 19, 1990.

56. In Chin T: Encephalitis, infectious. Wehrle PF and Top FW Sr, editors: Communicable and infectious diseases, ed 9, St Louis, 1981, CV Mosby.

57. Chin W and Coatney O: Malaria. In Wehrle PF and Top FW Sr, editors: Communicable and infectifous diseases, ed 9, St Louis, 1981, CV Mosby.

58. Cohen P: Primary care management of HIV seropositive patients, AIDS Clinical Care 1(1): 1-4, May 1989.

59. Cohen P, Sande M, and Volberding P editors: The AIDS knowledge base, Massachusetts, 1990, Medical Publishing Group.

60. Corbett J: Laboratory tests and diagnostic procedures with nursing diagnoses, ed 2, Connecticut, 1987, Appleton & Lange.

61. Corey L: Herpes simplex virus. In Holmes D and Mardh P, editors: International perspectives on neglected sexually transmitted diseases, New York, 1983, McGraw-Hill.

62. Des Prez R and Goodwin R Jr: *Mycobacterium tuberculosis*. In Mandell GL, Douglas RG Jr, and Bennett JE, editors: Principles and practice of infectious diseases, ed 2, New York, 1985, John Wiley & Sons.

63. Doenges M, Jeffries M, and Moorhouse M: Nursing care plans, Philadelphia, 1984, FA Davis.

64. Dunkelberg W: *Gardnerella (haemophilus) vaginalis*. In Holmes D and Mardh R, editors: International perspectives on neglected sexually transmitted diseases, New York, 1983, McGraw-Hill.

65. Edwards J Jr: Candida species. In Mandell GL, Douglas RG Jr, and Bennett JE, editors: Principles and practice of infectious diseases, ed 2, New York, 1985, John Wiley & Sons.

66. Evans A: Mononucleosis. In Wehrle PF and Top FW Sr, editors: Communicable and infectious diseases, ed 9, St. Louis, 1981, CV Mosby.

67. Fauci A: The human immunodeficiency virus: infectivity and mechanisms of pathogenesis, Science 239: 617-622, Feb 1988.

68. Feldman H: Toxoplasmosis. In Wehrle PF and Top FW Sr, editors: Communicable and infectious diseases, ed 9, St. Louis, 1981, CV Mosby.

69. Flaskerud J: AIDS/HIV infection: a reference guide for nursing professionals, Philadelphia, 1989, WB Saunders.

70. Fox J, Hall C, and Elveback L: Epidemiology, man and disease, New York, 1970, Macmillan.

71. Fraser D: Legionellosis. In Wehrle PF and Top FW Sr, editors: Communicable and infectious diseases, ed 9, St. Louis, 1981, CV Mosby.

72. Friedman S: Gastrointestinal symptoms in AIDS, AIDS Clinical Care, 1(3): 17-20, July 1989.

73. Fuerst R: Frobisher & Fuersts microbiology, ed 15, Philadelphia, 1983, WB Saunders.

74. Garner J: CDC Guidelines for prevention of surgical wound infections, 1985, Infection Control 7(3): 193-200, 1986.

75. Gee G and Moran T, editors: AIDS: concepts in nursing practice, Baltimore, 1988, Williams & Wilkins.

76. Gerber M and Markowitz M: Management of streptococcal pharyngitis reconsidered, Pediatr Infect Dis 4: 518-526, 1985.

77. Gershon A: Measles virus (rubeola). In Mandell GL, Douglas RG Jr, and Bennett JE, editors: Principles and practice of infectious diseases, ed 2, New York, 1985, John Wiley & Sons.

78. Gershon A: Rubella virus (German measles). In Mandell GL, Douglas RG Jr, and Bennett JE, editors: Principles and practice of infectious diseases, ed 2, New York, 1985, John Wiley & Sons.

79. Goodwin R Jr, and Des Prez R: *Histoplasma capsulatum*. In Mandell GL, Douglas RG Jr, and Bennett JE, editors: Principles and practice of infectious diseases, ed 2, New York, 1985, John Wiley & Sons.

80. Gorczyca K: Safe pet guidelines for people with HIV disease, AIDS Patient Care 3(1): 36, Feb 1989.

81. Gordis L: The virtual disappearance of rheumatic fever in the United States: lessons in the rise and fall of the disease, Circulation 72: 1155-1162, 1985.

82. Greenspan D: Oral manifestations of AIDS, AIDS Clinical Care 1(6): 45-48, Oct 1989.

83. Greer K: Papillomavirus (warts). In Mandell GL, Douglas RG Jr, and Bennett JE, editors: Principles and practice of infectious diseases, ed 2, New York, 1985, John Wiley & Sons.

84. Grimes D: Infectious diseases. In Thompson J, McFarland G, Hirsch J, Tucker S, and Bowers A, editors: Mosby's manual of clinical nursing, ed 2, St Louis, 1989, CV Mosby.

85. Grimes D: Potential for infection. In Thompson J, McFarland G, Hirsch J, Tucker S, Bowers A, editors: Mosby's manual of clinical nursing, ed 2, St. Louis, 1989, CV Mosby.

86. Grove D: Tissue nematodes (trichinosis, dracunculiasis, filariasis). In Mandell GL, Douglas GR Jr, and Bennett JE, editors: Principles and practice of infectious diseases, ed 2, New York, 1985, John Wiley & Sons.

87. Guyton A: Textbook of medical physiology, ed 7, Philadelphia, 1986, WB Saunders.

88. Hamilton, H: Amebiasis and primary amebic meningoencephalitis. In Wehrle PF, and Top FW Sr, editors: Communicable and infectious diseases, ed 9, St Louis, 1981, CV Mosby.

89. Hanshaw J: Cytomegalovirus. In Wehrle PF and Top FW Sr, editors: Communicable and infectious diseases, ed 9, St. Louis, 1981, CV Mosby.

90. Hart G: Chancroid. In Wehrle PF and Top FW Sr, editors; Communicable and infectious diseases, ed 9, St Louis, 1981, CV Mosby.

91. Hart G: *(1981).* Granuloma inguinale (donovanosis). In Wehrle PF and Top FW Sr, editors: Communicable and infectious diseases, ed 9, St Louis, CV Mosby.

92. Hart G: Lymphogranuloma venereum (LVG). In Wehrle PF and Top FW Sr, editors: Communicable and infectious diseases, ed 9, St Louis, 1981, CV Mosby.

93. Hirsch M: Herpes simplex virus. In Mandell GL, Douglas RG Jr, and Bennett JE, editors: Principles and practice of infectious diseases, ed 2, New York, 1985, John Wiley & Sons.

94. Ho, M: Cytomegalovirus. In Mandell GL, Douglas RG Jr, and Bennett JE, editors: Principles and practice of infectious diseases, ed 2, New York, 1985, John Wiley & Sons.

95. Holmes K: Introduction. In Holmes D and Mardh P, editors: International perspectives on neglected sexually transmitted diseases, New York, 1983, McGraw-Hill.

96. Hoofnaggle J: Acute Hepatitis. In Mandell GL, Douglas RG Jr, and Bennett JE, editors: Principles and practice of infectious diseases, ed 2, New York, 1985, John Wiley & Sons.

97. Jawetz E, Melnick J, and Adelberg E: Review of medical microbiology, ed 6, California, Lang Medical.

98. Jones T: Cestodes (tapeworms). In Mandell GL, Douglas RG Jr, and Bennett JE, editors: Principles and practice of infectious diseases, ed 2, New York, 1985, John Wiley & Sons.

99. King A, Nicol C, and Rodin P: Venereal diseases, London, 1980, Bailliere Tindall.

100. Krugman S and Katz S: Infectious diseases of children, ed 7, St. Louis, 1981, CV Mosby.

101. Larson E: Clinical microbiology and infection control, Boston, 1984, Blackwell Scientific Publications.

102. Levine M: Shigellosis. In Wehrle PF and Top FW Sr, editors: Communicable and infectious diseases, ed 9, St. Louis, 1981, CV Mosby.

103. Locks M: Tuberculosis. In Wehrle PF and Top FW Sr, editors: Communicable and infectious diseases, ed 9, St. Louis, 1981, CV Mosby.

104. Mahmoud A: Intestinal nematodes (roundworms). In Mandell GL, Douglas RG Jr, and Bennett JE, editors: Principles and practice of infectious diseases, ed 2, New York, 1985, John Wiley & Sons.

105. Maynard J: Hepatitis. In Wehrle PF and Top FW Sr, editors: Communicable and infectious diseases, ed 9, St Louis, 1981, CV Mosby.

106. McCabe R and Remington J: Toxoplasma gondii. In Mandell GL, Douglas RG Jr, and Bennett JE, editors: diseases, ed 2, New York, 1985, John Wiley & Sons.

107. McCance K and Huether S: Pathophysiology: the biologic basis for disease in adults and children, St Louis, 1990, CV Mosby.

108. Meisenhelder J and LaCharite C: Comfort in caring: nursing the person with HIV infection, Boston, 1989, Scott, Foresman.

109. Merck Manual, vol 1 ed 15, New Jersey, 1987, Merck.

110. Mogabgab W: Influenza. In Wehrle PF and Top FW Sr, editors: Communicable and infectious diseases, ed 9, St. Louis, 1981, CV Mosby.

111. Monath T: Flavivirus (St. Louis encephalitis and dengue). In Mandell GL, Douglas RG Jr, and Bennett JE, editors: Principles and practice of infectious diseases, ed 2, New York, 1985, John Wiley & Sons.

112. Muller M: Trichomonas vaginalis and other sexually transmitted protozoan infections. In Holmes D and Mardh P, editors: International perspectives on neglected sexually transmitted diseases, New York, 1983, McGraw-Hill.

113. Nahmias A and Kohl S: Herpes simplex. In Wehrle PF and Top FW Sr, editors: Communicable and infectious diseases, ed 9, St Louis, 1981, CV Mosby.

114. New York Statewide Professional Standards Review Council: AIDS Intervention Management System (AIMS). Criteria Manual for the Treatment of AIDS, New York, 1989, New York State Department of Health.

115. Oriel J: Genital warts. In Holmes D, and Mardh P, editors: International perspectives on neglected sexually transmitted diseases, New York, 1983, McGraw-Hill.

116. Otteson E: Visceral larva migrans and other unusual Helminth infections. In Mandell GL, Douglas RG Jr, and Bennett JE, editors: Principles and practice of infectious diseases, ed 2, New York, 1985, John Wiley & Sons.

117. Overturf G and Underman A: Typhoid and enteric fevers. In Wehrle PF and Top FW Sr, editors, Communicable and infectious diseases, ed 9, St Louis, 1981, CV Mosby.

118. Pizzi M: Occupational therapy: Creating possibilities for adults with HIV infection, ARC, and

AIDS, AIDS Patient Care, 3(1): 18-23, Feb 1989.

119. Ravel R: Clinical laboratory medicine, ed 4, Chicago, 1984, Year Book Medical Publishers.

120. Reese R and Douglas R Jr: A practical approach to infectious diseases, Boston, 1986, Little, Brown.

121. Rein M: Trichomonas vaginalis. In Mandell GL, Douglas RG Jr, and Bennett JE, editors: Principles and practice of infectious diseases, ed 2, New York, 1985, John Wiley & Sons.

122. Rein M. Vulvovaginitis and cervicitis. In Mandell GL, Douglas RG Jr, and Bennett JE, editors: Principles and practice of infectious diseases, (2nd) New York, 1985, John Wiley & Sons.

123. Robinson W. Hepatitis B virus and the Delta agent. In Mandell GL, Douglas RG Jr, and Bennett JE, editors: Principles and practice of infectious diseases, ed 2, New York, 1985, John Wiley & Sons.

124. Rudolph, A: Syphilis. In Wehrle PF and Top FW Sr, editors: Communicable and infectious diseases, ed 9, St Louis, 1981, CV Mosby.

125. Russell P: Dengue. In Wehrle PF and Top FW Sr, editors: Communicable and infectious diseases, ed 9, St Louis, 1981, CV Mosby.

126. Saah A and Hornick R: Introduction to rickettsiosis. In Mandell GL, Douglas RG Jr, and Bennett JE, editors: Principles and practice of infectious diseases, ed 2, New York, 1985, John Wiley & Sons.

127. Sande M and Volberding P: The medical management of AIDS, ed 2, Philadelphia, 1990, WB Saunders.

128. Sanford J: Lower respiratory tract infections. In Bennett JV and Brachman PS, editors: Hospital infections, ed 2, Boston, 1986, Little, Brown.

129. Schooley R and Dolin R: Epstein-Barr virus (infectious mononucleosis). In Mandell GL, Douglas RG Jr, and Bennett JE, editors: Principles and practice of infectious diseases, ed 2, New York, 1985, John Wiley & Sons.

130. Schumacher H, editor: Lyme disease. Primer on rheumatic diseases, ed 9, 1989, Arthritis Foundation.

131. Seals J. Nontyphoidal salmonellosis. In Wehrle PF and Top FW Sr, editors: Communicable and infectious diseases, ed 9, St Louis, 1981, CV Mosby.

132. Seidel H, Ball J, Dains J, and Benedict G: Mosby's guide to physical examination, St Louis, 1987, CV Mosby.

133. Sell S: Basic immunology, New York, 1987, Elsevier Science.

134. Simmons B: Center for Disease Control guideline for prevention of surgical wound infection, Infect Control 3(3), 1982.

135. So Y: Neurologic manifestations of AIDS, AIDS Clinical Care 1(5): 37-40, Sept 1989.

136. Sours J: Food poisoning, bacterial. In Wehrle PF and Top FW, Sr, editors: Communicable and infectious diseases, ed 9, St Louis, 1981, CV Mosby.

137. Spaeth R: Tetanus. In Wehrle PF and Top FW Sr, editors: Communicable and infectious diseases, ed 9, St. Louis, 1981, CV Mosby.

138. Stamm W: Nosocomial urinary tract infections. In Bennett JV and Brachman PS, editors: Hospital infections, ed 2, Boston, 1986, Little, Brown.

139. Stamm W and Bennett J: Nosocomial infections. In Wehrle PF and Top FW Sr, editors, Communicable and infectious diseases, ed 9, St Louis, 1981, CV Mosby.

140. Stites D: Laboratory methods for detection of antigens and antibodies. In Fudenberg H, Stites D, Caldwell J, and Wells J, editors: Basic and clinical immunology, California, 1976, Lange Medical.

141. Stites D: In Fudenberg H, Stites D, Caldwell J, and Wells J, editors: Basic and clinical immunology, California, 1976, Lange Medical.

142. Swindler L: Understanding the immune system, U.S. Public Health Service, USDHS. NIH Publication no. 88-529, Washington, DC, 1988, US Government Printing Office.

143. Thompson J, McFarland G, Hirsch J, Tucker J, and Bowers, A, editors: Clinical nursing, St Louis, 1986, CV Mosby.

144. Top F Jr: Rubella. In Wehrle PF and Top FW Sr, editors: Communicable and infectious diseases, ed 9, St Louis, 1981, CV Mosby.

145. Top F Sr, Johnson K, and Wehrle P: Enteroviruses: poliomyelitis. In Wehrle PF and Top FW Sr, editors: Communicable and infectious diseases, ed 9, St Louis, 1981 CV Mosby.

146. top F Sr and Wehrle P: Diphtheria. In Wehrle PF and Top FW Sr, editors: Communicable and infectious diseases, ed 9, St Louis, 1981, CV Mosby.

147. Tramont E: Treponema pallidum (syphilis). In Mandell GL, Dou-glas RG Jr, and Bennett JE, editors: Principles and practice of infectious diseases, ed 2, New York, 1985, John Wiley & Sons.

148. Underman A: Tapeworm disease. In Wehrle PF and Top FW Sr, editors: Communicable and infectious diseases, ed 9, St Louis, 1985, CV Mosby.

149. Veasey L, Wiedmeier S, Orsmond G, Ruttenberg H, Boucek M, Roth S, Tait V, Thompson J, Daly J, Kaplan E, and Hill H: Resurgence of acute rheumatic fever in the intermountain area of the United States, New Engl J Med, 316:421-426, 1987.

150. Wannamaker L, Rammelkamp C, and Top F Sr: Streptococcal infections. In Wehrle PF and Top FW Sr, editors: Communicable and infectious diseases, ed 9, St. Louis, 1981, CV Mosby.

151. Warren K: Introduction to diseases due to Helminths. In mandell GL, Douglas RG Jr, and Bennett JE, editors: Principles and practice of infectious diseases, ed 2, New York, 1985, John Wiley & sons.

152. Wehrle P and Mathies A Jr: Meningitis. In Wehrle PF and Top FW Sr, editors: Communicable and infectious diseases, ed 9, St Louis, 1981, CV Mosby.

153. White D and Fenner F: Medical virology, ed 3, New York, 1986, Academic Press.

154. Wilkins J and Bass J: Pertussis. In Wehrle PF and Top FW Sr, editors: Communicable and infectious diseases, ed 9, St Louis, 1981, CV Mosby.

155. Wilson R: Enteric infections. In Wehrle PF and Top FW Sr, editors: Communicable and infectious diseases, ed 9, St Louis, 1981, CV Mosby.

156. Wisseman C Jr: Rickettsial disease. In Wehrle PF and Top FW Sr, editors: Communicable and infectious diseases, ed 9, St Louis, 1981, CV Mosby.

157. Woodward W and Hornick R: *Rickettsia rickettsii* (Rocky Mountainj spotted fever). In Mandell GL, Douglas RG Jr, and Bennett JE, editors: Principles and practice of infectious diseases, ed 2, New York, 1985, John Wiley & Sons.

158. Wyler D: Plasmodium species (malaria). In Mandell GL, Douglas RG Jr, and Bennett JE, editors: Principles and practice of infectious diseases, New York, ed 2, 1985, John Wiley & Sons.

Index

HYPERTHERMIA (FEVER) related to Infectious Disease

DEFINITION: Hyperthermia is the state in which a person's body temperature is elevated above the person's normal range. Hyperthermia results from many interacting internal and external risk factors that act on or interfere with thermoregulation in the hypothalamus. Fever that accompanies infection is a distinct form of hyperthermia. Fever does not result from failure of the hypothalamus to regulate temperature as is the case with hyperthermia caused by external factors only. Rather, it is the result of an elevation of the body's thermostat in the hypothalamus to a higher set point. This causes conservation of heat and increased heat production. This whole process is initiated by the action of substances called pyrogens, which include the proteins and toxins of some pathogens and the extracts of normal leukocytes. These are the specific risk factors for hyperthermia associated with infection. However, many physiologic, behavioral, treatment related and environmental risk factors may interact to raise the temperature of a person with an infection. Nursing interventions may be directed at a variety of these risk factors to promote heat loss and lower the temperature. For these reasons all risk factors are listed.

RISK FACTORS

Pathophysiologic
  Circulating pathogens
  Inflammatory response
  Altered metabolic rate
  Cerebral injury or disease (CVA, tumors)
  Anemia
  Integumentary injury
  Neurovascular or peripheral vascular disease
  Dehydration
  Impairment in perspiration
Behavioral
  Vigorous activity
  Wearing excess clothing
  Bathing in hot water
  Failure to drink adequate fluids
Treatment-related
  Hyperthermia blanket
  Drugs (vasodilators, anesthesia)
  IV fluid and blood infusion
Environment
  Excess heat, humidity, or lack of air movement
  Exposure to direct sunlight

DEFINING CHARACTERISTICS

Body temperature above 100° F (37° C)
Flushed, warm skin
Increased respiratory rate
Tachycardia
Seizures/convulsions
Perspiration
Headache

GOAL: Body temperature will be maintained within the normal range; comfort and safety will be maintained for patient experiencing fever.

NURSING INTERVENTIONS	RATIONALE
1. Assess for signs of infection.	Infection is the most common cause of body temperature elevation.
2. Assess for the presence of risk factors in addition to infection.	Seriously ill newborns, elderly, immunosuppressed and persons with uremia may have serious infection without fever. Environmental risk factors may add to temperature retention during fever.
3. Monitor temperature q 2 h.	To detect extreme risk in temperature, patterns that may be associated with a particular pathogen, secondary rises associated with complications, and decrease in temperature associated with resolution of the infection.
4. Monitor other vital signs q 2 h.	Heart rate increases 15 beats/minute per degree C increase.
5. Monitor for signs of dehydration.	Significant fluid loss accompanies each degree C increase in temperature. Hyperventilation accompanies fever and may result in respiratory alkalosis.